GUARDIANS OF THE PEAKS

GUARDIANS OF THE PEAKS

Mountain Rescue in the Canadian Rockies
and Columbia Mountains

KATHY CALVERT

DALE PORTMAN

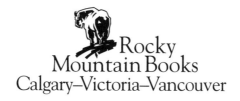

Rocky
Mountain Books
Calgary–Victoria–Vancouver

Rocky Mountain Books
#108 – 17665 66A Avenue
Surrey, BC V3S 2A7
www.rmbooks.com

Rocky Mountain Books
PO BOX 468
Custer, WA
98240-0468

Library and Archives Canada Cataloguing in Publication

Calvert, Katherine M., 1947–
    Guardians of the peaks: mountain rescue in the Canadian Rockies and
Columbia Mountains / Kathy Calvert and Dale Portman.

Includes bibliographical references and index.
ISBN-13: 978-1-894765-80-0
ISBN-10: 1-894765-80-X

    1. Mountaineering—Search and rescue operations—Rocky Mountains
(B.C. and Alta.) History—20th century. 2. Mountaineering—British Columbia—
Columbia Mountains—History—20th century. I. Portman, Dale II. Title.

GV200.183.C35 2006   363.14   C2006-905058-9

Library of Congress Control Number: 2006932789

Edited by Ursula Vaira
Proofread by Corina Skavberg
Cover and book design by Frances Hunter
Front-cover photograph of Mt. Louis by Brad White

Printed in Canada

Rocky Mountain Books acknowledges the financial support for its publishing
program from the Government of Canada through the Book Publishing Industry
Development Program (BPIDP), Canada Council for the Arts, and the province
of British Columbia through the British Columbia Arts Council and the Book
Publishing Tax Credit.

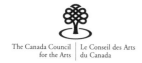

The Canada Council | Le Conseil des Arts
for the Arts | du Canada

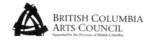

BRITISH COLUMBIA
ARTS COUNCIL
Supported by the Province of British Columbia

In Memory of

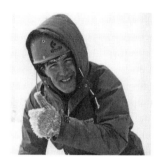

SIMON PARBOOSINGH

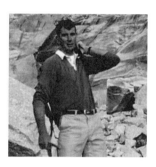

PAT SHEEHAN

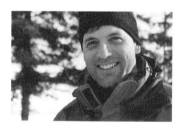

MIKE WYNN

Table of Contents

Acknowledgements

I wish to thank Peter Spear for pointing out that the story of mountain rescue in Canada needed to be written. Peter brought it to my attention in 2002 while doing an interview for the Don Forest book. Unfortunately the subject was too complex to complete for the bicentennial anniversary of the establishment of Canada's first professional rescue organization by Parks Canada in 1955. Despite the lapse, I sincerely hope the story does justice to the work of the dedicated men and women, both professional and volunteer, who have saved so many lives.

This story was too large to be done by one person, and I soon engaged the help of my husband Dale Portman as co-author. Without his unstinting effort and insight, this project would be many years behind the 2005 anniversary.

I wish to thank the two original alpine specialists, Peter Fuhrmann and Willi Pfisterer, who were the first men to give their time to interviews revealing the early years of public safety in the western national parks. Their stories revealed the early development of mountain rescue in Canada.

Many other people were instrumental in seeing this book to completion. First, I wish to thank Tim Auger, a leader of the Banff public safety team for over 30 years, who was behind this endeavour from the beginning. His interviews and editorial suggestions were invaluable. Other members of the public safety teams were equally supportive and unstinting in devoting time for interviews and editorial comments. Foremost of these individuals is Clair Israelson, former alpine specialist with Parks Canada in Lake Louise and current director of the Canadian Avalanche Association. His support was always encouraging.

This book would have been incomplete without the help of Lloyd Gallagher, the first public safety specialist for Kananaskis Country, who truly understood the value of teamwork and the need for supportive teammates. His example inspired the dedication of George Field and Burke Duncan, who followed him.

Other leading members of the parks' public safety teams were instrumental and unselfish with their time. They graciously opened up their rescue files and office space for the essential research to be done. I wish to thank the Banff public safety team led by Gord Irwin, Mark Ledwidge and Brad White. Gord Irwin also supervises the equally dedicated team in Lake Louise of Percy Woods and Lisa Paulson, who also gave of their time. The Jasper public safety team claim full share in this endeavour. Thanks to the time given by Gerry Israelson, Steve Blake, Rupert Wedgwood and Garth Lemke. The smaller parks have exactly the same job and also gave unstintingly of time and resources. Thank you Brent Kosechenko, Edwin Knox and Derek Tilson from Waterton. From Glacier I wish to thank Eric Dafoe, who oversaw the running of the public safety program there and his successor, my sister Sylvia Forest. Thanks also to Jordy Shepherd and Anna Brown who have worked in this field in Glacier.

Invaluable help came from Hans Fuhrer who spent many formative years running the public safety program in Kootenay National Park. Hans was also deeply involved with CARDA and the B.C. Provincial Emergency Program, for which he provided much insight.

For information into the role Glacier National Park played in the avalanche program, I wish to thank Fred Schleiss, Peter Schaerer and Hans Gmoser. Hans and Mike Wiegele also provided background on the heli-skiing industry that inevitably became involved in the development of avalanche rescue.

I must also give particular thanks to the helicopter pilots I was able to interview about their contribution to the mountain rescue program. Thank you Jim Davies, Lance Cooper, Todd McCready, Don McTighe, Matt Callahan and Gary Forman. I only wish I had had the time and perseverance to talk to all the dedicated pilots who worked in this field over the years.

I wish to thank Scott Ward for all his time and help with editing the rescue dog section. Gord Peyto, thank you for your stories. I also thank Alfie Burstrom and Earl Skjonsberg, who were instrumental in providing details of the early dog program. Thank you also to the new dog handlers Mike Henderson and Darien Sillence as well as Will Devlin, who bridged the gap between then and now.

Stories of mountain rescue are incomplete without the support of the volunteer program. For their help I wish to thank Arnor Larson, Ken Pawson, Gord Burns, Rod Pendlebury, Bruce Watt and Jay Pugh.

Many people came forward with critical recollections and insights that tied the story together. For their time I wish to thank all those identified in the bibliography under personal communication.

I thank also those who provided images for the book: Brad White, Cliff White, Mark Ledwidge, Steve Blake, Sylvia Forest, Jordy Shepherd, Greg Horne, Lloyd Gallagher, George Field, Hans Fuhrer, Dale Portman, Garth Lemke, Edwin Knox, Ken Pawson, Rob Jennings, Jim Davies, Todd McCready, Gord Irwin, Don Vockeroth, John Niddrie and Bob Sandford. Special thanks to Cathy Hourigan for the hours spent in the Banff library finding and scanning many pictures for the book. Although not all the pictures were able to be placed, the time spent by individuals was well appreciated, and the pictures not included will hopefully be used in the future.

Though the project did not receive any grant funding, we did receive support from Don Mickle in charge of Cultural Heritage for Banff National Park in return for oral history transcriptions now in the Banff Archives. Thank you Don for your enthusiasm and contribution to the stories in this book.

The last person to review the manuscript was Chris Stetham (of Chris Stetham and Associates), well-known avalanche protection consultant in Canmore, Alberta. Thank you for your considerable time for this last input into the manuscript and for earlier contributions for this aspect of the book.

I wish to add that people's recollections from many years past are selective to individual experience and do not necessarily encompass the full extent of rescue scenarios. The rescue reports were invaluable in confirming many details, as were collaborative interviews, but discrepancies often arose. I ask forgiveness if some of the events described in the book are not in accordance with people's memories. The stories selected for the book were those that were representative of a particular rescue situation or important in the development of the mountain rescue program. Regretfully many very interesting rescues were not included due to limited space and time.

Finally I thank Parks Canada staff for all their support throughout the years it took to write this book. In particular Gaby Fortin, former Parks Canada Director General of Western and Northern Canada, who provided the initial letter of support for the project.

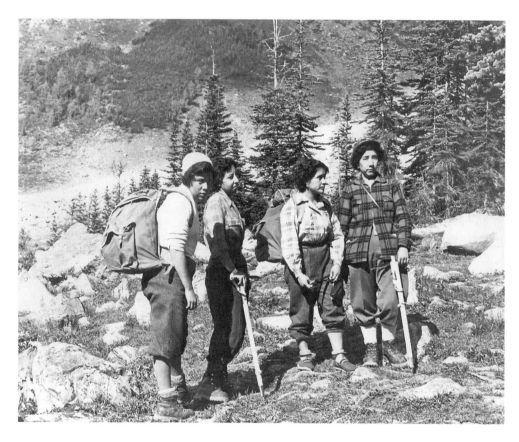

The Mexican women survivors of the Mt. Victoria tragedy, 1954. ROB JENNINGS COLLECTION

Introduction

On July 28, 1954, summer seemed to have finally reached the shores of Lake Louise after a particularly harsh winter. Guests at the Chateau Lake Louise took the opportunity to wander the lakeshore and smile at the seven young women who stood apart, distinguished by their exotic looks and suppressed excitement. They conversed eagerly in low tones of soft Spanish as they warily eyed the steep white slopes of Mt. Victoria at the end of the lake. They were part of the first all-women's climbing team from Mexico coming to test their ability on some of Canada's more challenging climbs—a most unusual event in the male-dominated sport of climbing.

They had also attracted attention in their native country—but in an un-anticipated way. The Mexican Alpine Club, which they had approached for financial assistance, was not at all sure the women were experienced enough for their chosen climbs in the Rockies. In fact, the choice of climbers was challenged vigorously by members of the financial committee who had debated the issue hotly with other members of the club. But the chosen guide, Eduardo San Vincente, supported the women and a second, more supportive committee was formed.

The choice of Mr. San Vincente was not really contested, as he was considered an outstanding climber after scaling some of the highest peaks in the western hemisphere including Huascaran and Mt. McKinley (Denali). The women—all gainfully employed in various careers in Mexico—had been chosen from various Mexican climbing clubs throughout the country and took the task seriously. They trained for seven months before departing and paid for some of the expenses themselves. Eventually the Mexican Excursionismo Federation approved the plans for the trip but withheld official sponsorship.

With the money in place and the wrangling over, they found themselves at the train station in Banff, where they were met by a reporter from *The Banff Crag & Canyon*. The leader of the group was an attractive young woman of 29 years who was less than five feet tall. She told the reporter that the women had set their hopes on Mount Victoria, Mount Eisenhower (Castle Mountain) and possibly Mount Lefroy. They had settled on these objectives after listening to the glowing reports of two of their compatriots who had visited the area in 1953. Their guide remarked that an international expedition of this kind was the first ever undertaken on the continent. He then cautiously added that the mountains back in Mexico were higher but not as difficult to climb as the Rocky Mountains appeared to be.

The Swiss guides who worked for the Chateau Lake Louise, with whom the women conferred about climbing Victoria, could not comment on the comparison, but they were certainly in agreement about the difficulty of the climb when the women indicated they wished to climb the East Face rather than the standard route. The face had been climbed only once before, and it was considered extremely dangerous owing to its steep pitch and its exposure to avalanches. San Vincente wanted to hire one of the Swiss guides to lead them up the mountain, but the guides turned him down. Ernest Feuz told the party: "The high mountains are in bad shape this winter. In all history we have never had such a hard winter, so much snow or so late a spring." The Mexicans were also told that if they were successful, they would be the first party to ascend the south summit that year.

Despite the guide's warning, the party left the manicured shores of Lake Louise on July 29th with much fanfare. On the way up to Abbots Pass, the group met Ernest Feuz's brother Walter, who warned them to stay on the rock ridge and to avoid the excessively snowy east face. But nothing deterred the determined group. After spending the night at the Abbot Hut, they headed for the summit the next morning minus one woman who was ill. They travelled in two roped groups, the first led by their guide with two of the most experienced women and a fourth less-experienced climber. The second group consisted of the expedition leader and the other two women.

The summer sun was soon warming the frozen snow, giving them good conditions. Before the snow got soft, they reached the skyline and headed for the south summit to spend half an hour taking pictures and resting before starting the descent. They had the choice of either returning down the ridge, which would have been much safer, or climbing down the route they had come up. They chose the latter with devastating results. Because the snow was so soft from the afternoon sun, their crampons continued to ball up. They also had to move quickly to get down before the snow began to avalanche. But that meant descending together without belaying to maximize their speed. With virtually no protection, it was impossible to hold a woman who missed a step. The leader of the rear group later reported: "I saw position three start to slip and drag the others down. They slid down, and then they tangled up together in a ball and rolled down very fast. When I saw them fall, I knew it was all over." It was 1:30 p.m.

Down at the Chateau Lake Louise, guests, with the aid of the hotel telescope, had watched the group's progress with fascination. Cliff Pethybridge, a mechanic at Brewster's Transport, happened to be looking through binoculars at the exact moment the accident occurred. He later reported: "I saw them sliding down and it looked as though they started an avalanche. I could see them easily for about half of the way, then they were covered in snow and then [they] dropped behind [Mount] Lefroy." The fall had occurred less than 91.5 metres below the south summit of Mount Victoria at about the 3,500-metre elevation.

Up on the mountain the three remaining women were paralyzed with fear. For more than two hours, they wandered aimlessly about in the rotting snow, sometimes waist deep, attempting to reach safety. Well into the evening spectators lined up to watch in fascination and concern as the three women attempted in vain to reach the ridge.

Ernest Feuz wasn't surprised when he got report of the accident. His immediate thought would have been centred on what resources he had at hand for rescue personnel, knowing this was the worst mountaineering accident to have occurred in the Canadian Rockies. The first to respond to the "Climber's Code" to help fellow mountaineers was a young 20-year-old medical student. Charles Roland, who had been at Lake Louise for the last five summers, had become an enthusiastic mountaineer during his tenure in the Rockies. Harry Green, a lawyer for the CPR, and two fellow bellhops Frank Campbell and Ray Wehner composed the rest of the team. A second party consisting of Corporal Ray Morris of the RCMP, Chief Park Warden (CPW) Herb Ashley and Dr. D.L. Tittamore left soon after but only went as far as the foot of Abbots Pass.

Once they reached the edge of the moraine, Ernest saw what looked like two bodies. Not seeing anything further, he wondered if the others had fallen into a crevasse. They soon found all the women and their guide tangled hopelessly together in their rope. There were no survivors. There was little they could do, so they carried on to Abbots Pass where they found the woman who had stayed behind. Leaving the other three rescuers to prepare food for the survivors, Roland and Feuz covered the distance to the peak in half the normal time. Later Roland recalled, "Ernest usually goes slow and steady. I've never moved so fast on a mountain in all my life."

From here Feuz belayed Roland down to the women, giving him time to cut good steps. He reached them shortly after 8:00 p.m. Once they reached the safety of the ridge it took two hours to guide the stunned women back to the hut, often showing them where to put their feet as they made their way down the ridge. The guides could only guess at what had happened, because none of the women spoke English. They had planned to spend the night in the Abbot Hut, but Ernest compassionately decided to bring them down immediately so that they would not have to see the shattered bodies of their companions. With the help of Green, Wehner and Campbell, they had little difficulty in getting the women down, though they slipped on the snow from time to time. Headquarters for the rescue had been set up at the Plain of Six Glaciers Teahouse about midpoint between the Chateau Lake Louise and the spot below Abbots Pass where the bodies had come to rest. It was here at 1:30 a.m. that the rescuers finally had a chance to take a break. The speed with which the rescue parties reached the victim was considered "fantastic" by the waiting press.

Though Ernest Feuz, now 60 years old and feeling the strain, left the group to return to the Chateau for the night, Roland and Campbell got only two hours of sleep before returning to prepare the bodies for evacuation. In the meantime, the survivors were cared for at the tea house.

The two bellhops spent four hours untangling the bodies from the rope, and wrapping them in canvas for the trip down. Throughout this entire operation the rescue party was exposed to avalanches which raked the approach to Abbots Pass at frequent intervals. One big slide from the glacier-hung heights of Mount Victoria actually forced them to run for safety. Later that day they were joined by

Ernest Feuz, Wehner and Green and two others. Before the bodies were removed, the rescuers wrapped the guide with a Mexican flag. From here, the recovery team worked its way down the steep pass and across the snowfield to the beginning of the moraine. There was little option but to carry the bodies by stretcher over the crumbling moraine—an arduous task for the sleep-deprived rescuers. The last obstacle was up a 50-metre near-vertical pitch of loose rock. The party was extremely fatigued by the time they turned the bodies over to the packer, who had arrived with a string of pack horses for the rest of the journey.

The guests at the Chateau were following the progress of the rescue and recovery with morbid fascination. Those who had witnessed the accident through the telescope pointed out to newcomers where the accident had occurred. This was slowly creating a fevered pitch of intense interest amongst the crowd. One guest showed a group of arrivals the track in the snow slope made by the victims as they slid down the mountain. Another fellow saw the first of the rescuers bringing the bodies out of the pass and shouted almost hysterically: "They're bringing the bodies down! They're bringing the bodies down! They've got them on sleds!"

Ernest Feuz, in an exclusive interview with the *Calgary Herald* after the accident said, "The Mexicans should not have used crampons on the soft rotten snow of the sun-soaked east face." The crampons could not reach the hard snow underneath the slushy upper layer, and the climbers therefore were supported only by the unstable surface snow. He went on to say that "Neither the Mexicans nor any other mountaineer should climb on the east face of Victoria. That's committing suicide especially in these conditions."

Seated on her bed in the Chateau Lake Louise, the expedition's leader sent her memory reluctantly back over the fatal climb, and with the aid of an interpreter told her story to the same reporter. But she no longer had to stare at the coldly indifferent mountain and the fateful skid marks of death. Blessedly, the weather moved in, obscuring the spot where the bodies had been recovered. Today it is known as the "Death Trap," and over the years it has more than lived up to its gloomy name.

The accident on Victoria occurred at a time when climbing in Canada was on the verge of expanding. It was singular in scope and revealed how inadequately equipped parks were to deal with a rescue of this dimension. The event catapulted the National Parks Service onto the path of developing a rescue organization that would one day be an equal member of the international rescue association founded in Europe.

1

Man and Mountains

THERE IS AN UNWRITTEN CODE amongst climbers that if one is injured or killed, their compatriots will automatically render all possible assistance. This was the case with the women on Mt. Victoria. But such accidents often lead to great controversy. The non-climbing public views extreme sports such as mountaineering a foolish waste of time that only leads to endangering others in rescues undertaken at great, unfathomable cost. It seems prudent, therefore, to briefly examine how mountain adventure arose and some of the ideology behind the adventures.

Why do men climb mountains? This was a question posed by James Ramsey Ullman in his book *The Age of Mountaineering*. The answer also applies to any other risky sport such as kayaking or deep powder skiing. He answered it simply by stating that "most men don't." An examination of history or anthropology reveals that ancient man did not climb, nor did primitive man. Mountains were greatly feared and thought to harbour demons of all sorts; they were a dwelling place for the dead. Dragons kept the shores of Lake Lucerne in Switzerland closed for eons till the myth of their existence was disproved. Many of the more accessible mountains were adorned with crosses to hold at bay the monsters that lurked in hidden valleys, higher peaks or within the frozen glaciers.

This changed dramatically between the mid-18th to early 19th centuries during the Age of Reason and the birth of science. There was an explosion of thought that directly challenged man's fear of the unknown, opening the way to exploration of all kinds. The European Alps were the first great mountain frontier. Two hundred years ago scarcely a peak in the Alps had been ascended, now there are no new ascents left. Ullman writes that "The history of mountaineering is not merely a story of the conquest of mountains, but of the conquest of fear. It is not merely the record of stirring deeds, but of a great adventure of the human spirit."

The men who pushed the early mountain boundaries were the scientists: botanists, meteorologists, geologists, biologists—all chasing plants, animals, rocks or weather phenomena at the elusive heights, guided by the only men who dared venture to these unholy places—the neophyte guides. These men were outcasts of society who made their living on the periphery of existence, hunting among the crags for chamois and crystals. Claire Engel, who wrote *A History of Mountaineering in the Alps,* observed that "These hunters were usually looked upon as erratic and notorious characters, dare-devils who risked—and often lost—their lives in courting danger."

But as the boundaries were pushed back and men wandered through the alpine without the fear and dread of former days, the spell of the mountains was cast. One of the earliest men to climb merely for pleasure was Father Placidus è Spescha, a Benedictine monk from Disentis. He made the first ascent of several peaks in the Graubünden in the late 18th century. For this he has often been dubbed "The Father of Mountaineering." He was actually in good company with another man who could easily have vied for that title. The inveterate alpine traveller and scientist Horace Bénédict de Saussure of Geneva was the first man to record a love affair with Mont Blanc, which he finally succeeded in climbing in 1787, but only after encouraging others to attempt the climb. He surreptitiously wrote: "It became for me a kind of illness. I could not even look upon the mountain, which is visible from so many points round about, without being seized with an aching of desire."

The spirit of the mountains spread like an infection, finding fertile ground among the British, who are generally held responsible for ushering in "The Golden Age of Mountaineering." The publication of Alfred Wills's book *Wanderings Among the High Alps* in 1856 was the driving force behind the English inventing the sport of alpine climbing. But even before Whymper's disastrous triumph and calamity on the Matterhorn, dissenters of the sport were raising their voices. Respected men of letters such as Charles Dickens were writing that climbing "contributed about as much to the advancement of science as would a club of young gentlemen who should undertake to bestride all the weathercocks of all the cathedral spires of the United Kingdom." John Murray, who wrote the first guidebook, *Handbook for Travellers in Switzerland,* thought climbers "were of diseased mind." The essayist John Ruskin wrote scathingly of young climbers as men who "fill the quietude

16

of the valleys with gunpowder blasts, and rush home, red with cutaneous eruptions of conceit and voluble hiccough of self-satisfaction."

Clearly there was suspicion cast upon the burgeoning sport of mountaineering (or for that matter, any adventure undertaken for the sake of adventure alone), even before it got off the ground. The fact that mountaineering in the early days was considered "a lark" and was only undertaken by the privileged upper class who could afford this "frivolous" activity, did not help. Whymper's misadventure on the Matterhorn only added fuel to the fire, particularly as it was to haunt him for the rest of his life, foreshadowing many future tragedies that would have lifelong consequences.

Nevertheless, growing controversy spurred thoughtful men to explore the inner drive behind their desire to seek out the remote high places and conquer the peaks. Claire Engel found that many writers struggled with the essential dichotomy of the alpine landscape, being "impressed by a constant opposition between its beauty and the sudden horror of which it is capable, between the love which mountains conjure up in many hearts and the feeling of hatred and despair which sometimes sweeps over the same persons among the same mountains." Nevertheless, she found it was a place "where divine inspiration comes more frequently than elsewhere." Essentially, mountains became a place where men found a sort of unconscious asceticism, a place to "win victory over oneself" which added "a moral charm to the manifold in the delight of a big climb."

Initially, it was the conquest of fear over an inherently malevolent environment that impelled men to climb. This conquest opened the door to inner self-knowledge and ultimately to a greater spiritual understanding of self and the mortal world. Ullman writes that climbing "in its essence, has been a struggle not of man against man, nor even of man against the obstacles of the physical world, but of man against his own ignorance and fear." He goes on: "It is a story of men and the spirit of men and the interplay of that spirit with the physical world in which they live. It is a story of the slow painful conquest of fear." Perhaps it was the reluctance of the detractors to face these fears that sponsors their vitriolic response to great endeavours.

Walter Bonatti, one of the finest climbers of the post-war era, felt obliged to marshal his thoughts on his many daring climbs in the face of scathing criticism. Bonatti reflects: "Contrary to what many people think, mountaineering does not consist of risking one's life for amusement." He elaborates: "Real mountaineering is quite another thing; it is above all a reason for struggle and for self-conquest, for spiritual tempering and enjoyment in the ideal and magnificent surroundings of the mountains. The trials, the hardships, the privations with which an ascent of the peaks is always studded, become, for that very reason, valid tests which the mountaineer accepts to temper his powers and his character. In the atmosphere of struggle, of close relationships with the unforeseen difficulties and the thousand perils of the mountains, that alpinist is shown in his true colours, ruthlessly laid bare, both in his qualities and in his defects, to himself and to others."

The emerging sentiments and discoveries of self-worth intrinsic to mountaineering were well established by the 19th century, and although often beyond the pale of most people, the sport was not about to fade from human endeavour. Unfortunately, not everyone who ventured into the mountains was as well prepared as Bonatti for the difficulties or dangers found there. With the advent of alpine sports, came an explosion of accidents and ultimately, the development of professional rescue services.

However, not all mountain tragedies can be laid at the feet of mountaineers. Indeed, mountain rescue in its purest form was well established long before the advent of climbing as a sport. Early travellers and pilgrims were the first people to encounter real difficulties in the mountains, and countless numbers perished in avalanches, in winter storms or by simply getting lost. But

help came to the wayfarer as early as 962 A.D. from an unlikely person. Bernard of Menthon, later to become St. Bernard (the patron saint of Alpinists), was a wealthy young man who decided on the eve of his marriage to renounce the world and join the Augustine Order. He founded a monastery on what was then called Mount Jove, at an altitude of over 2,400 metres for the sole purpose of saving the beleaguered traveller. This later became the Great St. Bernard Hospice after which several other hospices were founded on similar remote passes. Colin Fraser wrote in his definitive work *The Avalanche Enigma*: "So it is that from well before 1436 until 1885, not a single winter morning passed, regardless of how vicious the weather, on which men did not set out from the St. Bernard Hospice to guide travellers or to rescue those in trouble." Fraser adds: "Not only did St. Bernard found the first mountain rescue organization, but he also founded it in traditions of endeavours and self-sacrifice in the aid of all and sundry. And this tradition still inspires the better rescue organizations today."

The first non-ecclesiastical rescue organization in the Alps was founded by the Duchy of Savoy in the Middle Ages. The men were called Soldiers of the Snow and were essentially those excused from military service during the winter to form a group of guides and rescuers to assist travellers. Ultimately, these early efforts led to a comprehensive rescue network in the Alps, which became the blueprint for rescue organizations around the world.

Although early mountain rescue dealt almost exclusively with non-climbers, their expertise was honed at high altitudes where elements such as avalanches, bad weather, poor terrain and injured people were relevant factors. Many of the basic principles of rescue, which have only improved with technology (medical or mechanical), were established during these years. Climbers, however, propelled rescue into another realm. Cliffs and vertical faces or knife-edge ridges proposed different problems altogether. The fact that climbers chose to go to these places for no good reason that most people could fathom, brought into question the moral responsibility of going after them if they were in trouble. In the beginning no one did come to their aid. It was expected that if they got themselves into trouble, they could get themselves out or suffer the consequences. This was a harsh reality that early climbers accepted, giving rise to an independent spirit and a considerable measure of self-reliance. But other climbers realized it was not always foolishness or inexperience that got people into trouble, and the ethic of aiding others in distress soon became a code.

Hamish MacInnes, one of the foremost rescue leaders in the world, puts this clearly saying: "There are always objective dangers on a serious climb. It is a fact of life. You have to consider what you want to get out of the sport and just how far you are prepared to go." He also makes it clear that life in general demands that all people must accept the haphazard element. "If you are on a dangerous solo climb or a gentle Lakeland walk, there is a degree of inherent danger in both."

But every action has consequence which demands a measure of responsibility. Bonatti gave much thought to this, "For better or worse, our actions are in the last resort, never entirely our own, but are always subject to external influence. Persons and facts, circumstances and judgements, have often been motives and incentives to me in my ventures. Thus I am in debt to others at least to the extent that my deeds belong to them."

MacInnes pays tribute to the men and women who have dedicated themselves to the rescue profession by putting the work in perspective. He speaks of tales of tragedy and death that to many may seem to border on the macabre. But he cautions the reader not to see the stories in that light saying, "They are not intended to be so." Instead, he wishes the reader to "comprehend the self-sacrifice and the stark facts of a rescue operation. One of the greatest forms of human endeavour is to pit your resources against the odds stacked up by a mountain."

THOUGH PROFESSIONAL MOUNTAIN RESCUE did not come to Canada until the middle of the 20th century, well after climbing had been established, there were significant accidents that foreshadowed the need for such an organization. By the time the mountain parks were established, most of the major peaks in the Alps had been conquered, leaving ardent alpinists looking for virgin territory. The Canadian "Alps" offered huge challenges, not just because of the beauty of individual unclimbed peaks, but because of their often sheer inaccessibility. Local historian Robert Sandford acknowledges the challenges: "The high barrenness of these mountains, the hazards of crumbing and falling rock and the verities of moving ice combined with an almost unimaginable remoteness make the Rockies and surrounding ranges as dangerous and difficult as anything but the thin-air summits of the high Himalaya." Indeed, although the fur trade and later the railroad were responsible for opening up the west, most of that exploration was concentrated in the main valleys. It was the climbers who poked into hidden alpine passes and ventured across the icefields to find the secret treasures of the mountains.

The earliest recorded fatality related to climbing was that of Phillip Abbot on Mt. Lefroy in Banff National Park in 1896. Lake Louise with its spectacular peaks had become a prime focus for tourists and was the logical spot for a luxury hotel. It was from here that many climbers based their activity and attempted to climb the virgin peaks. Abbot set his sights on Mt. Lefroy but was killed attaining the summit. With his eyes firmly planted on the summit rather than the loose hold that broke free in his hand, he fell to his death. The rescue party that recovered the body consisted of fellow climbers Charles Fay, George Little and Willoughby Astley (assistant manager of Lake Louise Chalet). Tom Wilson, a packer, and a crew of railway bridge builders acted as backup. Unfortunately it was a costly way to learn about the crumbling frailty of the impressive mountains.

The news of Abbot's death sparked controversy—yet again—over the sport of mountaineering. The event ultimately prompted the Canadian Pacific Railway (CPR) to bring over the Swiss guides who led to a new era of climbing.

The guides brought with them the latest in mountaineering knowledge and equipment, but there was still a steep learning curve as they adjusted to the new land. They learned about the rock, the weather, the bush and the distances with the significant help of the local guiding and outfitting community, one of the most colourful and interesting set of characters to be found in the west. These local cowboys knew the bush well and were eager to help the climbers and their guides reach the remote peaks they sought, but they did not venture too readily to the summits themselves. Bill Peyto, one of the more renowned outfitters and later to be one of Canada's first park wardens, said, "If I can't ride there, I'm not going." Although the guides were the CPR's backup plan for any rescues that needed to be carried out, it was more often those at hand who provided aid.

After the arrival of the Swiss guides, climbing and exploration proceeded at a considerable pace but within the ability of the guides and their clients. There were exciting moments and certainly dangerous places to negotiate, but no mountain tragedies akin to that of Abbot's befell them. Those who tackled the mountains unguided were not always so lucky. One incident in 1907 showed the remarkable courage, determination and resourcefulness of two early climbers on the first real attempt to climb Sir Sandford, a major peak tucked well back in the Selkirk Range of B.C.

Two college students from the United States set out in July of that year (having made an earlier attempt the previous year with three others) by boat down the Columbia River and then on foot into the bush. Chic Scott writes in *Pushing the Limits*: "Merkle Jacobs and Edward Heacock were deep in the Selkirk wilderness just south of Mount Sir Sandford when a huge boulder rolled over on Jacobs' leg and broke his femur." Heacock made his friend as comfortable as possible and then set out for help. As luck would have it, upon reaching the railroad days later, he met a Dr. Charles Shaw, also exploring the Selkirk area, who was willing to return with him to help Jacobs. It was many days after the accident before they were able to set the leg properly. The rescue team (now including Jacobs' brother) were obliged to stay in camp for two months while the leg healed. Before they were able to get Jacobs out, Heacock drowned while canoeing across the Columbia River—presumably on a return trip for more help and supplies.

By late August, they could no longer wait as winter would soon be upon them and there was great concern to get out before the railway was shut down by snow. In a heroic effort, the team made a dash for the tracks carrying Jacobs, in what remained in one rescuer's memory as "a long nightmare … That dash was the awfulest thing I ever experienced." As Scott justifiably observes: "These men knew the meaning of self-reliance, and were willing to accept the consequences of their deeds."

No other significant catastrophes occurred in Canada within the mountaineering community or otherwise until 1921. The Alpine Club of Canada had been formed in 1906 and had sponsored yearly camps every summer in locations that provided many climbing and hiking opportunities. In 1921, this usually meant there were still unclimbed peaks to be gained, and the camp that year at Mt. Assiniboine was no exception. Although the camps were usually well attended, the climbing community in Canada was still very small, fostering deep friendships. The story of the first ascent of Mount Eon and the subsequent fatality as told by A.H. MacCarthy in the *Alpine Club Journal* is quite moving, not only because of its epic proportions, but because it is also the story of his loss of a lifelong friend.

MacCarthy described Mount Eon as a "magnificent virgin peak" which "stirred the ambition of many of them to make an attempt on it." MacCarthy and his wife Elizabeth were not surprised, therefore, to hear that their close friends Dr. Stone and his wife Margaret set out to climb the mountain. The Stones (Margaret and Winthrop) and the MacCarthys (Albert and Elizabeth) were unique in their friendship in that both women were avid climbers who accompanied their husbands on dozens of first ascents in the Purcells (including the fearsome Howser and Bugaboo Spires) with their guide, Conrad Kain.

MacCarthy's quite lengthy account in the *Alpine Club Journal* (1922) of the accident and the subsequent rescue reveals the amazing fortitude of Mrs. Stone and the tremendous presence of mind it took to endure her incredible ordeal. The climb itself was a considerable undertaking, because the base of mountain was some distance from the main camp and required a full day's approach. The Stones had planned to be gone from camp for several days to explore the area and attempt the peak. It was not until the third day after leaving Assiniboine Camp that they began their ascent.

After going well over steep ledges of good rock and a long firm snow slope, they reached a series of "short couloirs of unstable rock to a final wide steep irregular chimney that opens with dangerous sloping top sides on to the summit." MacCarthy continues: "Upon reaching the base of this chimney at about 6:00 p.m., they felt that they were near their goal; so after placing Mrs. Stone in secure footing at its base and clear of any possible rock falls, Dr. Stone ascended it until he could see over the top slopes but was still unable to determine whether or not a higher point lay beyond, and to answer Mrs. Stone's enquiry if they were near the top, he replied he could 'see nothing higher' but that he would go up and make sure; that the rock was very unstable and to be careful and keep under cover.

"Dr. Stone then climbed out of the chimney and disappeared for a minute or so, and shortly afterwards, without any warning, a large slab of rock tumbled off from above, passing over Mrs. Stone, and was closely followed by Dr. Stone, who spoke no word but held his ice axe firmly in his

right hand. Horror-stricken at the sight, Mrs. Stone braced herself to take the jerk of the rope, not realizing that her husband had taken it off to explore beyond its length." Mrs. Stone watched in disbelief as the doctor's body hurtled out of sight, striking ledge after ledge until it disappeared at "the bottom of the mountainside."

The shock and loss rendered her immobile as she fought for control, but by then it was too dark to descend. She spent her first night on the mountain only 12 metres below the summit, knowing in her heart that her husband was dead. She now had to contend with the trial of finding the body and going for help. With first light she began the descent, recognizing prominent features and staying close to the route they had taken up, but she was "unstrung" and "unable to reach the lower ledges before darkness set in." She spent her second night out still high up on the cliffs. On the third day she continued, keeping in view a prominent yellow-capped tower which marked the route, but now anxiety overwhelmed her, and in her haste to find the body she lost the route. Beyond all logic, she harboured the faint hope he might be alive and this kept her going. Unfortunately, Mrs. Stone now made the classic error of trying to reach safety by following a ledge that appeared to connect with a scree slope above the timber. This ended in a sheer cliff, forcing her to retrace her steps. But the tantalizing scree slope still beckoned, and she sought another way down. Seeing a broad ledge below her, she decided to use the rope she was still carrying to aid in descending a broken chimney. MacCarthy relates the heartbreak of this decision: "[She secured] her rope around a rock, let herself down a broken chimney until she was about three metres from the ledge. Here the rope ended and she was forced to drop to the ledge, soon only to find that it broke off at both ends in smooth faces, and did not connect with the scree slopes below, thus completely trapping her."

If the mountains could record cries, hers must be locked in the rocks for eternity. But Margaret Stone was not ready for death, and there was still

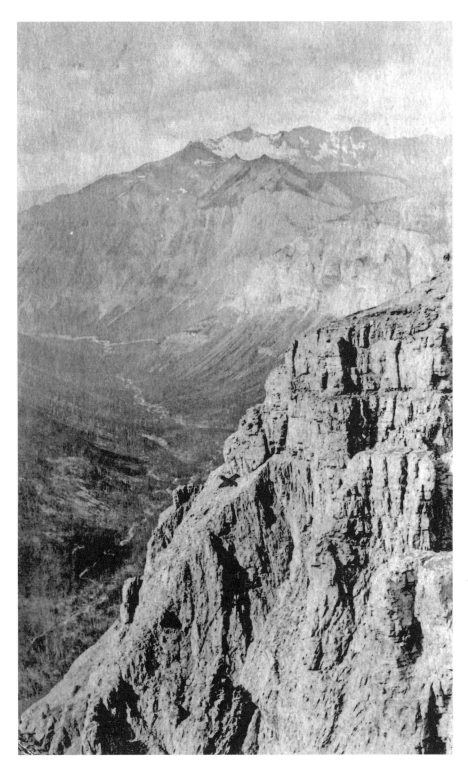

Mrs. Stone's location on Mt. Eon. WHYTE MUSEUM

the remote hope that a search party might find her. She attempted to reach the rope by building a pile of rocks but to no avail. Finally, she settled on the ledge, having providentially found a trickle of water, probably the first she had had in over twenty-four hours. She had only her flannel shirt and climbing pants for clothing, but fortunately the fine weather held. MacCarthy is most impressed with the presence of mind she showed once resigned to her fate. He writes: "By scooping out two small holes about the size of a watch and directing the trickle to them she was able to get a swallow from each every four hours. To this supply of water; the fact that her narrow ledge was on the south side of the cliffs where they and she received all the warmth of the sun during the daytime; and her firm balance of mind, causing her to wind her watch and to thus regulate her hours for taking her meagre supply of water, she can ascribe her coming through the terrible ordeal alive."

She may have wondered if help would ever come, for she was to spend another five days on this ledge before she heard the sound of another human voice. Because of the Stones' planned extended stay, concern was not aroused until the 18th, but it was not till the following day that it was feared an accident might have happened. Mr. Raiman of Brooklyn, N.Y., set out with some provisions but did not even reach Wonder Pass. He went on instead to the Trail Centre at the end of Spray Lakes and passed the tale of the missing Stones to Mr. Waterman (of Summit, N.J.) who upon finding no news of the missing couple upon arriving at Assiniboine, insisted they send for help. This was now the 21st, seven days after the Stones had first set out. Waterman left that day with a packer for Wonder Pass where they learned the location of the Stones' bivouac. By now they were certain that a serious accident had happened but had no idea of the route taken by the couple up Mt. Eon. They returned to Assiniboine Camp where they were relieved to learn that the packer had been dispatched to Banff to get the aid of a Swiss guide. Finally on the 22nd, Rudolph

Aemmer and warden Bill Peyto of Banff arrived after having made the 73-kilometre trip from Banff in one day. It was now four days beyond the time the Stones were to have returned, and the worst was assumed. It seemed most likely that both had succumbed to a fatal accident. With this in mind, Aemmer decided to take only a small party who were in good condition, leaving the trail crew to bring up supplies. The rescue party set out on July the 23rd for what they expected to be a body recovery operation.

After having located the Stones' bivouac site, they worked their way up Mt. Eon to the summit of the south spur from which they could command a good view of the south face. They searched the steep and broken terrain with field glasses and were about to return when, miraculously, they heard a shout to the westward. Astonished, they immediately fired a shot and were soon able to work their way around to Mrs. Stone's location. She had been out for eight days with only a small dribble of water and her amazing courage to sustain her. She was far too weak to move at all, so Aemmer carried her on his back over the broken terrain to the trees she had despairingly tried to reach. In total she had spent seven days alone on the mountain. Here they bivouacked for the night, then moved lower down where they rested with supplies brought up by the backup party. It was an epic journey to get her out. From this location they spent another two days not far from the original bivouac site while the trail crew slashed the trail from Marvel Pass through the valley and up to the Wonder Pass trail. From there, she was carried out to Trail Centre and the care of Miss Brown, the camp manager, and Mrs. Fred Bell.

The rescue had taken quite a toll on all persons involved but particularly on Rudolph Aemmer who had not spared himself in the work. Most of the rescue had been carried out in bad weather, which, most fortunately for Mrs. Stone, had held off till help arrived. During all this time the Director of the Alpine Club, A.O. Wheeler, had been on official survey work, but upon his arrival in Banff he took over the evacuation and set out on August 2 with a fresh party. The new party consisted of the ever-vigilant Rudolph Aemmer, Edward Feuz, Conrad Kain, Lennox Lindsay and the MacCarthys. They soon got to Trail Centre where Mrs. MacCarthy remained with Mrs. Stone while the rest set out to recover the body of Dr. Stone. They had a reasonable idea of where the body might be, but Mrs. Stone had never actually seen his final resting place. Therefore, they retraced the Stones' ascent route, until, just below the summit of Mt. Eon, Edward Feuz spotted the body "lying on a ledge about 300 yards [274 metres] to the west of us and directly below the summit."

The party now realized that recovering the body was going to be a momentous job. Before doing so, however, the party examined the terrain above the chimney and concluded that "in climbing out of the chimney and disappearing for a minute or so Doctor Stone had stood on the summit of the mountain and walked a short distance to make sure that there was no higher point beyond, then upon returning to the chimney he had stepped on a loose slab of rock near the edge that had slipped from under him and carried him over the cliff." Bringing out the body was a huge effort that took till August 9th.

This was the first major rescue undertaken in Canada after Abbot's death on Mt. Lefroy. It took 22 days and considerable manpower. Most of the technical work as well as labour was undertaken by the Swiss guides, whom climbers had come to rely on for safe climbing in the Rockies and now rescue work. Significantly, Bill Peyto, one of Canada's first park wardens—although the technical terrain was well beyond his ability—was part of the initial rescue team, foreshadowing the future role of this service. It was interesting that the Stones had undertaken the climb on their own, signalling a departure from heavy reliance on guides. They were the forerunners of the independent climber soon to change the landscape of climbing in Canada.

There would not be another climbing accident of this nature for another 33 years, but there would be deaths by avalanche in the mountains. The first avalanche fatality in the Canadian Rockies occurred in Yoho National Park near Lake O'Hara in February, 1933. This involved two local brothers Chris and Joe Daem, who were on a ski trip from Hector Station near the B.C./Alberta boundary via Lake O'Hara, Linda Lake and Duchesnay and Dennis passes. They had enough food for seven to ten days and with heavy packs set out to pioneer a new high route. It heralded a new phase of mountaineering that involved skiing and backcountry travel skills.

When they had not returned after 10 days, the boys' father, the road-master in Field, B.C., contacted the chief park warden, who immediately sent out two search parties. One group followed the boys' proposed route up toward Lake O'Hara while the other headed up from the Field side toward Dennis Pass. In the meantime a third rescue team was organized in Banff led by the well-known Swiss guide, Christian Hasler.

The first two parties soon returned, having found only ski tracks near the warden cabin near Lake O'Hara. The following day more tracks were discovered heading up toward Duchesnay Pass, disappearing into terrain now obliterated by wind and snow. When the Banff group arrived they proceeded to Duchesnay Pass. From there they had a good view of a narrow defile connecting Dennis and Duchesnay Pass. This alarmed them greatly as it required traversing steep, exposed avalanche terrain.

According to the *Crag & Canyon*, Banff's local newspaper, the search party stopped at the foot of the pass, hoping for better light to scout the route, when a huge slide thundered down the mountainside. This awe-inspiring sight convinced them it was too dangerous to proceed, and with little hope of finding the boys alive, they turned back. Indeed local mountaineers who had travelled the terrain in the summer stated that it was a very dangerous undertaking.

Another search a week later yielded nothing, and further efforts were put off until the beginning of June when a group of Swiss guides from Lake Louise resumed the search. They found evidence the boys had made it over Duchesnay Pass, but they could not determine if they made it over Dennis Pass. With late spring snow hampering the search, the guides postponed their efforts for another three weeks, after which they found the boys' bodies in avalanche debris on the Lake O'Hara side of the pass. The lads had reached the pass only to find out that conditions were questionable and had decided to abandon the traverse. On returning to Lake O'Hara, their luck finally ran out when they were caught in the avalanche.

The second fatality that winter is probably the best known in local lore because of the supposed haunting of Halfway Hut and Skoki Lodge by Paley's Ghost. This accident was the first of its kind from a commercial standpoint; the victim was a client staying at the lodge run by Catharine and Peter Whyte. Kim Mayberry, in her small book about the Whytes called *Romance in the Rockies: the Life and Adventures of Catharine and Peter Whyte*, writes that "tragedy cast a shadow over their idealistic happiness at the lodge in 1933" when the infamous guest came to ski early in the spring. He was "a brilliant mathematician who had recently been appointed to the Massachusetts Institute of Technology on a Rockefeller Scholarship." Perhaps this is why he turned out to be a "loner" who always "dashed off alone before anyone knew where he was headed" often to be seen "climbing the most dangerous slope you can imagine."

Mayberry relates: "After lunch on April 7, without the knowledge of the group, Paley left the lodge and made a beeline for the steep slopes of nearby Fossil Mountain—an area that had recently been deemed unsafe by more experienced skiers. The sky was heavy and grey as he neared the summit of the 2,900-metre mountain. Suddenly, violent gusts of wind whipped around the top of the mountain, creating a whiteout of blinding snow. Slippery patches of ice interspersed patches of crusty snow. A short distance from the summit, Paley's skis skidded. His 100-kilogram mass triggered the release of huge slabs of snow. The force of the slide sent Paley over a cliff in an avalanche of snow and rock." It was not till the next day that the body was recovered and brought to Lake Louise for the authorities to examine. The brunt of the interrogation was borne by Peter Whyte, who was nominal head guide of the operation. Although the investigation, also conducted by the Rockefeller Foundation, found that Paley was solely responsible for his own death, Peter Whyte was "haunted" by the tragedy for the rest of his life.

The death of Donald "Curly" Phillips and Reginald Pugh five years later brought a new awareness to the danger of avalanches. Curly was one of the few outfitters who had embraced the mountains completely by adding climbing and skiing to his repertoire. Curly Phillips became best known for his spontaneous journey with the Rev. G.B. Kinney on the disputed first ascent of Mt. Robson. It later became known that they were short of the summit by a mere few yards, but they claimed the summit in good faith. Later, Curly became a well-known guide and outfitter in Jasper and also an avid skier who sought to advance the sport locally. It was while searching for more ski terrain in the area that he was killed in an avalanche at Elysium Pass in 1938.

The accident report was filed by R.E. Baynes, a corporal with the Jasper RCMP detachment, who was the first to hear news of the tragedy. In the report he writes: "At 3:00 p.m. this date, I learned from warden Chas Phillips of the Jasper National Park Warden Service, that one Alan Pugh, aged 14 years, who resides with his parents near Jasper, had just arrived from the Elysium Pass and reported that his two companions, Donald 'Curly' Phillips and Reginald Pugh, had been caught by a snowslide and presumably killed about noon of March 21st. I interrogated Alan Pugh immediately and very briefly, as he was near collapse as the result of his experience and subsequent trip to Jasper.

"The lad's story was to the effect that in company with 'Curly' Phillips and his brother Reginald, the trio were making a ski trip in the district northwest of Jasper. They had been taking pictures as they travelled and when in Elysium Pass, it was decided that Phillips would take a snapshot of the two Pugh boys as they came down a small slope into a depression which lay underneath a large body of snow. Alan stated that he was carrying his pack when the suggestion was made, and his two companions were some little distance ahead of him. Phillips and Reginald Pugh proceeded on over the edge of the depression and almost immediately a snowslide started from directly above where they were presumably standing. Alan ran for safety, and when the slide stopped returned to where he had last seen his companions, but could find no trace of them. He said that he circled the base of the slide and could find no tracks; he then crossed the slide with the same result. He stated that he spent a short time shouting in the hope that they had escaped, and in receiving no answer, had returned to their camp one-and-a-half miles [2.5 kilometres] away and left a note to the effect that he had gone to Jasper for help. His trip to this point occupying about 24 hours to cover the 17 miles [27 kilometres]."

Two dearly loved people from Jasper were dead and the loss was immediate. Shortly after having received the news, a party of experienced men set out from Jasper to retrieve the bodies. Wardens Frank Bryant and Frank Wells, who went on this mission, again set the stage for the future role of the Warden Service in rescue and avalanche safety work.

That same year a woman also was killed in an avalanche on Mt. Schaffer, Lake O'Hara, in Yoho National Park.

ONE INCIDENT THAT DREW ATTENTION to avalanche hazard in the backcountry occurred in the Skoki area. In this case, Ken Jones, the first Canadian-born guide, was involved in recovering the body of Hermann Gadner who worked at the lodge. It turned out to be an ordeal of endurance for Ken, who had been out on a long trip with clients to the Bonnet Glacier that day, when he noticed that a huge slide had let loose on a ridge near the soon-to-be Whitehorn Ski Area of Lake Louise. He remembered saying that he hoped nobody had got caught in that one. Despite the already long day, his plan was to set out that evening for Lake Louise to meet another group of clients. He relates: "It was dark, but I had made that trip so many times I could do it in the light, or dark, or whatever. I went because I was to meet another group at Field the next day and take them into Yoho.

"I got to Temple Lodge about eleven o'clock that night—that was the old Temple Lodge—and I stopped in to say hello. They asked me, 'Did they get Hermann out yet?' I had come right by there but I hadn't noticed any activity. I had seen a light in the Halfway Hut but I assumed someone was spending the night there." It was then that Ken learned that his friend Hermann had been caught in the avalanche he had noticed earlier that day, and his response was immediate. "I'll leave my pack here and go back and see what I can do for them." Before he went, a member of the party Hermann had taken out that day gave him a shot of whisky saying, "This will help you along."

He was soon back at Halfway Hut speaking to a couple of people resting from the search. Cliff White, who was managing the search, told him they had just found the body and were digging him out. In the end, it was four-thirty in the morning before the body was recovered and taken down to Temple Lodge. By the time Ken had a chance to stop moving, he had been on the go for over 24 hours, and had added yet another tale to support the legend of his stamina.

BUT CHANGES WERE ON THE HORIZON. The national parks in Western Canada experienced a huge leap in park visitors after the Second World War with increasing use of the automobile.

Climbers were beginning to show more independence in the 1930s and wanted to climb without always using guides. The sense of accomplishment at climbing an unknown peak without a Swiss guide was becoming a more and more sought-after experience. The end of the war also saw the emergence of the middle class, in which the average family could afford to go to the mountains for a vacation.

However, the moderately well-off middle class were not rich enough to support the guiding community whose services they had no compelling need to use. R. Burns writes in *Guardians of the Wild:* "As these circumstances brought more people into the Rocky Mountains on their own, alpine guiding ceased to be a profitable enterprise." Seeing change in the wind, the CPR decided to get out of the guiding business altogether and abruptly discontinued the employment of the Swiss guides. The now well-established Canadian National Park system was suddenly without the rescue expertise of the guides they had so long relied on and "increasing numbers of people, often ill-trained and poorly quipped" were suddenly at risk in the mountains.

Soon climbing was no longer the sport of the rich. Places like Lake Louise and Skoki Lodge became very popular in a short period of time as backcountry use continued to rise. Parks personnel kept an eye on the rising tide of tourism and the growing numbers of people who required attention each year, but they were not ready to leap into professional rescue service. The Swiss guides were still the main resource for climbing accidents though wardens had no problem bringing a stranded tourist back from backcountry trails. At this time, the small number of serious accidents were seen as isolated incidents, but some men, because they had seen the changing tide in Europe, knew this would not last forever.

2

The Walter Perren Years

WALTER PERREN IS CONSIDERED the father of mountain rescue in Canada, but the door for this opportunity was opened before he arrived in this country.

Curiously enough, the first man to see the coming tide of social change and what it would mean to the burgeoning National Park Service was a cowboy from the ranching community of Bragg Creek just west of Calgary. Noel Gardner was the son of Clem Gardner, a world-class bronc rider who along with Guy Weadick and other local ranchers started the Calgary Stampede in 1912.

Noel was born in 1913, the same year that the CPR started construction of the Connaught Tunnel in Rogers Pass—a place that would ultimately figure largely in his life. But it was his skill with horses and his love for the mountains that soon had him guiding dudes around Lake Louise during the summer months in the early 1940s. With his winters open, he gravitated to Sunshine Ski Hill and the skiing activity there. Here, he met a gregarious Swiss mountain guide and photographer by the name of Bruno Engler, who taught him how to ski. Noel was talented and as strong as an ox, and not long after picking up the sport he qualified as a ski instructor at the hill. It was during this formative period that Bruno

introduced Noel to ski-touring and avalanche awareness. Together the two would head for untracked powder, and Noel soon excelled at this type of skiing.

Another job he picked up during this period was packing provisions into Skoki and Assiniboine along with Ken Jones and Cyril Paris. This cycle of guiding and packing on horseback in summer and teaching skiing in the winter led to a natural desire to become a park warden. In 1948, Noel achieved his goal and was posted to his first station at Flat Creek just west of Rogers Pass. Above the station was Mt. Fidelity, whose steep upper reaches had numerous open glades that provided great powder skiing. His exposure to this daunting terrain became critical in his emerging interest in snow-craft. He was also becoming aware of another issue looming ahead for the Warden Service.

With the rapid increase in visitors, national parks benefited from the lucrative post-war era, and increased the number of wardens to patrol the backcountry, now divided up into districts, often notable for their isolation. The men who gravitated to this work were often war veterans with a farming or ranching background. They usually had basic hunting skills, were all-round handymen and generally familiar with horses. Almost to a man, however, they had no mountaineering or skiing skills.

Noel realized that wardens, as guardians of the parks, would be called upon to save the hapless visitor who got in trouble. He was also aware that one of the greatest dangers in the mountains was the avalanche. Park managers, up to this point, were quite happy to leave rescues to the Swiss guides who seemed to come equipped with the expertise and the moral conviction to save anyone who needed saving. Noel apparently did not have much faith in this continuing. Well before the last Swiss guide said goodbye to Canada, Noel was urging his superiors to teach wardens to ski and to become familiar with avalanche hazards.

Noel Gardner was a large man with a fearsome personality. He dominated those around him with an intimidating temper and an equally intimidating physical presence. But he had vision and conviction with which to back his rogue ideas and set forth to enlist the unconverted. By 1951, he succeeded in gathering five new recruits to Glacier, where he drilled them with classroom lectures on the dangers of avalanches followed by strenuous basic ski exercises on slopes behind the CPR station at the pass. None of the men were really prepared for this aspect of the job, but they pitched in to do their best.

Ollie Hermanrude was one of the wardens sent on that first ski school, which he remembers with some asperity. He was sent over with Ed Carlton, John Romanson and Marty Allred by train to Glacier House where they were met by Noel. They lodged at the Wheeler Hut, which at that time was a good trek from the train station and an eye-opener for what was to come. Hermanrude commented laconically: "It was on that slide path above the CPR station that we used to tramp the hell out of first and practise our snow plow. That was day one. Day two we tramped the hell out of the slope and practised our snow plow—and that was over nine days."

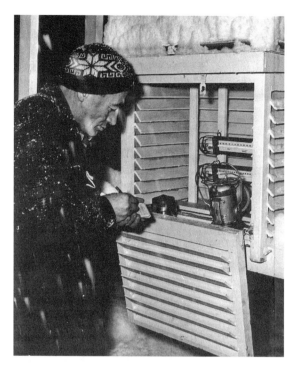

Noel Gardner. BANFF WARDEN ARCHIVES PHOTO BY BRUNO ENGLER

It was an inauspicious beginning but Noel was encouraged. Ollie, in hindsight, thought the school was "very good, very good" and Noel felt the men had advanced at a "satisfactory rate." Noel did have one observation, however. He felt that most wardens were fighting an uphill image battle when it came to skiing. He felt that: "Wardens feel a sense of inferiority when confronted by some of these ski teachers and guides when in all actuality [they] should be the [men] looked up to by these people."

Noel was quite committed to the idea of wardens becoming involved in rescue scenarios that he felt would inevitably become the parks' responsibility. In this he was considerably more far-sighted than some of his superiors, which must have been endlessly frustrating to a man of his temperament. After the nominal success of the first school, Noel realized that the task ahead was monumental and that the training required would be far beyond the scope of a small yearly ski school. His ultimate vision was to bring the district warden to a level of competence in rescue and skiing ability that "should the need for a rescue party arise at any time, [he would] be capable of leading the party efficiently, making the decisions and at all times be in command of the situation." In this he was well supported by his own superintendent in Glacier, R.J.J. Steeves, who also had a vision of wardens conducting rescues within the parks instead of relying on outside expertise.

In the early fifties, most wardens had no reason to think they would be involved with mountain rescue on any scale and were certainly not enthusiastic about adding it to their repertoire. Gardner's initial attempt to just get the men to ski was met with considerable resistance. It meant they had to learn to ski proficiently, which is usually accomplished at a young age after many years of training and practice. Most of the men Noel was trying to convert were no longer young, having used up their enthusiasm for adventure during the Second World War. As a result his suggestions received strong support but also considerable resistance. Superintendent Dempster in Jasper National Park agreed in principle with many of Gardner's recommendations but knew that the wardens in his park "would be in a rather bad spot" if it came to a rescue. Others pointed out that a warden travelling alone in the backcountry was safer on snowshoes and did not wish to see the potentially more dangerous skis introduced as a means of travel.

But an idea had been launched, and Gardner was not about to see it derailed. To succeed, though, he felt that the training should be given to men under 45 years of age and the schools limited to ten men. Banff Superintendent J.A. Hutchison saw the wisdom in this and wrote the regional director strongly recommending that Gardner be given the support he needed. Bryant went further saying, "There are a number of elderly wardens who would not 'go' for the ski, who will finish on snowshoes."

Noel was given the initial go-ahead to continue the training program, but not all was entirely to his liking. Jasper did not like the idea of sending wardens down to a school in Banff and elected to train their own men under the guidance of the local Swiss Army veteran Alex Neumann. Gardner's plans for a second school in Glacier were also thwarted by a "shortage of affordable accommodation" and the alternative in Banff was nixed by the sensitivity of the apprentice warden. The men were not anxious to be exposed as neophytes to the more sophisticated skier on the "public ski slopes of Banff"—realizing they were being trained to save the very people who could out-ski them. A compromise was reached when the school was held at Sunshine under a "modicum of privacy."

Despite concerns by some of the wardens of not lighting the slopes on fire with their alpine expertise, there were a few who already had some background in skiing and made excellent progress. Tom Ross in Jasper was already a proficient skier, as was Jim Sime from Yoho. Sime, in fact, had grown up in Golden under the tutelage of the Swiss guides and was fully aware of the need for rescue capabilities in the warden service. The school at Sunshine prompted Gardner to recommend him to be enlisted as an assistant instructor in future courses.

Things now began to move quickly. In the spring of 1952, officials from Yoho, Banff and Jasper convened to discuss the future of the ski/avalanche rescue program, and agreed that it should continue under the direction of Noel Gardner with two more ski classes to be held in both Banff and Jasper in 1953, but only for a two-week period. In the interim, one very successful course was held in Yoho in the Little Yoho Valley at the Stanley Mitchell Hut. The upside to this was that selected graduates would go on to advanced courses to be held in Glacier with the help of CPR's alpine guide, Walter Perren. Aside from Jasper using Alex Newmann (who was not a full Swiss guide) for outside expertise, Parks was now recognizing the need to employ someone of Walter's stature as a full guide. At the time, Walter was only on loan to the park and was not a park employee, but it was an excellent introduction to his talents as an instructor.

Other issues were aired at that auspicious 1952 conference as well. It was agreed that only those wardens who were eager to participate in mountain skiing and rescue would be asked to attend the courses. It was also agreed that a uniform be issued for the team consistent with both the service uniform and the clothing required for mountain travel. This meant boots, parka, slacks and ski cap all in requisite green. Though each park received the itemized list, only a few of the "eager participants" showed up with either gear or eagerness. But the new direction took root slowly; non-supporters saw the courses as a paid ski holiday and the keener participants as elitist. Gardner was quick to defend the work and the men who genuinely wished to excel in the new field. He wrote rather challengingly: "There has been in some quarters the popular misconception that ski and snow-craft courses are merely glorified holidays. This misconception I hasten to correct. All pupils have been worked harder by far than on any job that they possibly do in the regular course of duties with the possible exception of fire fighting. On these courses I have had strong men completely exhausted by three o'clock in the afternoon, and in many cases at the end of the course some men have lost as much as 10 pounds in weight. While I endeavour to make instruction as easy as possible to absorb, these courses cannot be considered as play periods by any possible stretch of the imagination. I should like to have a chief warden of any park concerned along during an entire course, both for his benefit and my own."

By 1954 Noel had succeeded in running several courses in skiing, avalanche rescue, terrain evaluation and glacier travel. The men were now familiar with the use of ice axes, pitons, carabiners, crampons, skis, poles, shovels, avalanche probes and ropes. Despite some resistance, in reality a budding mountain rescue function had been accepted in 1953 as a new role for the warden service.

It was fortuitous that Noel Gardner said in 1954: "Ski and snow-craft training for field personnel has made a fine start and will, I hope, go on to a fitting conclusion." For shortly thereafter, he resigned from the Warden Service. Although he would return to play a vital role in snow research, he would no longer orchestrate the development of the public safety program he had so assiduously launched.

WALTER PERREN, WHO HAD COME to Canada with Edmund Petrie on the last five-year contract offered Swiss guides by the CPR, was not immediately eager to work with the Warden Service. Burns reports that Walter had "exhibited a reluctance to join the park training program as a co-instructor with Gardner." Walter, who was a patient man, was never able to work easily with the more forthright, tempestuous Noel. They were physical opposites as well; Walter was a diminutive man barely five-foot-eight and 140 pounds when heavy. The more robust Noel was well over six feet and probably never less than 200 pounds when light.

Initially, they differed on the emphasis of the rescue program; Noel wanted most of the training to revolve around skiing and avalanche work while Walter knew that general mountaineering skills would soon be required. This disagreement may have been the cause of the dissatisfaction Noel felt for the national parks leading to his abrupt resignation after Walter was hired. Before Noel left the Warden Service, however, he saw that the next advance in the program needed to include general mountaineering. He also acknowledged it would have to be taught by someone more experienced than himself in this field.

THE YEAR BEFORE NOEL QUIT the Warden Service, he worked on a part-time contract with the Department of Public Works to identify avalanche paths through Rogers Pass that would affect the future building of the Trans-Canada Highway. This job, which would become full time when he quit the Warden Service in 1954, formed the foundation for later avalanche research at the Pass. The work that Noel accomplished during this period intrigued the U.S. Forest Service in Alta, Utah, and they invited him to attend a week-long avalanche course that winter. The following year they invited the Canadian Parks Service to attend a similar advanced snow and avalanche training session. The course was actually put on by the American National Parks Service, which wished to see what their northerly cousins were up to. The Canadian Parks Service, up to this point, had rejected suggestions to employ any American instructors, preferring to keep training and development within the Warden Service (which meant Noel Gardner), but Banff Chief Park Warden Herb Ashley welcomed the invitation. He saw it as a chance "to assess the existing programme and learn from the American experts."

But in 1955, the wardens chosen to go felt they had something to prove. The best of the best were picked: Jim Sime, CPW of Yoho, Bert Pittaway, Assistant CPW of Banff, and Tom Ross, the ski graduate of Noel's program. They were expected to "use 'spit and polish,' be courteous and dignified and create a favourable impression" of the Canadian Parks Service. Accordingly, they were outfitted with the previously recommended olive green uniform, and as Sime said: "We were all decked out like a million dollars."

They stood out immediately, impressing their hosts not only with style, but also with ability. In fact, they were put to a rather severe test according to head instructor, Monty Atwater, a leading figure in snow research. Atwater later wrote to CPS Director J.A. Hutchison, saying, "I hope you won't mind a little human interest story about these men. When they first appeared at Alta I recognized them by their uniforms. They were, of course, complete strangers to the area and everyone present. I took the opportunity to introduce myself to them, make them welcome and at the same time form some estimate of the kind of man Canada has as snow rangers. I suggested we take a little tour together of the ski area.

"Snow conditions were a bit difficult for anyone unused to the heavy snowfalls of Alta. The terrain I chose was the steepest and roughest we have, and I set the fastest pace of which I'm capable. You will understand that I thought this would be as good a chance as I'd have to 'get my bluff in first,' as we put it. The course was as familiar to me as it was unfamiliar to the Canadian snow rangers. If you are a skier yourself, you will realize how great an advantage this gave me and I exploited it fully. Some of the other instructors who saw this performance later accused me of most unfair tactics, and they were justified. Nevertheless, no matter how I forced the terrain, every time I looked back, those Canadians were right on my tail. I knew then that your National Park Service was going to be well represented, and it was."

Although it was a good beginning for the exchange of information between Canada and the United States on snow research, avalanche control techniques and rescue procedures, the development of mountain rescue in Canada stayed aloof from direct American influence. Canada's ties to Europe in this field were becoming strongly entrenched through the influence of climbers and guides who flocked to Canada from Europe during the 1950s.

It was on the verge of the departure of Noel and the Swiss guides that the tragedy of the Mexican climbers on Mt. Victoria occurred. The horror and the magnitude of the accident was unprecedented in Canadian alpine history but was fortunately dealt with expediently by the now-aging guides. It was quite evident that no one in the Warden Service had the mountaineering skills to march to the top of Victoria and bring down the stranded women from the upper reaches of the mountain. None of them had yet even gone climbing. The accident happened in July, and by the end of the summer, the Feuz brothers had retired, and Walter and Edmund Petrie's contract was up. Edmund immediately departed for the United States and was not seen in Canada again for some years. Suddenly it was apparent that looming throngs of inexperienced, guideless climbers were poised to besiege the mountains with their youth, enthusiasm and ignorance.

One of the men who recognized the problem was Sime, the new chief park warden of the small but significant Yoho National Park. His intimate friendship with the Swiss guides with whom he had grown up with in Golden, B.C., gave him an insight into the future for climbing in the Rockies on the basis of how it had developed in Europe. Edward Feuz was particularly adamant in airing his views to Sime about the potential for accidents in the mountains if no preventative measures were taken. Parks had taken a tentative step in developing a mountain rescue program, and in so doing, had made some commitment to the safety of the park visitor, but the terms of that commitment were as yet undefined.

Jim Sime had no reason to doubt the guide's ominous predictions, and soon after becoming chief park warden, he began a letter campaign to Ottawa outlining the problem. Sime was convinced that the new function needed a strong leader with impeccable qualifications and that the person for the job was Walter Perren. Walter and Jim had become good friends during the period that Walter worked for the CPR. Jim fondly recalled: "The Swiss guides had brought Walter over to our house … and we got to be good friends."

Finally, Jim's door-knocking produced results, just before the five-year contract Walter had with the CPR was up. But before a job could be put on the table, Jim had to do some fast talking with the Regional Director, Jim Hutchison. Rather than waste his own breath, he decided the director should be told the situation by an expert. Accordingly he brought him down to Golden to meet with Edward Feuz, who was blunt enough to convince Hutchison that action was needed.

With little hesitation Hutchison gave Banff Superintendent "Bim" Strong the go-ahead to hire Walter. There actually was no position open in the Banff Warden Service, so he was brought on temporarily as the Maintenance Supervisor, a title that was soon amended to Public Safety Maintenance Supervisor. Hence the function of mountain rescue in the Warden Service was ever afterwards referred to as "public safety." Walter's future had been dramatically shunted to the role of the "Father of Mountain Rescue in Canada."

Fortunately for Canada, no better man could have been found for the job. Walter Perren was born in Zermatt, Switzerland, in 1914 to a relatively poor family who had five children besides himself (three sisters and two brothers). His father was a guide and stone mason by profession, so it was not surprising that young Walter showed a propensity for climbing at an early age. Don Beers in his book *The World of Lake Louise* relates: "[Walter] always loved climbing. He had been a mischievous boy who hated school, and would run off to climb the cliffs instead. When his mother found out, she went up after him. Walter gave in, worried that she might slip and injure herself."

This did not last long, however, as he was already apprenticing to be a guide at the age of 14 when he made his first ascent of the Matterhorn. It was on this first trip that Walter came to famously "attend his own funeral." Walter was actually a porter on this climb, when the party became engulfed in a vicious storm that stranded the group on the mountain. Their failure to return was long enough for the villagers to give them up for dead and hold a funeral service, as was the custom, in a hut near the base of the mountain. But the party survived and arrived in time to attend the prayer services being offered up on their behalf. The experience did not deter Walter from the profession or the mountain—during his career in Switzerland he would ultimately climb the Matterhorn over 140 times.

Walter thrived in the calling he was born to, and soon worked his way up from an underprivileged apprentice, to a renowned guide able to attract some of the best clients in Europe. He kept himself employed year-round guiding in Zermatt in the summer and teaching skiing in the winter. Just prior to the war, Walter's reputation as a fine climber and excellent companion convinced the Swiss to invite him on the first expedition planned to scale Everest. The war defeated that prospect but opened up other avenues for Walter. He became very active in the French underground, smuggling refugees and allies over the Alps from France to neutral ground in Switzerland.

By the time he was 36 years old, Walter's reputation as a guide attracted the attention of the CPR, who offered him the guiding contract in Canada. The unmarried Walter was entranced at the prospect but probably would have been astounded had he known where it would lead. All he knew was that it was a very long journey by train across Canada to his ultimate destination in Golden, B.C., home of the Swiss guides. According to his son Peter, Walter finally got a chance to get some exercise at Lake Louise. It must have been a marvellous vision for him, and he took advantage of the opportunity to "stretch his legs" by climbing The Needle on Mt. Whyte before the train left. Obviously the journey had not impaired his stamina.

Walter soon settled into the life of a Swiss guide, setting high standards for climbing and entertaining his friends with his lively personality. He certainly gained the hard-won praise from the men he worked with. Beers writes: "Both Edward and Ernest Feuz had great respect for his ability and judgement, especially his route selection. Edward, a proud man who never gave unmerited praise, told warden Jim Sime that he was frustrated that he couldn't do as well as Walter." He goes on to say that "He was the last of the CPR guides, and was considered the finest climber of all; he was the only one to do difficult technical routes like The Tower on Eiffel Peak or the overhanging East Ridge of Mt. Whyte [a solo first ascent which he made in 1951, ten years before other climbers

began trying similar routes]." And, at the age of 39, he found a wife.

Pamela Hughes was a lovely young woman from England, with an unusually adventurous nature for the times. She was travelling with a friend across Canada, ostensibly heading to other destinations, but fortifying her expenses by working at the Chateau Lake Louise, where she met Walter. As guide in residence at the Chateau, Walter (and his compatriots) would often take the staff out climbing on days off and was entranced with her from the moment they met. It was not mutual, however, and Walter was challenged to gain her attention. His renowned good humour may have swung the pendulum in his direction when he inadvertently referred to her as a "bitch," through the corruption of his English. He actually said, "Pam is a peach," and fortunately held up the illuminating fruit to clarify the comment to the laughter of all. Their courtship was firmly grounded in the mountains, and when he finally had the confidence, he proposed to her on the summit of Mount Louis. Having her undivided attention, he added, with careful humour, that he would not take her down unless she accepted. Rumour has it the threat was softened by the graceful offer of a red rose. It was a fitting place for Walter to make such vows, as mountaintops "were sacred to him." His son Peter added a poignant insight into the day, saying he later found an old photograph showing Pam wearing a light blouse and a scarf around her head "as though she were just going shopping to Safeway," but with a rope around her waist and the blue sky behind her. They were married in the small Roman Catholic church in Field, B.C., in 1953.

As Walter cruised through the early years of his marriage and the final days of his contract with the CPR, events within Parks Canada were conspiring to keep him in Canada. He accepted with alacrity the post to "Public Safety Maintenance Supervisor," but with some reservations about the magnitude of the task ahead of him. Walter had no misconceptions of the challenges he would face in that regard and did not hold lightly his responsibility for the men who would be his charges. In February 1955, just months after he was hired, Parks Canada "agreed to support the establishment of a mountain climbing and rescue speciality" with the Warden Service under Perren's tutelage.

WITH A FEW GOOD SKIERS and literally no climbers in the ranks of the men working as wardens, Walter set out to create an effective mountain rescue portfolio, with competent rescue teams available to deal with all contingencies in each of the western parks. The base for the training would be at Cuthead Camp, a former warden station, later developed as an alternative workers' camp during the war. It was situated well up the Cascade fire road, about 32 kilometres north of Banff Townsite. The area was remote, but provided all the terrain Walter needed to introduce his inductees to the fine art of mountaineering and rescue. It was such an embracing centre of learning it was soon referred to affectionately by successive warden trainees as "Cuthead College." But before Walter was able to generate an effective rescue team, the worst accident on a mountain in Canadian history was about to unfold on the snowy slopes of Mt. Temple, the formidable monarch that dominates the vista of Lake Louise. It was the first time a custodial group of children (and not climbers in the remotest sense) were involved in this type of accident, but it would not be the last.

The accident involved a group of eleven boys who were part of a larger group that formed the "Wilderness Camp of Philadelphia." It was actually a private enterprise run by a lecturer from the University of Pennsylvania. The group of 24 boys (conflictingly reported to be as many as 30) had already travelled through Glacier, Montana, climbing a couple of small peaks, before heading to Banff and ultimately to Jasper to complete the trip.

Upon arriving in Banff, the leader sent the group up Mt. Rundle, which they ostensibly

signed out for, but it was here that they began to make poor choices. They were directed to the warden office to sign out and to obtain additional information on both the Mt. Rundle climb and on Mt. Temple, next on the itinerary. Despite receiving little information from two young girls in the office who knew nothing about either climb, they did not seek further help. In fact, no one went further to obtain information about either mountain, since the park "did not provide information when they sought it."

The party successfully scrambled up Rundle and then proceeded to Moraine Lake with eager eyes on the summit of Mt. Temple. A photograph shows a beautiful snow-laden mountain, far from being in condition for early summer climbing. They made base camp at the Moraine Lake campground but also decided to put in a supply camp higher up in Larch valley. The leader, probably run ragged by keeping such a large group operational, had left to pick up more groceries in nearby Lake Louise, leaving the trip up the mountain under the care of a younger supervisor who was no climber. In fact he admitted he did not even like heights. Only one of the boys had any real experience in the mountains, having gone on guided climbs in the Alps in the past summer. But to the inexperienced eye, the standard route on apparently benign snow slopes did not look that difficult—an opinion reiterated in the guidebook which did not rate it as a particularly technical climb. Once they reached the depot area, 18 of the boys convinced the supervisor to go higher despite the lateness of the day. They went on until six of the boys felt they had had enough. At the inquiry the supervisor related: "We had reached about 2,600 metres about that point, when I stopped. Travelling was satisfactory up to that point. I wasn't too keen on going on farther. I don't particularly like steep heights. I asked anyone if they wanted to stay. They had permission to go on if it looked safe on the basis of the leader's instructions." The supervisor and the six boys who stayed behind sat down to have a bite to eat. He had left a second boy in charge of the remaining nine, reminding them that the mountain was 3,536 metres high, well beyond what they might expect to do that day. None of the boys were concerned about the time. It was now going on to 4:00 p.m. on a south-facing, heavily laden snow slope heated through the day by the summer sun.

The boys carried on in single file across a large open snow slope becoming slushy with afternoon melt. They had reached 2,743 metres when the boy left in command noticed sluffs cascading down from above and "urged his companions to turn back." Before descending, however, they decided to take the precaution of roping up, revealing the extent of their inexperience. Using only a 3/8-inch manila rope, they tied together 1.5 metres apart with "slipknots" and proceeded back across the slope. One boy, upon being asked why they had roped up at all, said that "they knew this was incorrect procedure but put on the rope for practice." The most experienced boy was now the anchor man at the top end of the rope, which was appropriate as he was the oldest and also had the only ice axe they possessed. But any action was too late. The anchor man heard the avalanche coming like a freight train, but only had time to yell to the others and plunge the axe into the butter-soft snow. He managed to save himself by being braced just enough for the thin manila rope to break on impact, leaving him behind as it swept the remaining ten boys down 91 metres where they stopped just above a large drop. The boy at the other end of the rope was dragged down by the rope which he "felt tighten around his neck." With a desperate effort he pulled it free and broke away from both the rope and the avalanche. He was thrown clear when the slide stopped and found himself miraculously uninjured except for a few bruises on his face.

Not so the remaining boys. When the slide stopped, two were completely buried but five remained on top in varying degrees of shock and injury. One boy tried to help a second who was partially buried and screaming for help. Farther up the slope, the unhurt anchorman was trying desperately to extricate a second boy with little more success. The snow, which resettles upon sliding, solidifies like concrete, making extrication extremely difficult.

In the valley below, the supervisor had watched the party going up in "a thin vertical line;" then he saw what he thought was "someone rolling." Whatever or whoever it was stopped and all was quiet for a moment. Then he suddenly heard what he thought was a cry for help. This caused him to "perk up his ears" and start upward, still in confusion as to what had happened. He noticed people walking around but apparently did not see or hear the avalanche. By this time the survivors had given up trying to dig out their companions, and one went for help. He met the supervisor part-way down and hurriedly told him about the avalanche. Nothing in the man's short career as camp counsellor prepared him for what was to follow. Two boys pushed on to Moraine Lake to notify the main camp, while the supervisor proceeded to the accident site. What he saw must have been devastating—four bodies on the surface, not moving, and higher up he spotted the first survivor, now shirtless, still trying to dig out the second boy. He had given his clothing to another, but must have been near freezing himself by then. They were at an altitude of 2,700 metres in deteriorating weather with darkness approaching. None of the group had adequate clothing, let alone anything spare for the oncoming night.

The supervisor tried to comfort one boy whom he cut free of the rope, but then spotted another farther up the slope and moved on to him. He was unable to move this fellow either, and moved on to another sitting up but didn't approach him. "I didn't see what I could do to improve him." The supervisor did not hang around to take in much more. He decided that help should be brought up, and he "made for the lodge at top speed." He stopped momentarily to help one boy off the slide on his way by. Another boy was unconscious but alive, while his twin brother appeared to be dead, lying roped next to him. Now the boys were left on their own with no aid in sight and only the remote hope of a rescue party finding them in the deepening night.

The first person in authority contacted was warden J. Schauerte who, with Acting Warden Gilstorf and Dr. Sutton from the Chateau Lake Louise, formed the first party rescue team. They received news of the accident at 5:00 p.m. from the boys who had made excellent time getting back. The three men were on their way at 7:10 p.m., having notified Bert Pittaway, CPW of Banff. to organize a follow-up party. The second party under Pittaway left at 9:45 p.m. with 20 in the party, among them Walter Perren. Meanwhile, the first party had moved quickly and reached the accident site at 11:10 p.m., only two hours after leaving the trailhead. Pittaway recalls: "Perren and a couple of others went ahead. We spread out on the flanks searching for signs of the party." They soon ran into Gilstorf who "was climbing down the mountain with one of the injured boys on his back. He had carried him about a mile. It was a cruel thing to do, but I asked Gilstorf to come back up with us to lead us directly to the spot."

What alarmed and dismayed the rescuers was the obvious fact that five of the boys had lived well after the accident with non-life-threatening injuries. They might well have lived had simple precautions been taken. One of the boys was found "huddled in the snow, apparently trying to find warmth as the cold wind swept the ramparts of the mountain." Another boy who had no injuries was half buried and still tied to a second boy. Pittaway states: "If someone had cut that rope or dug him out, that boy might have been alive. There didn't appear to be anything wrong with him." The main plan of action was to take care of the living, though sadly in one case, one small boy whom they had put on a stretcher died in the short interval while they went to help another. Only two of the boys who had sustained injuries survived their ordeal. The rescue work continued

through the night aided only by the light of the moon. At 3:00 a.m., two boys were found buried about 61 metres above the rest. The five boys who died of exposure were within a 30-metre area, near or in a small creek flowing under the snow where the avalanche deposit had settled.

It was a long night bringing down the bodies, but the greatest shock was yet to come for the traumatized supervisor. When he had left for help, seven of the boys were still alive. Constable Al Moore of the RCMP recalls vividly his reaction when the bodies were brought out and he realized that only two of the boys had survived. "He turned around and started running toward Moraine Lake. I forget who was with me, but we ran down and tackled him. And the medic gave him a shot and put him out. Put him in the ambulance and took him to Banff. I think for two or three days he was sedated. You know, it was almost as though he was trying to jump in the lake or something." The seven bodies were packed out by horse, just as the Mexican women had been when they had fallen off Mt. Victoria. The horrific particulars of the accident, which occurred on July 11th, were covered early enough the next day in the *Calgary Herald*, but the full story did not emerge until the inquest was held.

So ended the second tragedy to hit Banff Park in less than a year. But the incident with the Philadelphia boys was not the clear-cut accident that had happened on Mt. Victoria. In the latter case, the party was experienced, if not adequately informed, and had made a serious error in judgment for which they held themselves responsible. Although the leadership of the boys' group was called into question, the controversy might have died down had the leader not tried to blame the park service for the accident. Suddenly Banff National Park was embroiled in an inquest that would last for years, although the immediate outcome of the preliminary hearings found no fault with the Canadian Parks Service. It would not be the last inquest that called into question the extent to which individuals are responsible for their actions, but it was the first and a benchmark in the mountain rescue saga. Although park personnel were exonerated, Walter felt the weight of the responsibility as did the men under his leadership, and training continued with that in mind.

WALTER SET OUT WITH DETERMINATION, patience and a remarkable sense of humour to cajole the Warden Service into learning to climb. Some questioned the need for this training as it seemed all they were doing was learning to risk their necks to save a lot of people they had little regard for. The warden background was one of competence in a diverse environment, but one that stopped short of high-level mountaineering. This contrasted starkly with most professional rescue organizations made up of the climbers who had the most to benefit from such resources. However Walter did have the support of two men who had great faith in his ability to accomplish this task, the first being Jim Sime, his original sponsor, and Banff Chief Park Warden Bert Pittaway.

Bert Pittaway had also seen the need for developing an effective rescue service and felt that general mountaineering and rock climbing had to be the core of the program. Pittaway began his career in Waterton Lakes National Park but transferred to Banff in 1954, where he became active in climbing and teaching what he knew to those around him. However he knew his boundaries when it came to rock climbing and advanced rescue. Any illusion he may have had about this was probably dispelled in an early incident instructing the boys in the proper use of the piton as a safety tool. Ollie Hermanrude, an early, rather sceptical apprentice in the program recalls: "He was demonstrating how a piton held, and he lurched back against his line and the piton came out. He had three metres to fall … landed amongst a boulder pile. I'll give him credit for this—he was tough. He bounced right back up on his feet and said 'that one didn't work!' He could have got killed." Pittaway was lucky that all he hurt was his pride, although he very likely sprouted some pretty severe bruises in the next few days.

Walter must have seemed like a godsend not only to Bert Pittaway, but to all the wardens, although it would be a while before that became apparent. Al Moore remembers being at one of the first schools that Walter taught. He noticed that "Walter at first may have felt a little out of place because all these wardens were looking to him for guidance. He was so unassuming and relaxed." Indeed, he was almost shy. He was a devout Catholic who did not smoke or drink. Warden Jack Holroyd noticed that if he went to a party he would nurse a glass of coke, hinting that he was drinking, and show up the next day pretending to have a massive hangover. The only problem with this was that the girls in the office often believed him. He not only did not smoke, but he disliked it so much he placed deactivated blasting caps in the ashtray of his car to discourage others from doing so as well. Swearing was not part of Walter's linguistic repertoire regardless of how extreme the aggravation. Holroyd relates: "Walter never swore no matter how exasperated or frustrated he became when fighting the paper bureaucracy to get his job done." Walter hated the paper war but nothing prompted more than a "gee whiz and eleven" comment from him, which was heard not infrequently. For brevity, Walter would limit himself to "gee whiz." But from the moment Walter came on board he inspired confidence in a group of men who needed a leader they could respect and rely on.

The wardens, to whom Walter would become devoted, were resourceful veterans prone to independence. They could be stubborn and inclined to be distrustful of new ideas, but as George Balding, a field warden destined to become Superintendent of Jasper National Park, recalled, "[they] were a bunch of extremely competent individuals in their own right. They might not have been great skiers, but they could survive in the bush on their own, without any difficulty. They also knew the benefit of co-operation. If it was too heavy to lift on your own, you got somebody to give you a hand."

Ollie Hermanrude remembers meeting Walter for the first time at Cuthead College at an early school. "Here's this little guy—very polite and we'd start at the bottom of a mountain. 'Oh yah. Ve go up now.' And he'd put his hands in his pockets and he was already at the top, but we were played out. He was a wonderful man."

Walter's greatest asset was his incredible ability in the mountains. He was extremely fit, and he had an extraordinary natural talent as a climber and an iron will to metamorphose the men into a professional rescue team. Peter Fuhrmann, who would later inherit Walter's mantle, recalls trying to keep up with him coming down from the Eisenhower Tower. Walter first said to him, "Let's have a look and see if you can walk. And he took off running down this gully over the ledge and down to the treeline and I had the darnedest time following him because he was so fast and so accurate through the boulders, it was just unbelievable … and in steep terrain."

Walter had to adjust to an increasingly complex administration system intensified by the dual tragedies on Victoria and Temple. It had been a source of vexation to the wardens to have no authority over the number of people heading for the mountains often with little training and usually no equipment. Burns states: "It was becoming all too evident that guidelines were needed for the supervision of alpine activities in the mountain parks. One immediate result of this spate of incidents was a renewed effort to enforce existing regulations calling for climbers to register with the Warden Service before setting out, giving their approximate time of return." Now, climbers were directed to provide a daily itinerary and to obtain a certificate of registration that had to be returned at completion of the trip. Failure to register or return the slip would result in prosecution. The district warden now had the authority to caution people about where they were going and what they would need. No one who was properly

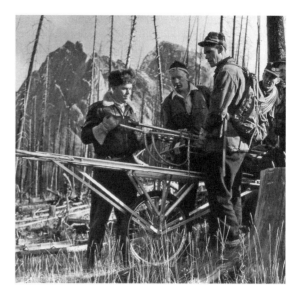

Early training with stretcher. BANFF WARDEN ARCHIVES

registered, however, could be turned back. It was a system that would come to haunt the wardens, but it was a place to start and an incentive to the wardens to wear the new hat with conviction.

Another of Walter's problems was acquiring adequate clothing and equipment for the men. When Walter took over training of the Warden Service, Western Region extended into the flatlands of Saskatchewan and Manitoba, where the men felt no compelling need to learn how to climb. But because there was exchange among parks within the region, it meant that a warden in Saskatchewan could be transferred to a mountain park and would need the expertise required there. Consequently Walter got men from many parks that had no interest in supplying their men with gear designed for high alpine country. They would show up with work boots, felt hats and blue jeans. Many early photographs depict farmers' sons and cowboys perched on a steep slab, possibly with ropes wrapped around their bodies as they descended a cliff face, looking up at Walter who had no less than a baseball cap on his head—head protection given by climbing helmets was still a thing of the future.

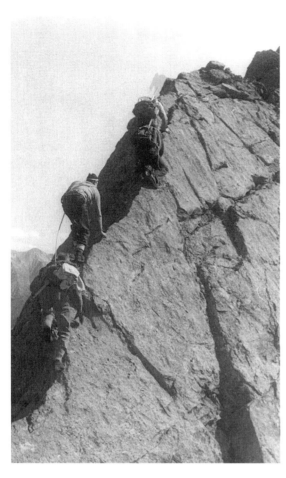

Early training at Cuthead College. BANFF WARDEN ARCHIVES.

Despite limitations, Walter asked them to go beyond their wildest dreams of what they were capable of. Often he used a carrot, saying, "Only a little farther and we will take a rest at the next rock." Or he would gently chastise them, saying, "You won't bump your head, it's only the sky." It was his favourite saying and he must have repeated it a thousand times. And when they were crawling along a broken ridge with hundreds of metres of exposure on either side, he would add, "You could bring a milk cow up here." Slowly, as a gently flowing stream carries its burden to the ocean, Walter brought the Warden Service to the role of saving lives.

Walter's main goal was to create an independent, reliable rescue service in each park. He simply could not be there when people were in trouble, which meant the wardens had to be sufficient unto themselves. In an incident on Mt. Field, just three days after the boys were brought down from Mt. Temple, Jim Sime had to contend with a small rescue on his own. The circumstance is related in *Guardians of the Wild*: "Chief Park Warden Jim Sime and Slim Haugen set out after dark in aid of a young bungalow camp worker who had gone missing on a climb of Mt. Field. Sime and Haugen found the woman just before dawn, trapped on a 30-centimetre ledge at the 2,500-metre level facing a sheer drop of 183 metres. Approaching from 40 metres above by rappel ropes, Sime was able to reach and reassure the young woman, secure her with a rope and then supervise her removal to higher ground."

Jean Lesage, the minister for Parks felt that "It was not difficult for us to see beyond the words of the report, the great courage, leadership and ability that you displayed in bringing this rescue to a happy and successful conclusion." Jim Sime dismissed the incident saying, "It was really nothing, but they made a big deal of it." This, of course, was precisely what Walter was looking for: independent thought, problem solving and determination to go when others without the training might not. Had the two men waited till daylight in the comfort of their beds, the girl would likely have perished.

But there were problems with communication and jurisdiction. Jasper and Banff share a shadowy section of wilderness that defies the thin line of a pencilled boundary indicating who is responsible for a rescue. In the early fifties, few people went into this domain of high peaks, glacial ice and snow—but the area's popularity was growing. Because of the increased amount of mountaineering activity, the superintendent of Jasper felt it was prudent to station one man with good mountaineering background at the Icefield Chalet to sign climbers out and to be on hand if an accident occurred. During the mid-fifties, that person was Fred Schleiss, who later went on to run the avalanche control program in Rogers Pass. Fred had come to Canada in 1955 from Austria, where he had been trained in mountaineering and rescue work with the Austrian Army. He was also an excellent ski instructor who had done a considerable amount of racing in his native country. Fred was a small man with piercing blue eyes and a fierce personality to boot. He commandeered the icefield area with all the authority of a Prussian general much to the relief of district warden, Mike Schintz, who was still a novice climber.

Mike's inaugural day in his new station at Sunwapta "was an indicator of things to come." While the moving truck was unloading his few belongings at the house, Mike decided to take a short patrol to the icefield area to acquaint himself with the most impressive part of his district. He had just stepped out of his truck at the chalet, when a group of people excitedly ran up to tell him that a skier had been caught in a small avalanche high up on the icefield. Mike had barely seen the highway, let alone the vast snowfields with the massive, looming peaks, but he was obviously the person in uniform and therefore responsible for any action to be taken. The enormity of his job settled heavily on his shoulders, sending a sharp pang to his stomach. He had no idea where to begin. What was apparent was that the victim, who had a broken thigh, would have to be transported over a series of broken ice-covered ledges lying below the glacier between Mt. Andromeda and Mt. Athabasca. His anxiety was soon relieved when he found out that Fred was already at the scene, where he had immobilized the victim and arranged for a rescue team to come from Jasper.

Unfortunately, because the Icefields are so vast, individuals who had accidents often did not know exactly where they were when things went wrong. It was understood that if an accident happened on the Saskatchewan Glacier, it was under Banff's jurisdiction. If it was on the Athabasca Glacier, it was to be handled by Jasper National Park wardens. Because the manpower at the Sunwapta station was very limited, it was usually necessary to call for backup from either Jasper or Banff, depending on the location of the accident. This resulted in a rather frustrating, somewhat humorous episode shortly after Mike arrived.

This unusual story concerned the early use of snowmobiles on the Icefield. In the mid-fifties the glaciers had not yet receded, and it was possible to drive a snowmobile to the top of the Athabasca Glacier and down the Saskatchewan, making for a fairly fast, very spectacular tour of the entire area. Snowmobile use was on the fringe of being banned for extensive backcountry travel, and this incident hastened that decision. A group of local snowmobilers from Jasper were doing the tour when one of their members went through a crevasse. The survivors came back to Sunwapta and reported the accident to have occurred on the Saskatchewan Glacier. Being of independent spirit, however, they proceeded to put together their own evacuation team. Walter meanwhile organized a substantial rescue party from Banff and set out the same evening, travelling through the night to save the stranded man. Unbeknownst to Walter, the snowmobilers had already returned and fished their buddy (who was up to his waist in water, but otherwise unhurt) out and returned to town. Sometime after midnight, Walter found the tracks, a hole in the snow on the Athabasca Glacier, and nobody around. The disgruntled team returned to Banff uncertain why they had even been called out. It did lead to better communications between the two parks, though the problem would continue to surface from time to time.

In 1957, an accident occurred in Jasper that the wardens handled quite well without Walter's help. One of the key persons who helped on this rescue was renowned climber Tony Messner, who was later recruited to help Walter at Cuthead College. Tony was a climber of international status known for major climbs in the Himalayas, and who had made his home in Jasper where he earned a living as a part-time guide and carpenter.

Two Hungarian men had apparently decided to climb Mt. Brule, a small, non-technical mountain at the east end of the park, but had opted to return by an enticing snow slope descending directly from the summit. The first man immediately lost control and shot down the mountain to plummet over an 244-metre vertical rock face. His body struck the ground some 15 metres from the foot of the cliff but rolled another 457 metres down a snow-filled gulley. The second man managed to stop before going over the cliff and descended to a point where he could yell for help. Unfortunately his garbled Hungarian led the people below to misconstrue the nature of the accident, and it was thought that the deceased was buried in an avalanche. When Messner arrived he realized that the follow-up party needed ropes and climbing equipment to bring the body and survivor down. He spent the night with the survivor, and the next day a party of "five experienced men" arrived to effect the rescue over difficult and unstable cliff bands above the railroad tracks.

Again, Walter had reason to be happy with the success of this rescue, particularly *because* he was not involved. It showed that Jasper could handle their own rescues without calling on Banff. This was critical and went a long way to establishing within each park an esprit de corps that sometimes bordered on friendly rivalry. In fact, it would become a point of pride within each park that teams could handle their own problems effectively.

Because the men were expected to be in their districts in the active summer season, Walter generally was only given about two weeks in the fall for the training sessions. Mike Schintz later wrote: "From the very beginning, proficiency in travel and survival in mountainous terrain and under all weather conditions were the foundation upon which the training was based." Walter was adamant that men who could not look after themselves could not help others, let alone rescue

them. The schools emphasized fitness, and early training tended to be route marches though bog, up steep deadfall-choked mountainsides to open scree slopes and broken cliff bands.

Once Walter was confident the men could handle themselves safely in mountainous terrain, he moved on to train for rescues. It wasn't long before problems inherent in pulling a body off steep, broken terrain became evident. Besides the risk of falling off, there was constant danger from rock fall that on several occasions almost cost lives. As much as he wished, Walter did not have eyes in the back of his head to monitor everyone's actions. Al Moore recalls one frightening incident while employing the cumbersome rescue basket to lower the "victim" on the first school he attended. On this occasion, they were trying to effect a traverse with the loaded stretcher to bring it into position for a straight lower. Walter had driven in two pitons on either side of the traverse, with the rope running on pulleys to ease the tension as the stretcher was hauled across the rock face. The hapless victim was an older warden named Glen Fagan. Moore relates: "So his body was hanging straight down and about halfway across—they were pulling it with a rope—it was sliding across and it caught on a rock and flipped over. And Fagan's nose was sort of rubbing across the rock. Fagan was screaming and hollering, but he always wanted to be the victim because then he didn't have to climb back down."

Fagan survived, but it must have been a relief when he was not the victim on a much more serious incident later on. Willi Pfisterer, who would soon play a principal role in the development of mountain rescue in the Warden Service, was one of the instructors on the school that day. He recalls the incident vividly, saying in his lingering Austrian accent: "We got this group and we were lowering a guy down in this mine basket and this guy was Smokey Guttman. We were coming down this little bit of a draw and there was loose rocks and so I sent anyone coming down to a ledge under a big face. Any time someone comes down,

I send them over there—so they be out of the rock fall. So they took Guttman over there in this basket. But it had started to snow in big flakes, wet flakes … and I say offhand 'He's lying there all exposed, let him out before he gets all wet.' And then down rappels one guy after another, and the last one down was a policeman. And I am the only one standing there when he knocks a rock loose—and it was a good one. It rolled down the gully, and it turned right across the gully in a big loop. But they just get the straps off and Smokey rolls over and gets up—and as he rolls over, the rock hits the basket."

There were many close calls by rock fall, which was particularly serious when the schools first started, because no one wore hard hats. Walter soon saw the folly in this and began to issue construction hats in lieu of proper climbing helmets, which were not yet on the market. Since Walter was officially in charge of public safety, he was able to obtain a few of these hats, and in two instances, none too soon. Warden Peter Tasker tells of the first time he ever wore a construction hat. "I was on a rope with Walter, and we were up on a glacier somewhere and a whole bunch of rocks came down. It was the first time I ever wore a hat and the rock knocked it off." Later, Joe Halstenson was on a rescue school on the cliffs at the end of Lake Louise when he got hit directly on the head by a large rock released by the cable he was being lowered on. The rock, which was about the size of a baseball, split the helmet in half and actually drove the hat band over his ears. Without a doubt the hard hat saved his life.

Walter set up serious and very realistic rescue scenarios, knowing that the men could very likely be faced with similar situations. Ollie Hermanrude described one practice where they had to cross a deep canyon. On this particular exercise, the rope was strung over the canyon (Tyrolean traverse style) to transport men and equipment across using carabiners and pulleys. The carabiners were attached to the climbing harness and then clipped to the rope. The first man went across hand over

hand trailing a second rope behind him. Once set up, they put a man in the rescue basket and brought him across. The first man across in the mine basket was warden Bill Hollingsworth, who fortunately had his hands free. He was poised over the canyon when the knot tying the head of the stretcher to the carabiner started to unravel. Hermanrude remembers that "Bill was watching because he reached up and just grabbed … the knot as it let loose … it was 200 feet below him where he would have dropped." They quickly hauled him across before he lost the rope and dropped head first over the torrent below.

Other problems surfaced. Ed Carlton did not want to trust anyone else tying the knots attaching his seat sling to the carabiner he went across on—which was fine, except that he left the tail on his seat harness way too long. Halfway across the canyon, the excess webbing twisted around the main rope and jammed in his carabiner. Hermanrude is not quite sure how Carleton extricated himself, but now everyone was jittery. Ollie decided to use two carabiners instead of one, which promptly jammed together, leaving him similarly suspended until he could free himself. Throughout the various trials, Walter remained calm, though his stress level must have been rising.

Despite the risks, the majority of the men did not give up. This had a lot to do with the reliance they had in Walter, who had an uncanny ability to assess a man's capacity for the work and to place him accordingly. Those who excelled at climbing and did not mind the exposure were put on the "point" or lead end of the rescue work or climbing schools. Others that did not function well under exposed conditions were given equally important tasks on safer ground. Schintz wisely observed: "Most important of all, they learned to take care of each other. Men who had been fiercely independent all their lives, if not outright loners, learned to work together as a team."

But the job was definitely not for everyone. Some men knew (as well as Walter did) that they should not be there. When a young fellow from Jasper was placed in the mine basket and lowered over a vertical cliff, he went white and almost fainted. At the end of the school, he marched into the office and turned in his equipment with a derogatory comment as to where Parks could put their climbing boots.

Although the accidents that occurred were still few and far between, there were enough serious ones to keep Walter challenged to assemble a reliable rescue party. Don Beers recounts a rescue of a friend on an ambitious attempt on Mt. Temple. It was a new route beyond the scope of the climbers, and after three days they were in trouble. Beers relates: "My close friend spent three nights on the face of Mt. Temple stranded with two companions as a result of a combination of calamities. One man could not go ahead on the rock route they had chosen, another lost a crampon and couldn't go back over the snow couloir by which they had come, and a sudden heavy snowstorm prevented them from finding an alternate way down. When conditions improved slightly, lack of food and sleep destroyed the confidence they needed to descend the steep cliffs." His friend remembers, "We began hallucinating simultaneously, *seeing* people who weren't there. We just couldn't go on. On the fourth day, Walter Perren arrived, and it all seemed so easy. I don't remember anything remarkable that he did. He offered to put in a fixed rope, but he gave us the confidence we needed, and going down was no problem."

Another more dangerous body recovery followed this rescue. The incident occurred on Mt. Blane in Kananaskis Country just east of the Banff National Park boundary. It also marked one of the first occasions that wardens began to extend their services beyond the park boundaries. A pair of climbers were climbing up a series of rotten gullies when one man was killed, leaving the other to go for help. When Walter realized how far up the mountain the accident was, he knew he would need considerable manpower to bring the body out.

The operation involved lowering the body down a series of steep slabby gullies which were natural funnels for every loose rock on the mountain. The awkward load was constantly jamming in small fissures or getting hung up on rock outcrops. Even moving men and equipment around was hazardous on the friable, unstable mountain. It soon became evident that the danger was becoming unacceptable, forcing Walter to make the difficult decision to expedite the recovery. As George Balding knew, Walter was concerned about the safety of the men. "Their physical comfort, well-being and safety was much, much greater than the indignity to some dead body." The body was very carefully wrapped in a tough canvas pack mantle, secured

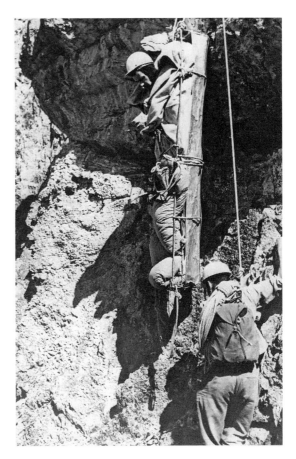

Bringing man off Mt. Blane. BANFF WARDEN ARCHIVES

43

with rope, and allowed to slide over the edge to the bottom of the cliff where retrieval was much easier and many times safer.

By 1960, Walter had been training men for over five years, and his reputation as an excellent instructor capable of moulding an effective rescue unit was spreading. He was now getting requests for men to attend from agencies outside the park service. Burns notes in *Guardians of the Wild* that, "The British Columbia government, for example, asked if its Mount Robson Provincial Park supervisor could attend the warden's fall climbing school. Later the headquarters staff at the Department of National Defence asked that three or four members of the armed forces be permitted to attend the next mountain climbing and rescue school. Permission was also granted to three U.S. National Park Rangers attend upcoming courses in Yoho—a feather in Director Coleman's cap, since it had not been long since the wardens had asked to go to their training schools in Colorado. Assistant Director Alex Reeve was happy to write: "It is apparent that our National Park mountain rescue training has gained favourable recognition in the United States as well as in our own country." Walter was also training the RCMP right from the beginning.

Walter was not doing the work single-handedly. From the outset he knew he would need help, and for this he turned to the swelling ranks of young climbers from the old country. Willi Pfisterer and Peter Fuhrmann, who would jointly succeed Walter, started out by being employed by him to help with the schools through the late fifties and sixties.

Walter divided the participants of the schools into three groups. He always took the A or advanced group, while Willi, who had climbed before coming to Canada, usually got the intermediate B group, and Peter took the beginners in C group. Walter also asked Fred Schleiss and Tony Messner to help with the training. Introducing these men to the Warden Service was of great benefit, because it provided continuity of training standards and rescue procedures that would become the core strength of the future rescue teams. To this end, Walter recommended each mountain park include two days of mountain rescue in its annual spring training program.

Walter himself spent most of the summer climbing with wardens in their districts. He was very familiar with popular climbs in the front-country, but this was a tremendous opportunity to explore the rest of the park and become acquainted with potential difficulties that might affect future rescues. For a while the wardens clung to ponies and often rode them to the base of a climb. Joe Halstenson recalls doing several climbs, riding to the mountain and leaving the horses tied up while they went off for the day climbing.

The skills they learned were put to the test on two significant rescues in 1960/61. An arduous rescue in Glacier National Park was an early testimony to the success of Walter's program in that it was carried out on difficult terrain by the wardens with no aid from guides or climbing instructors. The accident happened in July, 1960, on Mt. Avalanche, a fairly easy peak near the summit of Rogers Pass. A group of six inexperienced climbers reached the peak on the moderate rock ridges but decided to take an alternate route down that looked easy but which led into a series of snow gullies interspersed with rock ribs. They were inexperienced in the proper use of ropes and belay techniques which they haphazardly employed in their increasing frustration to get to safer ground. Inevitably one person slipped, pulling the others down, and the whole group fell some 60 metres. Miraculously, the greatest injuries were bruises and broken bones. The leader was able to go for help, which came late in the afternoon under the direction of Warden C. Thomas with eight park employees. Although a follow-up party of twelve led by wardens Bill Laurilla and L.B. Faggetter were hot on their heels, it unavoidably wound up being a night rescue. In total, the evacuation took over 14 hours and the efforts of 22 volunteers, but

Bert Pittaway found no problem with this. He wrote: "Considering the terrain they had to negotiate and the injuries reported plus the carrying up of baskets, deer-toter, first-aid supplies, extra ropes and food, I consider the number of men used were an absolute necessity." Their effort resulted in bringing everyone down alive, which was something of a record in those days and a huge boost to morale for the Warden Service.

The crowning epic rescue of Gordon Crocker on Mt. Blane, however, put everyone to the test. It was also the first time that the rescue team decided to use the controversial new machine available to the park—the helicopter. Walter probably decided to give it a try after Chief Park Warden Jim Sime and Bob Woods, another warden, found the helicopter to be "extremely valuable" in searching for a climber missing in the Purcell Range of B.C. Searchers covered a large area in a short time, which is of prime importance in a search. Unfortunately, the tracks which they picked up on one of the large glaciers were lost in a maze of crevasses and the person was not found.

On August 27, at 8:00 a.m. Walter got the call for help from Provincial Ranger M. Verhaege stationed at Canmore, requesting aid in rescuing an injured man on Mt. Blane. The accident was first reported by Dieter Raubach, who was climbing the mountain with Gordon Crocker, both members of the newly formed Calgary Mountain Club. From his report, it was apparent that Crocker was lying injured with a broken ankle and possible internal injuries at an elevation of 2,865 metres.

Walter's first concern was to reach the climber with supplies before nightfall. He writes: "This was achieved by D. Raubach and myself at 6:15 p.m. Mr. Raubach was left with the injured man, and I climbed back down to the high camp, elevation 6,800 [2,073 metres], which had been established by the rest of the party with the help of the helicopter."

Before Walter set out with Raubach, he had assessed the rescue requirements. He realized the evacuation would need a high camp and would probably take two days if the helicopter could be used. With some nervous anticipation, he requested a helicopter from Foothills Aviation in Calgary. From Raubach's description of the terrain, Walter knew he would need the assistance of some fairly experienced climbers. Accordingly, he immediately contacted fellow guides Hans Gmoser and Klaus Hahn from the Calgary Mountain Club.

Walter realized that the helicopter could only be used if a substantial platform was built on the steep hillside to support the weight of the machine for both loading and unloading supplies and men. He was able to commandeer the use of inmates from a local detention centre to build the structure, which was a feat in itself.

On August 28 a small party set off from high camp for the traumatized climber. Walter writes: "A party consisting of wardens Shepherd, Carlton, constables Kennedy and Bellman, G. Johnston [prevailing rate employee], K. Hahn from the Calgary Mountain Club, H. Gmoser, Banff, and myself left high camp with climbing and rescue equipment at 6:00 a.m. and arrived at the scene, 9,400 foot [2,900 metre] elevation, at 12:00 noon."

Possibly in deference to the wardens, Walter does not add in the report that only he and Hans Gmoser actually reached Crocker and Raubach at noon of that day. Hans recalls that the climbing, though not severe, was consistently steep and difficult enough that neither the wardens nor the RCMP could keep up a fast pace. Accordingly, Walter decided to go on with Hans, leaving the rest in Hahn's care to come up at a slower pace with the bulk of the rescue equipment. Hans relates: "I remember going up there … there was one little pitch where you had to climb … [and] we had to belay every warden up there and for some it was quite a thing. Then Walter and I just went on to go and find Gordon because we realized this wasn't going to work." They found both men in fair spirits and proceeded to set up a lowering system to bring Crocker down to meet the slower party. Hans was invaluable, because he was strong enough to carry the injured man on his back with an improvised rescue seat harness using a spare climbing rope. Hans relates: "In those days I was so strong, I could carry a man on my back … [we used] just the rope … you know how you coil it up? You split it in half and put half over your shoulders and then he [Crocker] puts his legs through the other half. It works really good. Walter was belaying me, and I was walking down, and he was just hanging [on my back]."

When the four men met the remaining rescuers, Walter recalls, "We transported and lowered the injured climber down the mountain with the help of a Gramminger seat carrier, to an elevation of 2,438 metres, arriving at 6:30 p.m. Climbing in the dark was considered too hazardous on account of loose rock, and it was decided to break up the operation. Warden Carlton bivouacked with the injured climber; the rest of the party climbed down to high camp arriving at 8:00 p.m." The following day the same rescue party without Gmoser or Hahn climbed back to the bivouacked party to effect the rest of the lower using a rescue basket. The operation was completed at 4:00 p.m. Walter also concluded that "the portable radios and helicopter were of extreme value."

Walter did not think the pair were prepared for a bivouac and questioned their ability to tackle the difficult climb. Robert Burns, in *Guardians of the Wild,* writes: "Perren complained that increasingly climbers were attempting new, more difficult ascents, often involving 'sheer vertical walls.' 'Climbers,' he felt, were 'taking chances knowing that they will be rescued at the cost of the department disregarding danger involved by the rescue team.'"

One of the principal persons pushing the limits of climbing on "sheer walls" was Walter's good friend Hans Gmoser. His climbing exploits marked the beginning of modern rock climbing in Canada. Young climbers soon followed, leading to the formation of the Calgary Mountain Club. Chic Scott, an early member, later wrote: "The membership was made up primarily of new Canadians from Britain, Austria, New Zealand and Germany. These men and women were energetic, resourceful and full of adventure. They had found that the existing clubs were stale and exhausted and sought to form their own group where fun and adventure were the bywords." On June 8, 1960, the CMC held its first official meeting and elected a slate of officers. From that point on, the club attracted the most daring climbers in the country, who rapidly pushed the envelope of climbing, giving Walter real grounds for being concerned. Although Walter kept the training standards as high as possible, it would be another generation of wardens who reached the benchmark of the climbers they sought to save.

ANOTHER DEVELOPMENT at this time was the creation of the Association of Canadian Mountain Guides (ACMG). Hans Gmoser was one of the principal founders. Hans had learned to climb in Austria before he came to Canada to visit the "Canadian Alps" he had heard about. "My background at that time was mostly climbing for my own enjoyment with just one friend, which was sort of the tradition back in Austria."

Shortly after Hans arrived in 1952 with friend Leo Grillmair, he went to work guiding for Lizzie Rummel at Mt. Assiniboine, but for this he felt it best to have a licence. He relates: "I went to the Parks office and got a guide's licence by filling out a two-page questionnaire and paid $2.00 for it." This went on until 1955 when Walter was hired. Walter was uncomfortable with how easily Hans had obtained the park licence and decided a more formal test was needed. Accordingly, he called Hans in and asked if he would be willing to take a test. This was no problem for Hans who was equally uneasy with such superficial requirements. Hans recalls: "It was a four-day test. One day rock climbing, two days mixed climbing and one day of oral examination—that was early 1956." Bruno Engler, also from Switzerland, and who would go on to record on camera some of the finest moments in mountaineering and rescue history, took the test with him.

Throughout the rest of the fifties, Walter continued to qualify different people for their guide's licence in this manner, including his successors, Willi Pfisterer and Peter Fuhrmann. But as the end of the decade approached, Walter became too busy to keep certifying guides when the applications piled on his desk. He finally suggested to Hans that the existing guides form an association and be responsible for qualifying their own members.

Hans and Peter were possibly the most enthusiastic about this prospect and called potential members together for a meeting at a small cabin owned by Heinz Kahl near Lac des Arc. It was an eclectic group of men, some excited, others more reserved, that gathered informally for the meeting that would establish a rigorous guiding organization. With a quiet smile Hans described that first meeting: "Oh, there were quite a few. There was Brian Greenwood, Dick Lofthouse, Hans Schwartz, Willi Pfisterer, Peter Fuhrmann, Leo [Grillmair] … about eight or 10 of us. Oh, yah, then Ken Baker, Dave Brewer and Heinz Kahl. At the time we were [divided] … some thought we should have a more comprehensive test and others felt whatever we had should be good enough. Finally it was left at that. Peter Fuhrmann was elected president, Leo was secretary and I was chairman of the standards committee. So I went to work and wrote out a training program—sort of a two-week course. Walter felt we should do something a little more substantial because it was just not a test any more. It was really for people to come and get training … and it was eventually a training course, but we expected people to come with a pretty good background."

The Association of Canadian Mountain Guides marked the beginning of establishing professional standards that would evolve as the sport pushed mountaineering boundaries. And it would be the standard that the Warden Service would adopt for leaders in the public safety field. But it was the climbers who remained on the leading edge of climbing, challenging the guides and the rescuers to keep abreast as they explored difficult routes in ever more remote country.

BEFORE THAT ERA SET IN, however, the wardens had to deal with rescues that would challenge their abilities and ingenuity. One interesting rescue that exemplifies the difficulties with ground evacuation over difficult terrain occurred in 1962 above Hector Lake just north of Lake Louise. On July 21st a party was registered out for one ambitious trip to ascend Bath Creek in Yoho National Park, cross the Waputik Glacier, and return via Hector Lake. The party of three (a doctor, his wife and a friend), had not returned their registration by the end of the day and a search was begun the next morning. Walter was able to contact local pilot Norman Genereux, who flew the area with Chief Park Warden Jim Sime. The tracks of the party were spotted leading to Turquoise Lake below the glacier and above a series of cliff bands. On a second pass they spotted the party waving a red shirt in the wind. The rescue party set off on foot with climbing equipment and food. Moving quickly they reached the stranded climbers three hours after setting out at 5:00 a.m. They found that the party had hunkered down to wait for a rescue after the wife had lost her ability to walk the afternoon of the previous day. No explanation was ever given as to why she could not walk. The wardens had to accept that, and the arduous process of hauling her out began. A second party under the leadership of warden Bill Vroom had come in to help with the task, and to everyone's relief, he also had a motorboat waiting for them once they reached Hector Lake. Once across the lake, the ever-resourceful Vroom also had horses for the rest of the trip to the highway. The lady was safely out by 8:00 p.m. that night.

It must have been some consolation to receive a grateful letter from the husband expressing his appreciation for the rescue and high praise for the men involved. He writes: "A brief episode in our lives, in ours and yours, but one in which I learned much. I have seen great difficulty before, but somehow, the spirit of the men involved made this different. The human element now was one of dedication, understanding—a matter-of-fact acceptance of a job to be done."

The following year, Walter put the helicopter to use again, this time stretching the flying limits of the machine. A couple were hiking and climbing in the Little Yoho Valley of Yoho National Park when the husband went missing. He wanted to climb The Vice President, the highest peak in the valley, but since his wife chose to stay in camp, he went alone. When he did not return later that night, help was sent for the next day.

Warden Bill Hollingsworth received the information which was immediately passed on to the chief park warden, Murray Dawson. Dawson realized a ground party would take 11 hours to reach the area, so he requested the use of an aircraft. Surprisingly, Superintendent Scott "was advised that the use of a helicopter was not warranted" but "he could perhaps obtain the services of a fixed-wing aircraft." It is interesting that the helicopter was so readily dismissed, but this was largely due to the unavailability of the machine. The closest helicopter at that time was in Calgary, and the cost was prohibitive. However, luck was with the rescuers on that day. When the park contacted the pilot of the fixed-wing aircraft, he immediately mentioned that a helicopter was due in Banff a few minutes later, and after further consultation with Regional Supervisor Coombs, the machine was sent for.

From that point on, things clicked into place. Hollingsworth was immediately dispatched by helicopter to do a hasty search of the peaks and surrounding glaciers and soon found the tracks. They led to the summit of The President, then to the summit of The Vice President. Here they stopped. The pilot, Ralph Hancock, landed on the summit at an elevation of 3,060 metres to confirm that the tracks were those of the missing climber. Continued flights revealed no signs of the man nor any tracks leading off the summit. Walter was now in charge of the search, and he decided to put two teams in.

Both teams were taken in by the aircraft: Perren and Rutherford to the summit of The Vice President to climb down to meet the second team of Hollingsworth and Dawson, flown in to the base of the mountain. The helicopter then flew Walter's party to the top of the Emerald Glacier, where the body was spotted by Rutherford at the base of a very hazardous chimney. It appeared that the man had descended directly from the summit down the open cliffs and had come to grief in the final chimney. The search concluded when the two parties were reunited by helicopter to move the body to a location suitable for pickup and airlift out to Takakkaw Falls, the base of the rescue operation.

The potential for this machine for use in rescue support was indisputable. They had been blessed with clear, hot, windless weather, perfect for flying; nonetheless, the machine had more than proven its versatility by being able to land the rescue parties in places totally unapproachable by fixed wing, thus eliminating a long ground search. Walter was very impressed that the helicopter could land on the summit of The Vice President at an altitude of over three thousand metres, a major feat for the underpowered craft.

ONE VERY SIGNIFICANT AREA of responsibility that Walter inherited was skier safety in the burgeoning ski areas within the national parks. The Norquay, Sunshine and Lake Louise (at that time called Whitehorn/Temple) ski areas had been developed in the 1930s. Noel Gardner, who had expounded earlier of things to come noted: "With the great increase in the popularity of recreational skiing, national parks with ski areas within their boundaries are faced with an entirely new type of problem ... the well-being and safety of the recreational skier, and it is thought that the Warden Service must handle the job." Noel had worked at Sunshine as a ski instructor and was quick to notice "the most flagrant disregard of all safety procedures." He also felt "if snow and avalanche hazard continues to be disregarded it will only be a matter of time until lives are lost." He was not wrong.

Shortly after Noel had uttered these words, Charles Dupre was killed in an avalanche at Marmot Basin in Jasper National Park after skiing into a closed area. The avalanche was triggered by the skier, who was carried to the bottom of the run after being hit by a second avalanche triggered by the release of the first. It was a massive slide witnessed by two wardens, Clarence Wilkins and Steve Kun (later superintendent of Banff National Park), who quickly organized a search party, finding the body only after extensive probing. If it is of any consolation to either the victim or the family, the slope is now in a controlled part of the ski area and has been named "Dupre Bowl."

Although the wardens started looking after the ski hills in the early fifties both as ski patrollers and in avalanche control, it was after Walter arrived that control work really advanced. And without a doubt it was avalanche control that caused concern—so much so that by the sixties the ski areas took over the ski patrol portion of the work, leaving the wardens free to concentrate on avalanche control.

Walter was also concerned with skiers travelling beyond the skiing areas into the backcountry, where avalanches were uncontrolled and very difficult to predict. He was also reluctant to post an avalanche warning hazard, because forecasting was not that advanced. Even so, Banff did put out an avalanche warning poster at Bow Summit in 1958, a popular ski area highly frequented by adventurous skiers. As Brad White ruefully wrote in an article on avalanche history: "The wording gives a good indication of the state of understanding of avalanche phenomena at the time:

DON'T ski on slopes of 22 degrees or more for at least three days after a fresh snowfall.

DON'T ignore a sudden rise in temperature. It may be the first hint of wet snow avalanches during rain or in warm weather. During a thaw, avalanches may occur more frequently in the afternoon than in the morning.

DON'T ski on slopes facing away from the direction of the wind immediately after a fresh fall of snow. (Soft and Powdery.)

DON'T be misled by a false sense of security. Slopes hardened by the wind will present a slab-like condition which may cause a fatal avalanche accident.

DON'T traverse a dangerous slope horizontally; if it is essential, remove your skis and cross high up.

DON'T cross a dangerous slope wearing skis. The chance of surviving an avalanche is greater when you are on foot and is less likely to cause slide.

DON'T travel within one hundred yards of your nearest companion when crossing a suspected slope.

DON'T cross a slope directly beneath a cornice. Should it break, an avalanche might result.

DON'T forget that the tip of an avalanche may travel over moderate slopes and even over flat ground.

DON'T take chances and don't let your skiing companion take chances."

This wordy warning—though basically good advice—did little to prevent the deaths of two skiers in a ski-triggered avalanche at Bow Summit in November of that year. The wardens had actually placed closure warning flags on the upper slopes, but the skiers had strayed too close and had caused the release of the avalanche. Wardens Neil Woledge and Hal Shepherd responded immediately, but there was little they could do. It was one of the few areas that the wardens tried to control outside of the ski areas proper, and the accident left a bad taste in Walter's mouth. In his report of the avalanche he states: "In my opinion, marking avalanche areas away from lift facilities in alpine country is not practical, the conditions change very rapidly, and the hazard cannot be tested and controlled." He went on to note: "When avalanche accidents happen ... it is usually due to either inexperience, ignorance or failure to ascertain the conditions of the area." In a prescient adjunct to that message he also makes the judgement that "it is the responsibility of all those who undertake to ski on alpine slopes to be sufficiently educated in ski lore to understand all hazards involved." With one bold statement he clearly places the responsibility for safety with the visitor—a notion that would be seriously challenged in years to come.

Walter's main avalanche control focus, aside from the ski areas, was the system of roads and highways within the parks. Neither the Norquay nor Lake Louise access roads presented much of a problem, but the road up to Sunshine passed under huge avalanche slopes, as did the Banff-Jasper Highway and the Trans-Canada Highway through Yoho. There were also large avalanche paths along the highway through Kootenay National Park, but it was lightly travelled and could be closed if needed. This was also true of the Banff/Jasper Highway which was, in fact, closed through the winter during Walter's era. Brad White reports, "Up until the mid-1960s very little active road control was undertaken. During the big snow winter of 1965 several large natural avalanches blocked the highways, and the need for active control work on the roads became evident." It was not till after Walter's death, however, that dedicated control work was applied to the highways, and that largely because of the increasing use of the helicopter for such work.

The Sunshine Road occupied most of Walter's time and concern because of the very steep avalanche paths and slow-moving traffic. It also had to be done on foot and much of the work was quite dangerous.

Ollie Hermanrude was the warden at Healy Creek in 1952, when people accessed the Sunshine ski hill with a small bus. At that time he ran the ski patrol, the communications and the first-aid hut for the few people who came up. The buses brought only about 8 to 10 skiers on weekends and two to three on weekdays. When Hermanrude left in 1966, this number had increased to a couple of thousand, and the road had a very rudimentary avalanche warning system. He recalls: "There was some avalanche control. Walter Perren started that up ... about 1964. We started putting avalanche triggers in up above the second and third slide on the Sunshine Road. When the avalanches started, it would trigger these lights ... the lights would come on at the road and you stopped. That was it. It could tell you an avalanche was coming—red light and it meant stop. And it would come right down in front of you!"

The wire was strung across the path early in the season, and when the avalanche released, the wire was ripped out, tripping a switch at the side of the path, closing an electrical circuit that switched on the red light bulb at the road. A minute later, an avalanche would sweep by. There is no record of the bus being in the middle of the path after the light had gone on, and no accidents occurred with this elementary warning system. However, after the first avalanche of the year went by, the wire would have to be restrung and the switch reset. This meant climbing into the trigger zone well above the road and working in the avalanche path. This was not very effective during a storm cycle when even small avalanches that did not reach the road would trigger the light.

They needed a method which would eliminate the need to crawl up to reset the trigger every time a sluff occurred. Walter had seen avalanches triggered by artillery and decided to see if mortars could be used in avalanche control. On the first occasion, Hermanrude remembers, "The army came in with the mortars, and they mortar bombed it to test it out. And they thought—well. They'll have a couple of minutes to get out of the way. It took less than 50 seconds for the avalanche to hit the road after the bomb exploded." In the end, it was not very successful because of the inaccuracy of the guns. There was always the possibility of lobbing the shells over the low mountain shoulder onto the Trans-Canada

Highway—a risk the park was not willing to take, no matter what the avalanche hazard.

George Balding, who also worked at Sunshine, recalls that using detonation cord in the trigger zone usually gave the best results. If the avalanche was set off by controlled means, the results were infinitely more predictable. Walter experimented with detonation cord to set off a small explosion within the snowpack when the hazard was high enough to threaten the road. Again, the drawback was that it meant laying new cord every time—which meant crawling back into the trigger zone.

The avalanche control on the Sunshine road would plague the wardens for years to come. Effective control meant stabilizing the slopes in the early hours of the morning so the road could be opened for daytime traffic. The problem is now solved by using two Gazex stations that allow nitrogen gas to be exploded over the top of the snowpack at the trigger zone, effectively releasing the avalanches.

Walter never turned down a good idea. He was very amenable to using hand bombs thrown into the snowpack to trigger the slide. But this method relied on hitting a weak layer in the snowpack to trigger the avalanche and was not always successful. Chief Park Warden Andy Anderson recalled: "At that time the Swiss had been playing around with explosives, and in the States they were using TNT in a jam can. But they were always trying to get a bit more shocking power."

Andy had picked up some knowledge of explosives during his career, and he worked with Walter to see if they could come up with a better control system. Andy convinced Walter to talk Chief Park Warden Bob Hand out of $50 to take a representative from Canadian Industries Limited (CIL) out for lunch. Andy got first-rate advice from the man. "I ended up with a box of seismic powder and a spool of Primacord. I also got some caps and some fuses. I went back to Sunshine with Walter and [one other] and just threw a 10-pound stick of dynamite onto the slope, and we had good conditions and good results." Andy

soon got a blasting ticket through the Workers' Compensation Board and they were in business.

Walter was also responsible for Norquay and Whitehorn/Temple ski areas where more traditional control methods were often used. These consisted of ski cutting the slope or cutting off snow cornices that overhung loaded slopes. The cornices were cut using a very large crosscut saw, or were blown off using Primacord strung along the natural break with the cliff edge. Both methods were fairly dangerous, because it would be easy to lose a man when the cornice was released. Andy recalls that "one guy would have a rope on and be out on the cornice … sawing away, and the other guy held him from above."

Slopes were also ski stabilized by keeping them packed down by constant skiing after a heavy snowfall; a method which is common practice today. Such work can be dangerous when the fresh snow is heavy enough to avalanche when skiing the slope. More than one patroller or warden has taken a frightening "ride" with a surface sluff that could easily have buried him. Joe Halstenson remembers getting caught in a slide at Whitehorn when he was skiing with Andy Anderson and Walter Perren. In a semi-humorous recollection he forces a smile saying, "Walter said to Andy: 'Gee whiz. There goes Joe. Keep an eye on him.' Anyway I only went so far then stopped … but that was a close one."

Other unforeseen hazards popped up from time to time during this work. On another occasion that almost seems like a version of the Keystone Cops, Halstenson relates: "We were with Walter again up in those chutes [at Whitehorn] with a stick of dynamite, and we had our skis off, because it was hard to get into this one area. Andy lit it, and we were climbing back out when he got his boot stuck in the rocks. The dynamite was lit and buried in the snow not far away. He was pulling away and when I said 'Hey, quite fooling around—we got to get out of here!' And Andy said 'No! I'm stuck!' Walter was on the other side watching all this, and he knew there was a

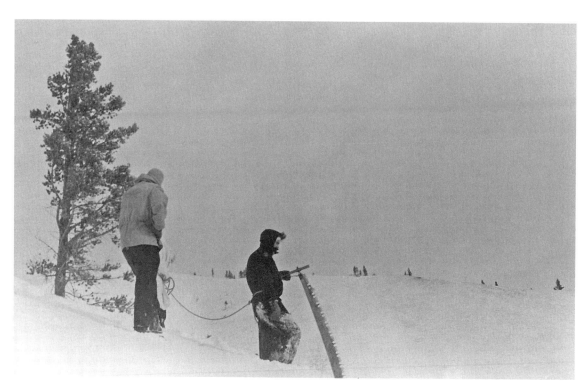

Sawing cornice with swede saw. BANFF WARDEN ARCHIVES

problem. But finally Andy got loose and we got out of there."

Another important thing the men learned was that the dry snow sometimes created enough static electricity to set the charge off. This quickly led to using safety fuses. Static electricity is also created around whirling helicopter blades—it became an important consideration when the machine was later used to drop bombs on avalanche slopes.

Mt. Norquay had few control problems until a new run called the Wishbone was created for the 1968 Winter Olympic bid. Warden John Wackerle helped clear and slash the steep slope that was never used for the event, but which became a major avalanche hazard every winter. Controlling the hazard was quite difficult as the trigger zone could only be reached by climbing to the top of the run to ski cut it. John recalls they also tried to tramp it down by foot (boot packing) but first they would attempt to undercut the snow slabs with a

ski pole by climbing a tree and poking the surface as far out as they could reach. This was largely unsuccessful, and eventually they would just ski it. Hand charges were eventually used, which more or less exchanged one risk for another. To this day it remains the biggest man-made hazard in the area and is usually closed for skiing.

MOUNTAIN RESCUE TRAINING (later called public safety training) schools were also becoming more important. They not only allowed the wardens to achieve new skills, but also provided a way to experiment with new rescue techniques and equipment. Robert Burns writes: "By 1962, the wardens were experimenting in the use of both a stretcher and a type of bosun's chair (now called the Gramminger seat) for moving injured climbers down vertical surfaces. By mid-decade the open stretcher had evolved into a body-length basket, its upper portion caged to protect the immobilized victim from abrasions during the descent."

One major leap forward was the introduction of the steel cable and winch system used successfully for some years in Europe. Substituting a steel cable in place of rope came about after a near-tragic episode when a group of schoolchildren got caught in a severe snowstorm on a big face in the Alps. Peter Fuhrmann heard the story of the rescue first-hand from Ludwig Gramminger, famed leader of the Bavarian Mountain Guard in Germany (the Bayrische Bergwacht). Gramminger, with his crew from Munich, went up the other side of the mountain and knotted a bunch of climbing ropes together and had himself lowered down—15 times—into the face. And every time, they pulled him up hand over hand as he brought up each child. On the 16th lower he brought up the teacher.

Gramminger did not think this was a very effective way to rescue people and soon got together with other people to find a solution. They realized that everyone in the construction industry used cables to lift loads, so why not use a cable? The first cables to be used for rescue work were 100 metres long and had a hemp core. Subsequent to that, systems were developed to either bring the victims up or lower them to a place they could be brought out safely. The cable itself ran over a tripod perched on the edge of a cliff. Other equipment was developed to enhance performance as different problems of raising and lowering arose with different rescue scenarios.

When Walter first brought the cable over from Europe, he did not have all the component parts. All the Warden Service had to start with were the spools of cable, the frog clamps and the brake block. Raising systems were identical to those used with ropes where victim and rescuer were brought up using simple pulley systems giving a mechanical advantage of 2:1 or greater, depending on how many pulleys were used. The disadvantage was that it took a lot of operating room. The rescue line had to be strung well back from the edge of the cliff so that several men had room to

manoeuvre. When winches were introduced, the system could operate in smaller spaces with fewer men. When Walter first started working with the cable, winches had not yet been perfected, and he made do with what he had.

As with all evolving systems, a certain amount of experimentation was needed to work out the bugs. Walter was a careful man, but he knew he had to test the ability of both men and equipment in different rescue scenarios. To this end, Walter tried his new tool in every conceivable situation. This led to scenarios where the cable was strung across gorges, over roaring canyons, from cliff faces to the ground, or from the ground up to an anchor above the cliff and back down again.

Mike Schintz remembered with a small shudder one occasion when they had a practice at the Weeping Wall on the Banff/Jasper Highway. "We were working there one day, and we had the cable anchored at the bottom of the cliff, and Walter and I were working at the top. Walter came up and set an anchor—he used a little bit of a scrubby spruce tree that was growing above the cliffs in the scree. We tested it, both he and I pulled on it and it seemed solid, so we anchored the pulley to it for the cable to pass through. So the braking apparatus was at the bottom where the guys were … and the cable runs up through the pulley at the spruce tree and then down to the basket on the edge of the cliff where Alfie [Burstrom] was in the basket and another warden—I think Wally McPhee—was the out rider taking it down. Now in the early days of the cable, we had a problem because when we set up a thing like that, there was always a sag in the cable. We could not get it completely tight … and when the weight of the rescuer and the victim first hit the end of the cable, when they went over the cliff, there would be a short fall. For a while we couldn't figure out what to do about it. Anyway, this day, Alfie is in the basket, there's another warden bringing him down, and Walter is at the edge of the cliff. I was up by the tree watching that the cable is running smoothly through the pulley. Well—they stepped off and the weight came on the cable and the tree began to move and I couldn't stop it. I tried but I couldn't. So I hollered at Walter, and I can still remember Walter looking up at me like that and his mouth formed a little round O … and he came running up the hill and both of us grabbed on to that tree and put our heels into the scree, and we managed to hold it until they got down to the bottom. Fortunately there was nobody up there but him and me and we made a pact to each other—it was unspoken—that we would never tell a soul about this. When we knew that they were safely down and the tree had stopped moving, we walked back to the edge and said 'Ohhh … everything's cool now.'"

WALTER STILL HAD TWO of the most serious rescues ahead of him, one which was tragic, the other an unqualified success and a landmark in Canadian rescue history. The first accident, in 1965, resulted from a sad chain of events that led to the death of a vibrant young woman experiencing the early joys of ski mountaineering. Peggy Telfer was a talented young ski instructor from Banff out for a spring ski break in Glacier National Park with a group of good friends and fellow ski instructors, also from Banff. The group was skiing on the vast Illecillewaet Glacier easily seen from the Trans-CanadaHighway. Their objective on the 15th of May was a remote mountain near the top of the glacier. As it was late spring, they travelled early in the morning to catch the early corn-snow skiing on the return trip.

Somewhere just below the névé, Peggy got separated from the main party, possibly because she was slower or was having some trouble with her skis. The main party did not notice her absence until they reached the top of the glacier. By then a severe storm had blown up, greatly reducing visibility. Peggy was deemed a strong skier by all members of the party, and they may not have been initially concerned, thinking she had returned to the Wheeler Hut on her own. Alarm set in when she had not returned by mid-afternoon.

Terry Gibbons, a warden stationed at the east end of the park, was one of the first to be notified around 1:30 p.m. He immediately collected his gear and headed for the pass, where he found fellow warden Gordon McPhail preparing for a possible night out on the glacier. The more experienced Fred Schleiss, who was now working at Rogers Pass on avalanche control, was also called, and he went with the first party consisting of three wardens. Fred recalls: "It was 3:00 p.m. in the afternoon in the May long weekend. We took off, but unfortunately the wardens were not skiing very well and not in shape. So I get up to the place where I suspect she is—in one of the crevasses. That's the way they explained it. So I sent one of the wardens [Bob Lehmann] to the Steps of Paradise." Gibbons writes in the rescue report that he helped Schleiss search the crevasses with Fred while McPhail was left to set up camp. Fred remembers: "It snowed already and was blowing quite badly … but we went up and looked all over the glacier but we couldn't find anything." Gibbons writes: "By 8:30 p.m. these [crevasses] had been checked. We then returned to our camp. Saturday night was spent in the snow hut that was erected by McPhail."

The crew was off at 4:30 a.m. the next morning to renew the search, but again was hampered by bad weather. Gibbons writes: "The weather at this time was not the best. Visibility was limited and snow was falling lightly. As we proceeded up the glacier, the weather and visibility deteriorated rapidly. The wind which was gusting up to 60 m.p.h. [97 kph] made it extremely difficult to face into it. Ice was forming on the faces of all members of the party and it became apparent that we would be unable to continue."

The rescue party tried to sit out the storm; "tarps were wrapped around members of the party [but] this afforded little shelter." Finally they went down with "visibility so bad that at times vision was restricted to around 4.5–6 metres. [They] reached the road at approximately 12:00 noon." They were, in fact, very glad to have got down at all with the severity of the weather and realized they could not continue till the storm was over. The regret over having to turn back is reflected in the words of Bob Lehmann who later wrote: "The survival of the rescue party was rapidly becoming questionable. If we encountered difficulties, the search for the missing skier would become greatly complicated. To continue the search was considered foolhardy. To remain in the face of the storm was impossible."

By this time Walter Perren had come over from Banff with four wardens (Bill Vroom, George Balding, Gerry Lister and Chief Park Warden Bert Pittaway) to help with the search, but the bad weather continued. By now, few believed that Peggy could have weathered the storm if she had not made it down to tree level. The members of the party she was travelling with confirmed that she was carrying only a small day pack with possibly a light jacket for added clothing. On the 16th Walter sent out a second party under the direction of Noel Gardner, but they got no further than meeting up with the first party. On Sunday the 17th, Gibbons and McPhail were sent to check some of the wooded valleys in the hope she had wandered down to the safety of the forest, but they found nothing.

Tuesday the 18th dawned cold and bright, finally allowing searchers to use a helicopter to search the upper glacier. Fred Schleiss and his brother Walter were flown up to the névé area but found nothing immediately as the wind had blown the snow free of any tracks. They were flown back to base where Walter Perren and Bill Vroom were picked up to search along a ridge leading to the Steps of Paradise. It was here they found Peggy Telfer. They were actually searching on foot when they saw a pair of skis set vertically in the snow, piercing the blue sky like a beacon of fortitude and hope—but all they found was a pale rigid hand, thrusting from the snow, beckoning them forward. The storm had completely buried her where she sat down to wait for the returning skiers, trusting they would see the crossed skis and bring her back to safety.

The second rescue, in 1966, ended much more favourably for two men daring enough to push the limits of alpine rock climbing on the north face of Mt. Babel near Consolation Lakes. It was the first real test of the cable equipment that the wardens had worked so hard to become familiar with, but it was not actually the first cable rescue as is often thought.

One year earlier, a couple of young men, Dale Portman and Rick Crosby, who worked at Deer Lodge, had decided to climb the cliffs at the end of Lake Louise. Halfway up the route, Portman had to complete a long traverse to Crosby along a thin ledge of friable rock. In an attempt to negotiate the delicate holds, and with his climbing ability stretched to the limit, he peeled off. He went penduluming down about 24 metres and was held by belay anchor and by Crosby. In his valiant effort to hold the fall, Crosby sustained severe rope burns to both hands. Portman broke his hip when he smashed into the rock on the way down. It was late in the day, and neither man could continue. Crosby's hands were so badly burned from the rope that he couldn't climb. Fortunately for Portman, there was a small ledge nearby that he could scramble to. They were just above the popular "Plain of Six Glaciers" trail, and their predicament was quickly passed on to the Warden Service.

At eleven o'clock that night, Walter Perren, belayed by Ollie Hermanrude, climbed up to Portman precariously perched on the ledge and set up an anchor, then lowered the injured man to the base of the cliff. It was difficult to reach Crosby from below in the dark with only a headlamp, but once Walter realized he was in a secure position, they decided to wait out the night. At first light a cable-raising system was used to bring up Crosby. Dale Portman, who joined the Warden Service several years later, remembers Ollie coming up to him during his formative years as a seasonal warden and teasing him to keep the incident "under wraps." "It's probably better you keep it to yourself if you want to go anywhere in this outfit."

Walter always knew the cable system worked admirably, but the accident above Consolation Lakes was the first real test of both men and equipment in a very serious situation. The two men, Charlie Locke and Brian Greenwood, were both guides attempting to establish a new route on the difficult, overhung face of Mt. Babel. They were very near the top of the 610-metre face when Locke, who was leading, fell off and smashed his wrist, making any further progress impossible. Neither could they retreat, as Locke's injury made it impossible to establish anchors on the way down. They would have actually been better off if he had broken a leg.

It was the second day after they had signed out for the climb when a group of hikers passing by the end of the lake heard cries for help. The hikers immediately reported to Wally McPhee, who was in charge of the Lake Louise District, and his heart sank when he got the news. He had signed the two men out the day before and knew exactly what route they were on. McPhee quickly sent out his assistant, Jay Morton, to verify the nightmare, and it wasn't long before "Morton came back ashen-faced" to report: "They're on a ledge maybe 400 feet [122 metres] from the top." He added, "The whole bloody mountain is overhung above them." Wally notified Banff, then went to look for himself. With the aid of binoculars he spotted two tiny figures clinging to the mountain on a small ledge where they had tied themselves in. What appalled him was the fact that they were so far up a face that ended in a series of black overhung cliffs, through which he could see no way to reach them.

Walter Perren arrived soon after with several men from Banff. It was immediately clear that a rescue would take a lot of manpower, even with a helicopter to fly men into position. Jim Davies was now flying a helicopter in Banff and was eager to help. Flying rescue missions in the mountains was a skill he would soon pioneer, and this was an excellent beginning.

McPhee thought a rescue was impossible, but the decision to try was made and soon instructions were flying. Jay Morton was told to bring up as many rolls of toilet paper that he could find. If Jay was puzzled, he didn't say much, but all became clear when he was then told to lay out a message on the valley floor saying: WAIT HELP COMING TOP A.M.

Walter's only choice was to lower a man down at the end of the cable and hope he could make contact with them. He asked Bill Vroom, the most experienced man, if he would go. Bill saw the enormity of what was required but didn't hesitate. But just to be sure of backup, Walter also asked Andy Anderson to ride in from his district at Cyclone. Then he flew the face with Bill and Jim to work out the details.

The first obstacle was the extent of the overhanging rock. Jim found a broad saddle to land on, from which men could carry gear to the summit. Walter needed to place a tripod pulley on the cliff edge so the cable would clear the cliff face and not cut into the rock. The problem was, he did not have one. He did, however, have the services of Stan Peyto, the government garage supervisor, whose genius with a welding torch and steel pipe was a thing to be respected. Stan set to work immediately upon hearing Walter describe what he needed, and by morning the apparatus was ready for first flight.

Bill Vroom probably did not sleep that night either, for he was about to do something he had spent years training for. But he had never been in a spot so fiercely overhung or exposed.

The other man who definitely did not sleep was Andy Anderson, who was having his own problems riding through the night to be available first thing in the morning. Andy first had to catch a horse, and he wound up riding a young colt that had been hanging around the cabin. He had a 20-kilometre ride ahead of him in the dark. By the time he got to Ptarmigan Lake, he could see little and was relying on the horse to find the trail. Suddenly there was a loud woof "in his ear" from a grizzly they had startled. The inexperienced colt leapt sideways down a steep bank onto a boulder-strewn slope six metres below, somehow not losing Andy, who rode it out and finally managed to calm the jittery horse, taking a long detour back to the trail.

He was greeted by a bustling team of men busy with mounds of gear, equipment and food being sorted for transport. Andy was impressed. "Walter had quite a crew. His selection was pretty canny. He had everything he needed. Had Paul Peyto, strong as an ox. For every chore, he picked the right guy. He could picture everything that was going to happen—which was great because it was a new thing."

It took a while to line up the cable equipment, establish the anchors and set the tripod, but when the sun was on the face they were ready. Bill could not see the stranded pair, and it was agreed that the first trip down would be reconnaissance only. Bill would have to give directions for raising and lowering by radio, since he would be out of sight during the whole operation. Bill's heart was in his mouth as he hung above the dizzying void, but it was nothing compared to what he experienced once he hung free with his weight on the end of the cable. Bill suddenly began to spin dangerously out of control, and it was all he could do to get the radio to his lips and shout "Spinning badly! Speed up the descent!" All he wanted to do was get down low enough to have contact with the rock and stop the nauseating spinning before he blacked out. Finally his boots struck rock and he stabilized himself. He was about 15 metres below the climbers and a little to the left. It took a moment to clear his head and try and figure out what was going on.

None of the men had worked with cable in a freefall situation; they did not realize that the twisted strands would start to unravel when hung free with a loaded weight. Later, they would remedy the problem by attaching a swivel that would allow the load to move independent of the strands. Unfortunately for Bill they had no such device, and there was no choice but to put up with it throughout the rescue. It was also unnerving to

watch the cable strands pull free of each other as though disintegrating.

Greenwood was able to throw a rope to the sick-looking rescuer and pull him over to their tiny ledge where he heard the story of the accident. The upper overhangs were quite technical, and they had had to resort to "aid climbing" to finish the route. Charlie was leading, when a critical piton failed and he fell, pulling all the other pins with him. He landed on his wrist, immobilizing him for any further climbing—up or down.

Other than the broken wrist, the climbers were fine, just hungry and dehydrated. Bill was hauled back up and soon returned with the Gramminger seat, water and chocolate bars. He manoeuvred Charlie into the seat and soon had him back on top. The work was exhausting, however, much to Walter and Andy's concern. Andy was sure that Walter had brought him to help Bill out if things got tough, which meant going down if Bill was too tired. Walter told him he could quit, but Bill said "no" he had been there and knew what to expect. After a half an hour's rest, Bill was ready to go back for Greenwood. He had him up in short order, thus ending one of the most daring and remarkable rescues in Canadian history.

Bill was nauseous for some time and finally wandered off by himself to take it all in. The outpouring of adrenalin alone was enough to have him feeling wasted. Bill was a relatively competent climber by warden standards, but it was part of the job, not a vocation he pursued beyond work. Where he had been asked to go was not a place he would have attempted to climb to on his own. The psyche for that belonged to an entirely different world. But he went, and he would go again, on other challenging rescues in the next decade before a younger generation took over. Walter said only a few simple words to Bill in acknowledgement of what he had done: "Good job Bill … good job!"

Two other noteworthy rescues under dramatic circumstances took place in 1966 and 67. The first, in Rogers Pass, was also one of the

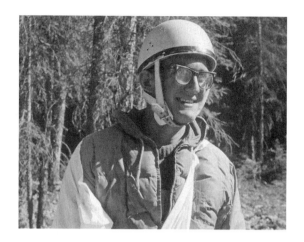

Charlie Locke after Babel rescue. DON VOCKEROTH
COLLECTION

last Walter would actually participate in. The accident occurred in late summer when two Americans decided to try the ridge route on Mt. Sir Donald. Bad weather on the descent caused them to get off route. Fred Schleiss was the most experienced climber around, so he responded to the call for help and took two wardens with him. Unfortunately the rescue party ran into trouble when one of the wardens slipped, badly injuring one arm. Fred suddenly had his own rescue to contend with, and it was all he could do to get the man safely down. Knowing he needed help to do anything for the Americans, Fred soon had Walter on the way.

Walter brought in Don Vockeroth, who was then working at Lake O'Hara as a patrolman. Don was well into establishing his own climbing career and was more than capable of assisting. But even with his experience, Don found the conditions quite tricky. He recalls "We got out there and the rescue was in progress but was getting more complicated and the weather was *just* a blizzard. Very bad weather. So we were flying up to the Uto/Sir Donald col in bad weather and the helicopter goes up the west side and the updraft sent the winds ripping over the col … he has to tip the blade and hold it just to stay there."

Walter and Fred felt they could speed up the approach by jumping out at the col. But getting out of the gyrating helicopter was much trickier than they thought. Don remembers that "there was actually a little slope, not flat but about 15 or 20 degrees and only about eight square feet or something … and Walter says, 'okay you get out.'" The "little slope," however, that hung innocently above the looming void below, was covered in ice. Don was a bit shaken, wondering how to make the transition from the helicopter to the ice with no protection. He laughs: "I had to put a crampon on. Then I was sitting on the skid … Walter is hanging on to me and the machine is just bucking there. After I get that [crampon] on I got onto the verglas which was about one inch of ice. Then I drove in a piton. It felt good!"

From that point he was able to help Fred and Walter out of the helicopter and retrieve enough gear and food for the stranded climbers. The Americans were actually working their way down the ridge when the team reached them. The hot food improved their outlook, but the hardest part of the rescue was still ahead. They now had to get the injured climber into a stretcher and lower him to a location that was accessible by helicopter. Don is quick to point out that these were the early days of helicopter assistance before standards were set. He remembers, "You're just learning how far you can push it … you don't consider the risk factors. There was no 'risk management.'"

Despite the difficulties, the climbers were brought out safely. It was a major rescue accomplished by personnel working together from different parks and aided significantly by a brave pilot willing to take a chance. Don was hugely impressed by the young pilot's ability but saddened when he died when his helicopter ran out of fuel a few years later on a routine flight.

The following winter, a young Jay Morton had just started with the Warden Service and was working at the Lake Louise ski hill. One day he was supervising the ski patrol—and learning to ski—when Ron Hall came roaring up on a snowmobile to report a man caught in an avalanche at Deception Pass en route to Skoki Lodge. It was the end of the day and most of the staff had gone down the hill leaving Jay to close up shop. Gord Brockway and Hall, ski-hill staff out breaking a trail for the snow machines, had met a young man skiing at breakneck speed down the pass to report that his friend had been buried by an avalanche.

Brockway was experienced in the mountains and proceeded directly to the avalanche with the survivor and began searching from the last seen point. Jay immediately sent Hall back in with probes and a hasty search kit. He then rallied a rescue team from Banff, which headed in shortly thereafter with more equipment. By this time the man had been buried for over two and a half hours.

Once Hall returned with the probes, both men started searching in earnest. The reporting victim was in poor shape and unable to give much assistance except to try and point out where his buddy might be. He was successful in that, because soon after the men began probing, Brockway yelled "I've got him!" The two rescuers then dug up the unconscious victim who, to their shock, was still alive. They were digging him out when the rescue team arrived. It was one of the first live recoveries from an avalanche in Canada, and it earned the rescuers a merit of honour award from the Canadian Ski Patrol System.

By 1965, WALTER'S INTENTION of having wardens conduct rescues on their own was becoming a reality. He felt it was very important to have good personnel stationed at the Columbia Icefield. Hans Fuhrer, who arrived to fill this position in 1965, already had quite a lot of climbing experience, but he was relatively new to rescues. But that was part of the job, and he was fully prepared to participate in any emergency. Still, he was taken aback on one particularly difficult accident that taught him never to judge a person by his outward appearance.

He received a call from the manager of the snow-coach concession operating on the Icefield, asking him to respond to an accident involving one of the workers. He was taken to the scene in one of the small coaches in the company of a young fellow who "looked like a hippie." The young man immediately asked Hans who he was and what he was doing there. With some reserve Hans replied that he was responsible for the rescue work in the area and who the hell was he anyway? The somewhat scruffy individual replied that he was a doctor.

The freak accident turned out to be a particularly gruesome one involving the ice cutter used to prepare the snowmobile road for the summer operation. The ice cutter had jammed when the cat pulling it had gone a little too fast over a particularly rough area. The assistant had stepped

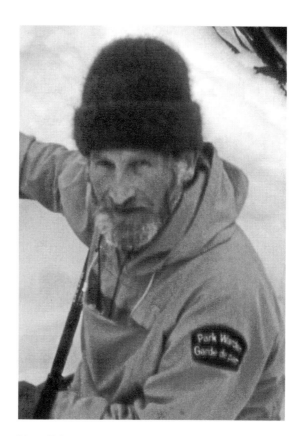

Hans Fuhrer. HANS FUHRER COLLECTION

59

off to loosen the ice from the axle that held the ice cutters, but instead of using a probe, he had used his foot. An untied shoe lace was caught up by the cutters which lurched forward upon being freed and dragged him bodily under the churning machinery. Hans and the young doctor were greeted by the sight of the poor man lying under the cutter "totally pinned" with one of the cutters imbedded in one leg. Hans later recalled, "I was so happy the doctor was there!"

Although it was his first medical emergency, the young doctor knew instantly that the man had to be freed right then if they were to save his life. With some incredulity, Hans recounted what happened next. "The doctor looked at me and said, 'In order to free that man we have to amputate his leg.' I said 'Oh, that's bad!' I mean, that's all you could do. The whole cutter was on his leg." And that is what they did. But first, "He asked me if I had a knife. I said 'Yah, I have a Swiss Army knife—that's all I got in my pocket.' And he said, 'Is it sharp?'" It was, but to have more leverage, they sent the driver down to get a few kitchen knives from the mess hall at the snowmobile station.

They applied a tourniquet above the knee and proceeded to cut the leg off. "And so we finally got his leg loose—everything separated. The guy was totally conscious because we talked to him to tell him that he would have to lose his leg in order to free him." At last they disentangled him from the cutter which had to be started up again to free the remaining leg from the blades caught in the clothing. "Since then," Hans said, "I have thought about hippies and all that. I started to think differently about guys with long hair. Was I ever glad to have that guy with me!"

Another episode that Walter Perren left up to the local wardens to handle happened in the spring of 1967 on Roche Perdrix, a small, cliffy mountain near the east entrance of Jasper National Park. A labourer working at the pulp mill in Hinton, Alberta, had lost his father in a plane crash the year before. Whether this had unbalanced him or not, by the spring of 1967 he was convinced that he had to climb the mountain to meet both his father and John F. Kennedy. He tried to get a permit from the warden at Pocahontas Warden Station, but could not convince anyone he had the qualifications or equipment to go. He then finagled a registration, saying he was going with a guide.

Although the day he left was bright and clear, the weather quickly deteriorated. It was still early when a young woman appeared at the station. She was in tatters, with multiple bruises and evidence of frostbite. More alarmingly, she claimed over and over again: "He is gone. He is on the mountain!" It turned out she was the wife of the missing man, who had insisted she go with him. She said that when they got to the steep part, she was sure he would kill them both, and she managed to escape.

A search party quickly followed up the normal approach to the mountain. After leaving timberline, the group split into two; one party continued on the normal route while the other followed the faint track left by the woman. Here they found evidence of where she had dragged herself over the rocks and places where she had curled up to rest. By now it was late in the day, making further progress treacherous in the worsening weather. The lower party preceded to a point below an ugly-looking chimney broken by low cliff bands before returning for the day. Just as they were about to turn back, the story took a bizarre turn. The RCMP from Hinton had done some checking into the man's background and passed on the unsettling information that the man was considered a manic paranoid. He had a record of violent behaviour, including the use of firearms, but more disturbingly, he hated anyone in uniform. Fearing the man might be armed, the wardens quickly got out of their orange anoraks and tried to become as inconspicuous as possible.

The following day the mountain was covered with over 60 centimetres of snow which did not depart completely for over a month. Despite continued search efforts, the mystery was not cleared up until much later in the spring when conditions had improved. Warden trainees attending the regional training school at the Palisades spotted a body that matched the description of the missing climber. Piecing the evidence together with the woman's story, rescuers surmised that he had gone partway up the ugly chimney her trail had led to the first day, but for some reason, he had traversed around to the exposed west side. He had obviously lost his footing, probably about the time the weather turned making the rock treacherous, and he had fallen to his death. He had probably died within an hour of the time his wife had left him.

AS THE SIXTIES WOUND DOWN, Walter Perren may have felt he had made significant advances in revolutionizing the Warden Service into a workable rescue unit, but he also knew he had much more to do. It was a life's work that he hoped would continue with succeeding generations, and in that he was right. But he would not live to see the incredible changes to come. He died on a dark December day in 1967, in the Foothills Hospital at Calgary, Alberta, at the still-youthful age of 53. It was December 29th to be precise, when Walter could no longer see the mountains that had cheered his view from his hospital bed. If it were possible for the small man to become smaller, he had done so fighting the wasting disease of leukaemia that had hollowed out his body. Peter Perren was only twelve years old, and puzzled about what was happening to his father. In those days, death was not talked about with children, and he did not realize the significance of his father's illness until just before he died. Later Peter became a warden himself and continued the climbing tradition of his family.

One event that helped Peter understand his father was an early climb up Mt. Hector with fellow warden Terry Skjonsberg in 1973. To his surprise he found an entry in the summit register written by his father and dated on the day of his birth in 1954. He told his mother about the note and learned that it still bothered her that Walter had missed the birth of his first son because he had gone climbing. Later Peter had another insight when he attended a reunion at Chateau Lake Louise. Here, he met someone also listed on the summit register that day in 1954. He had been a young bellhop working at the Chateau who had participated in the rescue of the women on Mt. Victoria. He had been badly shaken by the event, as were other members of the staff—it had left a bitter taste in their mouths about climbing until Walter organized the trip to Mt. Hector. Walter took the young people under his wing and reintroduced them to the joyful side of being in the mountains—a feeling that never left him. He did the same for Peter too, when he knew in his heart that he was sick. His last climb with Peter was up on the Needles of Mt. Whyte, which Peter only later found out was that first climb in Canada where he went "to stretch his legs."

Walter had never been sick a day in his life. Walking to Banff from Lake Louise because he couldn't hitch a ride was not uncommon for him. He had the strength and stamina of a wolverine, and when he suddenly started getting tired in the summer of 1967, he thought it was due to an adverse reaction to the dynamite he had been working with. Fred Schleiss recalls helping him out with a warden school at Abbots Pass that fall when Walter turned back halfway saying he was tired but would join them in the next day or so. He never returned. He was admitted to the Foothills Hospital shortly thereafter and was dead within months.

The funeral service was a solemn affair for the men who were unable to show their feelings too openly for a man they so dearly cherished. It was especially heartbreaking for Jim Sime when he saw Pam throw one red rose on the coffin as it was lowered into the ground.

Walter's legacy with the Warden Service was one of service. He dedicated himself to the profession and wholly embraced the concept of creating a rescue organization that would be equal not only to other organizations, but to the challenge of the mountains. He had a genius for working with people and determining the core of their potential. Mike Schintz said there were three types of people Walter could place immediately: the person who could not handle climbing at all and was a liability to everyone; the many who were scared silly but learned to cope; and those whose natural talents soared to the summits. He had a place for all of them. The ones uncomfortable on the side of a mountain became indispensable in organizing gear, communications or food. Those who learned to cope with their fear were used for carrying gear, operating equipment or belaying the point man. The less fearful were selected for the exposed part of the operation. No one was left out or felt left out. The men became a team, and that was what Walter wanted.

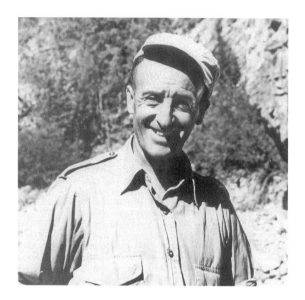

Walter Perren. BANFF WARDEN ARCHIVES

3

The White Dragon

During the last years of Walter's work in public safety, he began to devote greater effort to avalanche control. During the sixties, most of the concern was with highways and ski areas, since recreational backcountry skiing was still evolving. Though he recognized that forecasting avalanches was still a new field, he left much of this pioneering work to his old friend and rival, Noel Gardner. The study of avalanches (known to some as White Dragons) was an intrinsic part of mountain rescue training. In fact it was primarily danger from avalanches that led to the formation of the earliest mountain rescue operations—in Europe and in North America.

Viewed from a safe distance, an avalanche is a symphony of motion. Being caught in one, though, is a terrible and frightening experience— and only recounted in the unlikelihood of survival. Two thousand years ago, Strabo, a Greek geographer, was the first to record an attempt to recover people buried in an avalanche. He used the term "sounding rod" when describing the staff travellers carried in the Caucasus. He incorrectly assumed that a buried person would push the staff up through the snow to show his location. With the vice-like clamp that snow has, the staves were more likely used to probe for the victims.

Staves, in fact, were probably the forerunner of the modern collapsible avalanche probe.

The modern study of avalanches started with Robert Haefeli, a civil engineer who became one of the great avalanche experts in the world. His training as an engineer began in 1926; he soon applied it to the study of snow after the Swiss approached him to study the "shear strength of snow." Soon a small group of scientists and engineers were working out of a tiny hut above Davos, Switzerland, that would eventually evolve into the most renowned avalanche research centre in the world. In 1939, this team published the book *Snow and its Metamorphism,* which became the foundation for snow research throughout the world.

In North America, Alta, Utah, became the centre for avalanche research on this continent because of the great depths of snow the place was blessed with each winter. The ski area—previously an old mining town—inherited a history laden with the deaths of hundreds of miners caught in avalanches. That same winter the first U.S. Forest Service "snow ranger" was given the responsibility of observing avalanches and collecting weather data. This was the first step in the development of data collection and the understanding of avalanches in North America which would blossom into an industry. Monty Atwater arrived in Alta as a snow patroller in 1945 and stayed to pursue this new career, influencing not only fellow researchers in the United States but in Canada as well.

Snow research in Canada developed not from avalanches affecting mining operations—though there were a significant number of these—but from pushing a route for the Canadian Pacific Railway through the mountains. The route through the avalanche-plagued Rogers Pass was by far the most costly in terms of money and lives; it is alleviated today by a rigorous avalanche control program. For forty-five years the CPR waged a relentless campaign in the pass to defend itself from the peril that threatened the tracks. They built 30 kilometres of snow-sheds for the tracks, and kept them open with a huge rotary snowplow specifically built for dealing with the millions of tonnes of avalanche debris that was deposited on unprotected track each winter.

Rogers Pass would ultimately become the largest centre for snow research in Canada, precisely because of the huge avalanche threat it posed to the CPR and later to the Trans-Canada Highway. John Whelan, a freelance writer and historian, noted that employees such as James Ross found the snow-slides to be far more serious than anticipated. Many travellers doubted that the line could be kept open during the winter, but "with the largest investment in Canadian history and national pride, the CPR set out to prove doubters wrong."

Though they built snow-sheds for the tracks, they gave no thought to protecting the living quarters located three kilometres south of the pass, and on January 31, 1899, the station/boarding house was hit by a massive avalanche. The day operator, his wife and their two young children were killed along with a Chinese cook and the night operator who was asleep in his bed. The seventh victim was inside the engine-house; he was crushed when avalanche debris toppled one of the engines. Only two in that building survived. Nearby, two boarding cars full of Chinese labourers were tossed about like stones in a tumbler, but miraculously no

64

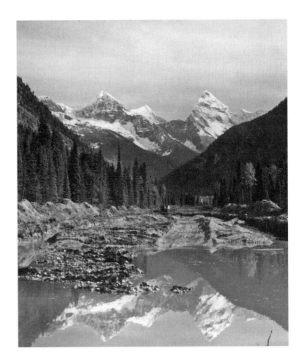

Rogers Pass in 1958. BANFF WARDEN ARCHIVES

one was killed or seriously injured. Along with the fortuitous Chinese, two dogs and a caged canary also survived the devastation. But this was only a hint of what was to come.

An often overlooked, but devastating tragedy unparalleled in the history of mountain avalanche accidents in Canada, occurred eleven years later in Rogers Pass. This was the great avalanche of 1910 that killed 62 people. Ironically, the slide came down at a location that once had the protection of the longest shed (over 600 metres) in the pass. Shed #17 had run through some of the most spectacular scenery in the park, enticing the railroad to build an unprotected parallel summer track. But in twenty-three years of operation, no avalanche had touched the snow-shed, so it was abandoned altogether. Nothing was known back then about the cyclic nature of avalanches. On March 4th, a small slide came down from Mt. Cheops around 6:00 p.m., forcing a large crew out to clear the tracks. As quoted in *Mountain Heritage Magazine*, "Utilizing shovels and a rotary plow, the crews succeeded in uncovering a long section of track by digging a deep trench through the debris of snow and ice. The cruel irony was that they were digging their own graves."

Throughout the evening, the storm continued with ever-increasing intensity, building up the hazard on the previously dormant slide paths on Mt. Avalanche across the valley from the site. Without warning the second slide hit at midnight, burying the unsuspecting workers. The huge avalanche struck so suddenly that many workers were entombed standing up. One man who was eventually uncovered appeared to be rolling a cigarette. An inquest absolved the CPR of any blame, saying the men volunteered to work at night and were not forced to be there. The jury recommended "The CPR withdraw their workmen from all slides in future during stormy nights."

In 1913, in response to the tragedy, the CPR began building an underground tunnel that would eliminate eight kilometres of snow-sheds and 35 kilometres of track. The Connaught Tunnel was completed in 1916.

Canada had another major industry that was threatened by snow in winter. Unknown to many was the danger posed to mines in British Columbia. As these operations grew, their access roads increased the threat of avalanches where they bisected major avalanche paths. According to the mining industry, between 1870 and 1979 there were 114 avalanche fatalities associated with mining.

In 1948, the National Research Council of Canada invited Marcel de Quervain to spend a year in Canada to make recommendations for development of snow and ice research. Dr. de Quervain was a senior scientist at the Federal Institute for Snow and Avalanche Research on Weissfluhloch/Davos in Switzerland. He was one of only a few men who could classify themselves as internationally known experts on the subject back in 1948.

He arrived by train at Glacier Station just below the pass in early February, 1949. He immediately checked the local snow profile, which showed a consistent increase in the density of the snow. This, fortuitously, was just after Noel Gardner began working as a park warden at Flat Creek. One may assume that Noel was present when Dr. de Quervain began his studies, which may have fuelled his own interest in avalanches.

Noel was already showing considerable confidence in his travel skills when he first climbed up Mt. Fidelity to explore the upper avalanche paths. At that time, few wardens ever left the valley to explore the backcountry, and none did so in the winter on skis. By 1950 his confidence and ability were such that he thought nothing of skiing from Mt. Fidelity to Rogers Pass through some very formidable terrain. From the beginning of his tenure at Glacier, Noel began making notes of avalanche activity in his district. He also kept meticulous notes on weather observations, which eventually allowed him to see the relationship between the two phenomena. It was during this formative era that his superiors recognized his skills as a skier and his understanding of snow.

In the summer of 1953 the Federal Department of Public Works had Noel guide them on a preliminary reconnaissance of Rogers Pass with the idea that it might be a route for the proposed Trans-Canada Highway. Noel pointed out the many avalanche paths on the route and explained the frequency of activity. The Department of Public Works contracted Noel to spend parts of the following two winters maintaining his readings and conducting monthly surveys. During this period Noel transferred to Yoho National Park, but despite the distance, twice a month he would board a train to the Glacier National Park boundary, strap on his skis and skins and head up toward Rogers Pass. He followed the proposed highway route, recording the frequency and size of the avalanches he encountered. Once he got to Flat Creek on the west side of the pass, he would turn around and head back. Though the wardens at Flat Creek, Glacier and Stony Creek stations helped out with data collection, he did most of the work on his own.

In 1954 Noel's work attracted the attention of his counterpart, Monty Atwater in the United States, and he was asked to attend a week-long avalanche course in Alta put on by the U.S. Forest Service. Here the two men discovered a common bond. It must have been an eye-opener for Monty, who for so many years felt he was the only one doing work in this field. It's revealing what he had to say about it in his book *The Avalanche Hunters.* "Now the parallel becomes very close. Like myself at Alta, no one told Gardner to do avalanche research. He simply had the itch to know when and why and began to make observations on his own. And just as it chanced with me at Alta, he appeared at the right place and moment."

Years later when Noel had established the research station on Mt. Fidelity, Art Judson, a snow ranger with the U.S. Forest Service and a long time friend, recalls arriving at the station for the first time. "There was someone doing ground-breaking work in avalanche forecasting up there … I was impressed with what I saw. He had a first-class system. I had never seen anyone integrate snowpack profiles with weather patterns." Judson also remembers a man who was obsessed with avalanches. "He thought snow 24 hours a day, often waking up in the middle of the night with new ideas on research techniques."

An oft-repeated story about Noel during this period sheds some light on the ranger's observation. Warden Keith Everts, who worked in Rogers Pass in the early 1970s, was the one who carried the story in his repertoire of amusing anecdotes. He passed it on to fellow warden Tim Auger who said, "Anytime I'm swapping stories with other avalanche people who may not have heard this, I always have to truck it out. It's such a classic. Noel is up at Mt. Fidelity and it's a dark and stormy night gripped in the jaws of a major blizzard. There is someone else up there with him … they're drinking Irish whiskey and playing cards … most likely crib. Noel has his dog there. It was a little mutt with long hair that looked like a mop without a handle. In the middle of this session

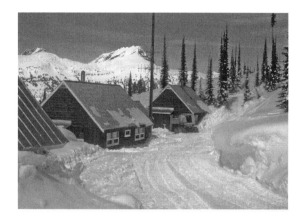

Mt. Fidelity in winter, 1970. DALE PORTMAN COLLECTION

Noel calls the dog over to him. The dog comes over and Noel tips his chair back, grabs the dog by the scruff of the neck and picks him up. Then he leans over and pulls the door open, heaves the dog out into the blizzard and slams the door and plays his next hand of cards—just like that. A few minutes later there is a whining and whimpering at the door. With the wind howling in the background, Noel tips the chair back again, opens the door and the dog comes scampering in. He slams the door against the howl of the wind and the curtain of snowflakes, picks up the dog again and plunks him in his lap. He reaches over his other shoulder to a shelf, gets his hand lens (magnifying glass), leans over and takes a closer look at the dog's back. Then Noel sits back and makes the pronouncement, "Yep … dendrites!!!" (which is a scientific term for star-shaped crystal flakes of snow).

In 1956, when the federal government decided to put the Trans-Canada Highway through Rogers Pass despite the avalanche problems, it addressed the dilemma of avalanche protection right from the start. That summer the Department of Public Works gave Noel the responsibility of organizing all the snow, weather and avalanche data into a workable method of predicting avalanches from which he could develop a hazard index. He received funding from both the National Research

Council and the Department of Public Works for building a Pan-Abode residence at Glacier along with two smaller observatories at Mt. Abbot and Mt. Fidelity. He also received weather instruments and up-to-date snow observation equipment from the National Research Council along with man-year salaries for experienced support personnel.

Canada was now starting to become a major source of avalanche research, slowly garnering a credible international reputation. Many who admired the facility came to observe while others came to learn. Monty Atwater was one who came to observe, for he envied the research being developed there. As he later wrote in his book, "The area of critical danger in Rogers Pass is fifty miles [80 kilometres] long, within which Gardner identified seventy-four avalanche paths. Through this gauntlet of snow-slides, the Department of Public Works proposed to push a four-lane all-year highway. All things considered—the density of traffic, the extent and severity of the hazard, the design of the highway—Rogers Pass qualifies as one of the most difficult problems in avalanche control ever undertaken. It is certainly the best researched and the most elaborately defended."

Avalanche research in the United States was a stepchild of the Forest Service and not a particularly welcome one either. Hence avalanche research there has never had the whole-hearted support of the sponsoring organization. Ironically this was also becoming true of the burgeoning national rescue organization developing under the Parks Canada umbrella, compared to the many splintered rescue groups forming independently in the United States.

When the Department of Public Works gave Noel Gardner the responsibility of developing an avalanche safety program, it did so with the qualifying stipulation that an engineer help with the development and location of avalanche defences. A Swiss engineer by the name of Peter Schaerer, destined to become the "Father of Scientific Avalanche Research" in Canada, was thus loaned to the Department of Public Works.

Peter Schaerer, a slight, gentle, easy-going man, was a total contrast to the boisterous Noel, and again personalities clashed. Peter displayed a quiet self-confidence, tackling his work with single-minded determination. But he had a great capacity to accommodate those around him both as teacher and mentor, always with an attitude of deferential politeness. Noel, by contrast, was a tough task master—a loner who grew restless with the confinement and restrictions of government bureaucracy. His moody disposition and independence often led to confrontation with his superiors, and he bridled at the position Peter had in his work at Rogers Pass.

Peter was born at Berne, Switzerland, in 1926 and graduated as a civil engineer from the Federal Institute of Technology in Zurich in 1950. One of the courses he attended at the university included snow mechanics and avalanche control by the world renowned snow scientist, Dr. Robert Haefeli. He had a strong interest in ski mountaineering and had taken courses in that field to hone his travel skills. After graduation he served as research assistant with the professor of road engineering at the Federal Institute of Technology. He carried out tests on snow removal and ice control on roads. His work brought him in contact with the Snow and Avalanche Research near Davos, where he acquired a good knowledge of snow physics. In 1956, while visiting his brother in Ottawa, he learned that the National Research Council was looking for snow researchers. Two months later he had a job.

According to Peter they offered him several projects, but the one that interested him was working on the avalanche control program at Rogers Pass. The actual work was still with the Department of Public Works (DPW) to whom Peter was loaned for the interim. And so started an illustrious career which was later crowned with the Order of Canada. In the meantime he familiarized himself with all aspects of avalanche control and research and with the relatively new study of the shear strength of freshly fallen snow at the research centre in Davos.

He arrived in Canada in March 1957. After travelling by train from Ottawa, he was picked up by car in Banff by Noel. As Peter later described it, "Noel Gardner picked me up for the drive to Golden and a train ride from Golden to Glacier … Noel, who had been kind and attentive during our travel together changed into a gruff mood as soon as we had arrived at Glacier and boarded the Sno-cat for the drive to the camp."

Here Peter met Noel's wife Gladys as well as the crew of snow observers including Howard Srigley and Bruno Engler. Noel's abrupt change in disposition may have been in response to discovering his home was about to be invaded. In the spring Noel had found out that he would be sharing his house with DPW highway engineering staff, and he was none too pleased about it. He was looking forward to a relaxing summer after a busy winter schedule when this was dropped on him.

Peter remembers his first discussion with Noel about snow. "On my second day at Rogers Pass we were out doing a snow profile, and Noel asked me what methods we used to forecast avalanches in Europe. I thought—what methods? We did not have a system. I realized quickly how things should be done." Until then the transfer of knowledge travelled north/south between Canada and the United States instead of east/west from Europe. Though Peter recognized the value of the work Noel was doing, he soon learned that little could be done to mitigate the avalanche hazard along the proposed route. So, in consultation with Noel, adjustments were made to the location of the highway wherever possible.

The relationship between Noel and Peter and his supervisors in DPW became poisonous in June when the engineers moved in. It was further tainted when Noel was instructed to take orders from Peter and assist with the highway survey that summer. Noel had been his own boss for too many years and felt no one was his equal in the field. It was more than he was prepared to accept, and after short reflection he abruptly quit when an opportunity arose to work with the glaciological survey of the University of Washington. He also refused to turn over his accumulated data, insisting he must submit it to DPW headquarters in Ottawa in person.

But Noel was not able to take separation from his beloved Rogers Pass for long. At the end of 1958 he was back working as a consultant surveying avalanche paths between Albert Canyon and the west boundary of Glacier National Park. He had gained valuable international experience and recognition during the time spent in the United States; it was a move that would ultimately pay off for him in subsequent work with the Canadian Parks Service.

While Noel was at the University of Washington, the Canadian Parks Service looked into the use of artillery to artificially stabilize avalanches. Artillery had been used successfully for avalanche control in Switzerland for about 20 years; in the U.S. for the last 10. Investigation into its use in Rogers Pass had already been explored early as 1957. In November of that year, an army reconnaissance team from Calgary, Alberta, arrived in Glacier with a 106 mm recoilless rifle. After touring the proposed firing positions, the army concluded that the steep firing angle needed to reach the high targets would require the gun to be mounted on a tower to provide room for the back-blast.

Over the next year, trials were carried out using a 75 mm and a 105 mm howitzer with very good results. Because of the consistent positioning of the howitzer at the gun placement, a set of bearings and elevations could be recorded for each target. With this established, the gun could be fired with a high level of accuracy during storms without the target being visible. The weapon of choice in Rogers Pass was the 105 mm howitzer.

That year the Director General of the Canadian Parks Service decided that national parks staff would take over the responsibility of avalanche safety and forecasting through Rogers Pass. The new function's ambiguous and long-winded title of Snow Research and Avalanche Warning Section was unique to the park and had no counterpart in any other national park. The NRC continued to do research in the park, remaining quite distinct from this new department of administration. To his surprise (or ultimate satisfaction) Noel Gardner was brought back to SRAWS, and two Austrians, Fred and Walter Schleiss, were hired as his assistants. The snow observers with DPW, Howard Srigley and J.P. Priollaud, were offered work on Noel's crew, but they refused. They had worked with him back in the winter of 1956–57 and wanted nothing to do with his tyrannical style.

There seems to be some controversy surrounding Noel's hiring, but there is little doubt they had the most experienced man. What no one knew was how he would adapt to working in a structured environment. At least there was no overlapping of responsibilities. Peter Schaerer worked for the National Research Council and concentrated on engineering and scientific matters, while Noel Gardner under the Snow Research and Avalanche Warning Section, confined his work to field applications of avalanche control and data collection. The transfer of equipment and responsibility was settled in October, 1959, when Noel arrived at Glacier Station and took over the residence and office. Peter noted that "Irish whiskey, Noel's favourite drink helped out our mutual understanding."

The Department of Public Works, however, still retained responsibility for the design and construction of avalanche control works, and because they needed reliable observations for another year, they kept the original avalanche survey crew on for the winter. Besides, they were not sure Noel would be successful with the operation of the program, and with his history of walking out suddenly and dramatically, they felt much better with an experienced backup crew of their own. Noel, of course, would have much preferred to have all avalanche observation and data collection firmly under his control. As could have been predicted, the two avalanche crews did not get along and this resulted in much friction between them. Finally, at a meeting in Ottawa

in the summer of 1960, the untenable situation was put to rest when it was decided that DPW would discontinue avalanche studies in Rogers Pass altogether. Gardner would now take on all responsibility for avalanche work at Rogers Pass under the auspices of the Canadian Park Service.

The hiring of Fred Schleiss in the new position of Assistant Forecaster, and later his brother Walter, came at a very fortuitous time. With the volatile Noel in charge, there was concern about having trained staff in place who could take over if he quit. Fred Schleiss had the potential to take the lead job if that need arose down the road. Before emigrating to Canada, Fred had earned a degree in engineering that had led to avalanche work in Kaprun, Austria.

Fred was also asked to oversee whatever public safety work cropped up in the park, and he had his hands full with some of the earlier rescues. Fred's brother Walter Schleiss also had a background in mountaineering. As Fred said, "We knew we needed another man, and I knew Walter was a hell of a good skier and he had mountain [skills] and we brought him in." Noel now had a good team, and there was mutual respect between the taciturn Canadian rancher turned "Snow Guru" and his Austrian assistants. They wasted little time putting together an avalanche forecasting strategy for Rogers Pass. Mt. Fidelity became the centre for all the field investigation of snow conditions in the park.

Avalanche forecasting was not an exact science at the time—and will not likely ever be—but in 1960 much of the substantial database so essential in present-day forecasting was non-existent. The goal was to establish forecasting on a less subjective basis. Fred observed: "I always said forecasting was 60–65 percent technical and the rest intuition. Now I would say personally [when] I was in my prime and I went out a lot in the field—that is one thing that is very important—I would get to 80 percent, I would think at times. When I was a manager and not able to get out into the field as much and spent more time in Revelstoke,

I lost a lot of that and it came down to 65 percent. But the 65 percent was definitely accurate, and what I normally say with most forecasting, if it's not done on the right lines … it's 50/50."

In May of 1961, Peter Schaerer completed his work in Rogers Pass, and he decided to move back to Switzerland. He visited the park in April before leaving. Noel was quite amiable with Peter on this occasion, and they shared a drink of Irish whiskey. Noel may have felt that he and Peter would not be bumping heads again, and it was a fitting way to wish him bon voyage.

During the summer of 1961 a new road accessed the observation post on Mt. Fidelity, and the facility was expanded. Now that it was accessible year-round, it became the centre of snow research and avalanche forecasting in Rogers Pass. From here Noel and Fred collected data, while Walter and an assistant monitored readings in the valley bottom.

Finally, with much fanfare, Prime Minister John Diefenbaker opened the Trans-Canada Highway in September of 1962. The hard-fought battle to conquer the avalanche problem was considered accomplished—at least well enough to declare the road open for business. Before this, motorists travelled the Big Bend route of the Columbia River on a tedious gravel road that was dangerous in places. The loggers for whom the road existed were relieved to see this unpredictable traffic rerouted. The Rogers Pass route reduced the travel distance to Revelstoke by half, offering spectacular vistas, and it remains to this day one of the prime destinations of tourists.

By 1963, with the road now in year-round use, the staff at the pass settled in to do daily battle. This meant continuing to get the people required for the daily tedium of keeping the research stations functioning in a smooth manner (lots of shovelling) during the winter. The pass became a source of work for laid-off summer seasonal wardens. It also proved to be a training ground of inestimable value for those who sought future work in avalanche control. One of the first of those destined to go far in the Warden Service was Don Mickle, the son of a Lake Louise outfitter and later a park warden in both Yoho and Banff national parks.

He worked for Noel Gardner, Fred Schleiss and Peter Schaerer (who returned to Canada) between the years 1963 and 1972. Don's father Bert knew Noel Gardner from Bragg Creek and so managed to get Don a job working for him at Rogers Pass. Upon receiving an offer, Don wrote back to say he would take the job—it was good money in those days. Noel told him to buy his own ski boots— they would supply the skis and skins. (Don wondered what skins were.) He bought the boots at the Hudson Bay Co. store in Banff for $10 and showed up at Mt. Fidelity. That first day of work, he had to put his skis on and follow Noel up to the top of Roundhill Mountain. His bafflement over the skins was soon answered when Noel produced a long strip of seal skin that attached to the bottom of the skis to prevent slipping back when they walked up the hill. Copying Noel, Don soon had his skins on, then up they went. He was run quickly through his duties, which included maintenance, snow measurements and weather readings. Then, offhandedly, Noel pointed to a skinny 30-metre-high pole that had some revolving cups sitting on top and told Don to climb up and clean the rime out. Don reluctantly slithered up the shaky thing using everything for questionable grip. To his dismay he suddenly realized he had a great view all the way down to Schuss Lake, some 600 metres below. Now terrified, he realized he had to let go with one hand to clear the hoary things. He used the side of his face to stop the twirling cups and stabilize them while he cleaned them with his free hand. Thinking he had survived the worst when he at last reached firm ground, he was now confronted with the ski down. Mt. Fidelity is not a good place to learn to ski. Noel was busy taking his skins off when Don asked if he should do the same. Noel replied sardonically: "It up to you." So he took them off. By now the fog had rolled in, and all Don could do was follow in Noel's tracks.

He fell a lot on the way down. Actually he fell a lot that winter. This had been Don's second time ever on skis and Gladys, Noel's wife, decided she would teach him how to ski.

Don continued with his main job of shovelling snow, checking the light plant and on occasion taking some readings. The job gave him good insight into the duties of the avalanche observer and assistant observer in the control program back then. Observers were there to train staff in safe travel procedures, take all the critical readings and help out with avalanche control. They also did snow profiles and managed the data. Assistants did mostly grunt work: shovelling snow, running around and occasionally helping with observations on avalanche shoots.

As Don settled into the routine duties he came to know the people he was working with. Unlike many others, he candidly remembers Noel as a "really charming guy—really interesting to talk to." To Don's happy surprise, he also discovered Noel loved to teach, and soon he learned a lot about the avalanche program and the basic principles of avalanche behaviour. "Noel had a temper. He was tough. He learned by the school of hard knocks. He certainly didn't pamper you." Despite this, Don adds, "Noel was fair and I really liked him, but when you earned his wrath you wanted to hide." Don continues, "Noel's nickname was 'old snowflake,' but he had a lot of power on what was going on. People jumped when he said jump." He also felt that Noel was good to Fred and Walter Schleiss.

"Noel was spending a lot of his time sorting out where to shoot and doing a lot of testing. He was also doing more observations and trying to perfect the forecasting. He had a lot of visitors and this is where he first met Hans Gmoser. Hans was just getting his heli-ski business going in the Bugaboos and was a good friend of Noel's." Gmoser in later years praised the control work of Gardner and his team. "The best example is what has been done at Rogers Pass, starting with Noel Gardner, who identified the avalanche paths— trigger zones—and set up the program with the armed forces to shoot them down with artillery. Under Freddy Schleiss, I think it was developed to perfection or as close as it comes to perfection."

In the summer of 1964, Peter Schaerer was made an attractive offer by Dr. Legget of the National Research Council to resume work in Canada. So in October of that year Peter immigrated to Canada for the second time, but now with a wife and two children. His job was to develop snow and ice removal techniques for roads. But they probably really needed him as a backup in case things fell apart in Rogers Pass.

Throughout 1964, the relationship between Noel Gardner and the staff of the Canadian Parks Service at the local, regional and national levels had reached a critical juncture. Parks officials were concerned that Gardner would quit his position in the middle of the winter, leaving no one to oversee the avalanche control program. Fred and Walter Schleiss had been working with Noel for five years, but Noel maintained that they were not experienced enough to forecast hazards reliably. The Canadian Parks Service officials were in a quandary as to whether or not this was true. The regional director of the CPS quietly approached Schaerer about the matter. He assured the regional director that Fred and Walter were capable of assuming the duties of avalanche hazard forecasting and being responsible for the safety of the highway. As Peter later observed, "In the years following, Fred and Walter lived up to and exceeded this expectation."

The Canadian Parks Service approached the NRC about Peter's availability in case Noel should suddenly quit. In January 1965, Peter moved into the new maintenance compound at the summit of Rogers Pass and resumed his duties with regard to avalanche defences and observations. It turned out the CPS management had grounds for concern throughout this period. Noel not only threatened to quit, but he obstinately moved up to Fidelity, where he dug in his heels for the rest of the winter until he finally resigned that spring.

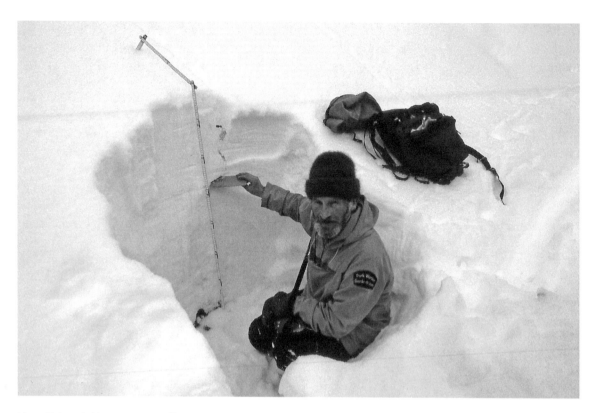

Hans Fuhrer taking a snow profile. HANS FUHRER COLLECTION

Because Noel did not move from Fidelity, Fred moved the forecasting operation to the pass while continuing to obtain prime data from Fidelity. It is interesting to note that the location of Mt. Fidelity as the main field post for data collection was always a bone of contention between Noel and Peter Schaerer. Don Mickle remembers that Noel and Peter argued a lot about this. Peter always felt it should be located closer to Rogers Pass near the concentration of problem avalanche paths. For several years, however, Fred maintained the Mt. Fidelity Station as the prime source of data collection, probably because he was familiar with the area and the infrastructure was firmly in place.

The adjustment to forecasting from the valley was not easy for him. Fred was used to forecasting from Mt. Fidelity with test slopes close at hand and all the instrumentation he needed. More important, when he was there he didn't need to rely on the observations of other people. Though they had telemetry that sent down valuable information, it wasn't the same—Fred lost the direct *feel* of what was happening at that altitude during a storm. He now had to rely heavily on his snow observers and the information they brought back from the field. For this reason he insisted that observers stationed at Fidelity be well trained with a minimum of a couple of years' experience behind them. He knew he was often a tyrant, but he needed accuracy, neatness and consistency if he was going to be successful in forecasting avalanches. As Fred put it: "And that's why I developed so much reliability on my guys because I couldn't be up there anymore. The system had to work or I would have ulcers all the time. But when it's a stormy night and you have 150 targets, and any one can hit the highway, and you got a good eye on that guy up there on the mountain—to tell you how stable the snow is—you got to know the guy is part of a system that is iron bound and you can sleep with that."

The winter that Fred Schleiss took over from Noel Gardner, two snow plow operators for Parks Canada were killed in an avalanche, which led to a change in the chain of command for the avalanche program. According to Fred, it was either the 6th or 7th of January, 1966, when the roof of his trailer blew off. It was at night, and he was in bed when the wind hit. When he got to the office, he found the wind measured 160 kilometres per hour. Walter had shot avalanches that night and had had reasonably good success, but with a real tempest blowing in the valley and with no visibility, they decided to close down the highway. They shut down both the east and west ends, but there was still traffic caught between the gates. The only thing they could do was send a warden through to sweep the highway. A half hour after closing down the highway, an avalanche came down just west of the pass. Without knowing where the cars were, wardens had to assume a vehicle might be caught in the slide. In desperation they called out all available staff to search the deposit while the wardens blocked each side to prevent anyone from plowing into the frozen wall of snow. The wardens had their hands full parking oncoming traffic in areas safe from other slide paths that were still running under the onslaught of heavy precipitation. The crew, meanwhile, probed the deposit that had crossed over the highway and run part way up the other side of the valley, constantly aware that fresh snow was accumulating in the nether regions of steep slopes above.

All of a sudden Fred spotted a front-end loader and grader heading to the slide. Fred was alarmed and demanded; "What the hell are you guys doing out here?" He found out the wardens had let them through. Fred asked the wardens why they had let the machines through and the response was, "Well they have authority to go through to plow slides." Fred retorted, "Nobody goes through out here—

there's danger of another slide!" After failing to reach the foreman or anyone with authority, he jumped in his truck and drove to the closure site. He yelled at the wardens, "Look, I don't care what, nobody goes through! … and I want those two guys off the slide." But it was too late. As he turned back to the site another avalanche roared down the mountain. With a sinking feeling, he radioed to his own crew to get off the slide path. They had pre-established an escape route and they followed Fred's cry of alarm—all except the two machine operators who had no escape plan and no communication with those who had.

It was unfortunate that it took an accident like that before Fred got the authority to run his own operation. From that point on Fred dictated when and where the closures were and inveigled the Warden Service to operate the road blocks. With the authority of the badge and with permanently assigned staff, he kept unauthorized people out of closed areas from then on.

It was at this time that Willi Pfisterer got his foot in the door with the park service when he was hired as an observer for the winter of 1965/66. He was happy to get steady work and soon moved his family up to Mt. Fidelity for the season. Willi spent three seasons in Rogers Pass learning the technical aspects of avalanche forecasting and data collection, which helped enormously with his role later as an alpine specialist in Jasper National Park.

Willi was an independent man, which made the sometimes abrasive direction he received from Fred difficult to take. But he recognized the value of what he was learning, because it gave substance to the art of avalanche prediction. He recalls: "I grew up in an avalanche area. We had all kinds of troubles and accidents. Being out in the field I had a real gut feeling for the whole thing, as a guide you know. I am still sitting here after 50 years of it. But, scientifically, I knew nothing. So at Rogers Pass, I was there for three years and learned all that. You cannot phone down to the forecaster and say, "I have a bad feeling—you should close

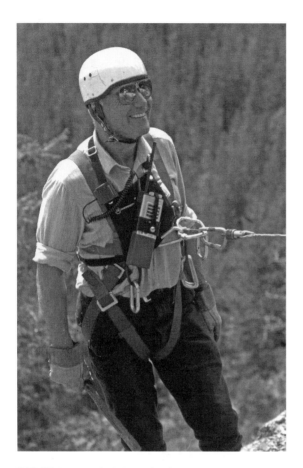

Willi Pfisterer on training school. GREG HORNE COLLECTION

THE YEAR 1965 was pivotal in avalanche awareness; this was the year of the largest avalanche accident to occur in Canada since the CPR disaster in 1910. In February, 1965, an avalanche buried a mining camp at the Granduc Mine near Stewart, B.C., and the aftermath of the accident had a major effect on how seriously the province of B.C. began to view such events.

In 1964, work had commenced on developing a copper mining operation near Stewart at the head of Portal Canal, one of the most spectacular fjords on the west coast. A large camp had been built next to the Leduc Glacier on a moraine at the junction where the north and south glaciers met.

Excerpts from Murray Lundberg's web site dedicated to the accident provides riveting details. This area traditionally gets some of the heaviest snowfalls in the world, up to 2,540 centimetres per year. So when four-and-a-half metres of snow fell during the second week of February, 1965, it meant more work to keep things operational, but there was little concern about what was developing above them. On February 18, at 9:57 a.m., the avalanche struck. Lundberg writes: "Radio operator Innis Kelly managed to get a brief Mayday message out before his equipment faltered, and within hours, a massive rescue force from across Canada and the United States was battling storms to reach the scene, where 50–70 mile per hour winds were reported. While nearby helicopters and fixed-wing aircraft waited for the weather to ease, four cat trains ground through the drifts at top speed, the U.S. Coast Guard cutter *Cape Romain* got into position to move the injured to hospital as quickly as possible, the huge Alaska ferry *Taku* was equipped as a hospital and sailed for the harbour closest to the disaster, and a wide array of other military, police and civilian aircraft and boats from both countries sped to the area."

Of the one hundred and fifty men who were working at the camp, sixty-eight were buried. According to the official records outlined in *Avalanche Accidents in Canada,* the others were in

the road. You have to come up with some facts and that I learned at Rogers Pass."

One thing Willi appreciated was the opportunity to travel to other avalanche control centres in both the United States and Europe. Observing avalanche forecasting in different locations gave those involved in the Canadian avalanche industry access to development of avalanche research in other parts of the world. It also gave Canada the opportunity to become a leader in the avalanche business. Pfisterer noted, "Rogers Pass avalanche control really had their act together. This was the biggest avalanche control centre in the world. We went to Switzerland and to America to the ski hills to look at what everybody was doing. We took the best of them all and applied it at Rogers Pass."

buildings that were untouched or were working in safe areas outside. It goes on to say: "Twenty-one men were working underground. The men caught in the avalanche were shovelling roofs, bulldozing pathways, digging out equipment and working on construction and machinery in the area of the mine portal."

The lack of proper equipment, the intensity of the storm and the state of the survivors, who were "injured or in shock," meant the rescue progressed slowly. With some searchers reduced to digging with their bare hands, 41 men were saved that day. Of the men outside the mine portal, all were found fairly quickly with six being recovered alive. Rescuers uncovered the last man five-and-one-half hours later. By 17:00 hrs, regular communication had been established, a helicopter pad had been built on the debris using a cat, and operations at the camp were fairly well organized.

Soon helicopters arrived with equipment, rescue personnel and search-and-rescue dogs. But poor weather and high winds continued to hamper the operation. Complicating the search was the enormous amount of material and debris scattered on top and throughout the deposit that had to be dug through. The rescue dogs were often confused and distracted by the amount of debris with human scent on it. Despite this, one RCMP dog had some success finding bodies. On February 21st, after abandoning any hope of finding further survivors, rescuers used bulldozers to trench the area. They operated carefully, shearing off debris only a few centimetres at a time.

Eino Myllyia, a carpenter, lay in his icy tomb listening to all the activity above. According to official records, "For three days between fitful comas, Myllyia could hear helicopters landing and taking off above him." That afternoon while a cat worked in the location of the active helicopter pad with spotters on the bulldozer blade watching for any sign of clothing, a large section of snow sheared away. Looking up at the astonished spotters was a blinking Myllyia. "Don't move me, I think my legs are frozen," he called

out. He was carefully extracted from his tomb and immediately flown to Ketchikan, Alaska. Amazingly, a team of U.S. doctors saved both his feet and hands. He lost only the toes on one foot and some fingers. His astonishing reprieve from death, however, was short-lived. Six months later he was killed by a vehicle while crossing a street in Vancouver.

The last body wasn't recovered until June. Officially the death toll was 26, with a further 20 people injured. The rescue operation must at times have been an organized chaos. With the sheer number of casualties, the hideous weather, the many diversified international rescue groups involved, the lack of trained staff, its remote location and the complexity of the terrain, the search was praised, "as a massive effort on the part of many."

The camp on the glacier was never reopened because of the avalanche hazard, and a permanent camp was set up on the shore of a nearby lake. A 50-kilometre all-weather road was eventually built to connect the camp to the town of Stewart, B.C. There had been no avalanche control program in use at the mining operation prior to the accident. A large-scale avalanche program was introduced immediately after the accident to protect the new access road to Stewart during the winter.

The Granduc avalanche disaster is also credited with introducing the helicopter as a means of controlling avalanches. Many important people in the avalanche industry got their start working in the avalanche control program at Granduc. Many experts were brought in from North America in the aftermath of the accident, including Monty Atwater and Norm Wilson from the United States. The mining company also consulted Peter Schaerer and Fred Schleiss. But it was Noel Gardner, now free of the Canadian Parks Service, who benefited considerably as an avalanche consultant for developing future avalanche programs, thereafter used by other companies. The fallout from the disaster slowly led to a whole new awareness of avalanches that in turn created a small but lucrative industry in training, education and avalanche control programs.

But now interest in avalanche safety began to grow in Canada. The National Research Council decided that Schaerer should do research more in line with avalanches rather than with the snow removal project he was working on at the time. When Peter returned to Rogers Pass, he brought with him a young technician by the name of Keith Everts. The focus of their study was based on the characteristics of avalanches, instead of the protection of the Trans-Canada Highway. Some years later Keith would join the Warden Service and move on to Banff where he would become a major force in creating a sound avalanche control program for that park.

By 1968 the Warden Service was using Rogers Pass as a training ground for park wardens with good results. It was a period when a number of wardens from other parks learned about avalanches from the best. They were able to take this experience back home to aid in developing viable avalanche programs tailored to their needs.

After Willi became the alpine specialist in Jasper, he decided that Rogers Pass would be a good place to introduce wardens to deep-powder skiing. But though it was a great experience, it had to be accepted into the training curriculum as a school. The Deep Powder Ski School, based out of Mt. Fidelity, was held every winter for several years and was looked upon by the stronger skiers as a great reward, while some of the more inexperienced dreaded attending. But just to keep a "school" aspect to the week, one day was dedicated to snow observations while another day ended up being a mock rescue scenario.

The wardens with poor skiing ability had cause to worry about getting down alive, because the snowfalls during the late sixties and early seventies were record-setting. Indeed, the winter of 1971/72 was referred to as the "the season of the hundred-year avalanches," because the avalanche activity was almost unprecedented,

wiping out large tracts of one-hundred-year-old timber. The school, which was nearly cancelled that year, became an epic of survival. One of the wardens who took part was Mike McKnight, who remembers how desperate things were in Rogers Pass that year.

As the snow fell and the avalanche hazard grew, the group continued to ski off Mt. Fidelity in deepening powder until Willi decided it was time for the obligatory training day. When they got up the next morning Willi went around and had them all draw straws to see who would get to be the victim in the rescue toboggan. Mike says, "Yah it was a training school so we trudged up onto the Roundhill carrying this toboggan that breaks in two pieces and packed it up there and I of course was the lucky one that got to ride it. Pfisterer was bound and determined he was going to strap me into this toboggan, and I said if nothing else I got to have my hands free. I was all covered in a big tarp, but I had my arms up over my head and Gord Peyto was on the front of the toboggan and Joe Halstenson was on the back. Well they skied down over this pitch on Roundhill and the whole slope broke loose and started to slide and all I can hear is 'Oh, shit here we go,' so we kept going over these little rollers and we get on to a bench and then the avalanche would take us down over the next roller and it would break loose again and I would hear these guys yelling and they were hanging on to this toboggan trying to keep everything upright. Finally everything came to a stop and we were on this little bench. I'm laying in this thing and I knew that I was buried. Finally the rest of the guys got down there and dug us out. Both of these guys hung on to the toboggan, but they were buried up to their chest."

In the end there was too much snow to ski with any degree of safety as even the most innocuous slope was sliding under the vast accumulation of deep, powdery snow. Things got critical at the station when the group began to run out of food. Finally, they had to chance taking the Sno-cat down the road to resupply. Mike recalls: "Skiing behind the deep ruts plowed out by the cat tracks was a serious challenge for even the best skiers. You'd get going down these ruts and of course you would pick up quite a bit of speed. So you'd try and dig your knee into the bank to slow yourself down and of course every once in a while your knee would grab in the bank and you'd go for a horrible header and away you'd go."

Once they got to the valley they found that only four or five kilometres of the Pass was left open, and it would remain that way for the next five days. From here the group pitched in to help. The army continued to shoot down avalanches, but its mobility was quickly being compromised by the snow. Mike remembers: "A lot of the avalanches coming down were natural … it was natural releases that closed the highway on both sides. It was just one of those things when the gun crew got behind in the program and the avalanches started coming down bigger and bigger and then they just lost it. They couldn't move the gun fast enough to keep up. The snow intensity was unbelievable."

Jay Morton was also on that school and remembers details of the ordeal at the summit. "There were a bunch of people marooned at the summit. They even had horses there. So they kept sending feed up on the train, and we would go down with the Sno-cat cat and pick up this hay and bring it back to the pass for these horses. The roads were blocked, and they couldn't get the guns out to shoot … so they brought in a gun from Calgary. Oh yah. There was a trucker stuck in a snow-shed. He couldn't move. The superintendent kind of freaked by this time, because the guy had been in the shed for three days. I think he had one Charlie Pride tape in his eight-track. Willi and I skied down to get him out, and that was pretty hairy, because it hadn't been shot, and there was tonnes of snow. Willi turned to me and said, 'Morton do you have an avalanche cord?' Yah … like that will help! So anyway they sent this gun out from Calgary, but the lieutenant in charge of the outfit couldn't ski, so he had to teach us [wardens] how to operate the gun. Yah, a warden

gun crew … that was quite a thing. The slides were just terrifying! I can still smell the needles of the trees snapping off as they went by. Shoot one target, and about six of them would come down."

Don Mickle remembers the same incredible winter. He was working for Peter Schaerer recording measurements of avalanche deposits shortly after they had run. "It was dangerous everywhere," he said. "Sometimes slides came down after Peter and I had just finished measuring snow density up in the middle of the slide path. Some of the truck drivers, cat operators and road foremen had nervous breakdowns that winter. There was too much stress from the threat of almost always being caught in an avalanche. One cat operator's father was killed in the 1966 avalanche, and the son had a breakdown trying to keep up with the clearing of the highway and the avalanche deposits. There were times when you would drive by an avalanche path and in the rearview mirror you would see the dust from an avalanche that had just missed you. It was wild."

Dale Portman, who also worked in Glacier, recalls what it was like to be an avalanche observer at one particularly exposed gun position, shooting avalanches in the middle of the night. "It was a typical night shoot with the Canadian Army at the Lens avalanche shed. The gun location to shoot this particular avalanche, however, was 100 metres up the road from the safety of the snow-shed, right in the middle of the avalanche path. It was not originally located there, but avalanches had widened the path over the years until they had exposed the gun position. At night the practice was to shoot the gun and then stay silent, as the only indication that the shoot was successful would be the sound of the detonation then the subsequent avalanche. Because it was so dark, everyone's senses were heightened. We had no idea how far the slide would come."

The first audible sound in the encompassing blackness was the woof of the exploding shell high up on the mountainside. After an indeterminable time the next sound heard by the crew was the distant bellow of rushing air, followed by a slight hint of stirring trees, and the sharp sound of snapping branches. They dared not wait until they saw the avalanche as it would engulf them. Once they confirmed that they had released an avalanche, the only thing to do was run for the protection of the shed. He recalls: "We ran like hell, hoping we hadn't lingered too long or missed the subtle sounds of warning back at the gun position. When you do get to the shed, it's exhilarating because you've managed to cheat a bit. Then we'd hear the sound of the avalanche roaring overhead like a freight train. One time we got back to the gun position and found everything covered in snow and pushed around like dinky toys. This happened on more than one occasion until Fred relocated the gun position."

Don Mickle also remembers one of the worst storms, which brought down a new slide at Cougar Creek. "It had never been down before—there was one-hundred-year-old timber up there. It was amazing." The huge avalanche came down and covered the highway as well as the railway tracks. Don shudders remembering that he and Paul Anhorn had just been there the day before taking measurements from a National Research Council snow gauge, thinking it was one location they did not have to worry about. Because the slide was not the result of a shoot, there had been no road closure, so once again there was no way of knowing if any vehicles were buried. The night the slide came down, warden Gord Peyto was on duty and was free to help Don check the slide for vehicles. Before they arrived, a cat operator had been sent down to begin the clearing process. The operator, happy to see someone else, came down on foot to meet them, leaving the machine on top of the slide, now some six metres above the road. The CPR workers had their hands full as well and had another crew working on the tracks below.

The two men began searching the debris with a magnetometer (for detecting metal) when, to their horror, they heard the timber cracking and snapping well up the creek valley, trumpeting the rushing onslaught of another slide. The three men stared at each other in that brief moment of paralyzed panic; then they realized the slide deposit was over 900 metres wide and they were in the middle of it. Fortunately only the dust from the wind blast settled gently on their shoulders from the snow above. All they could feel now was relief as they listened to the groan of the compressing slow-moving mass above them.

Gord immediately shut down all the work on the slide, retreating to the sanctuary of the Northlander Hotel at the summit of Rogers Pass. Here they were unceremoniously received by a pack of angry motorists trying to get through the pass on delayed journeys either east or west of the snowy hell they found themselves in. The men were both so pumped full of adrenaline from the slide experience that when a kid's toboggan accidentally fell over they both nearly jumped through a window. Ignoring the crowd, since they could not help, they made their way to the hotel bar.

By the end of the sixties and early seventies mining exploration and logging began pushing deeper into open avalanche terrain. In 1969, after the mining disaster at Granduc, Mr. J.W. Peck, the Chief Inspector for Mines in B.C., approached Peter Schaerer and Fred Schleiss about conducting an avalanche safety course for his mining inspectors. They agreed and put together a two-day course in Rogers Pass—the first of its kind for people working professionally in a field outside the small world of the select few studying avalanches.

After the success of the 1969 avalanche safety course, Schaerer and Schleiss received requests for more avalanche safety courses. They could teach the principles of avalanche behaviour and how they were forecast, but they felt that a third component of search-and-rescue techniques should be added for overall safety. With this in mind they approached Parks Canada about sending someone to teach this aspect. The alpine specialist Willi Pfisterer, now in Jasper,

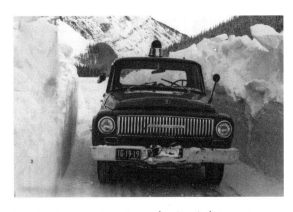

Warden truck in plowed road (avalanche). JASPER WARDEN ARCHIVES

was chosen, and he became an integral part of avalanche training workshops and courses over the next several years.

Prior to 1969 small individual courses had been held for recreational skiers and climbers in both Alberta and on the west coast by individuals who felt they had some understanding of the dangers of avalanches. Noel Gardner, of course, had been putting on avalanche awareness courses for his fellow wardens and other interested parties (usually recreational skiers in Alberta) in Banff during the early 1950s, but it was an American who immigrated to Canada who started reaching out to more recreational skiers and mountaineers.

Brad Geisler came to Canada in 1955, and shortly thereafter joined the CSPA. The CSPA is a volunteer group of men and women who help the professional ski patrollers in various ski areas on weekends, patrolling the slopes and providing first-aid to injured skiers. It is a very successful program that has provided valuable assistance to ski areas across Canada over the years. Geisler arrived with a background in skiing and mountaineering. Brad had trained in Canada at the Columbia Icefield in the early 1940s with the U.S. Army where he picked up an appreciation for the Canadian Rockies. He teamed up with Russ Bradley, another ski-patroller and ski mountaineer, in putting together avalanche

education programs geared for mountaineers and recreational skiers. They were one of two providers of public avalanche education courses in Canada, the other being the Federation of Mountain Clubs of B.C. In conjunction with Banff National Park, Geisler and Bradley were the first to put out an avalanche bulletin to the general public.

But Geisler saw the need for a much expanded public avalanche service for the increasing number of recreational mountain users in the years to come. In her history of the Canadian Avalanche Association, Christine Everts writes, "At a 1969 Conference on Snow and Ice at the University of Calgary, Geisler proposed the establishment of an avalanche information and research centre, which would serve as the headquarters for research and up-to-date information. He suggested that the centre be supported by the National Research Council and interested universities. In addition to advising ski instructors, mountain guides and patrollers on how to establish standards and set up snow-craft programs, he reinforced the importance of offering avalanche safety programs for the public." Geisler warned that, "Western Canada is a country of mountains and snow and its mountains are being utilized more and more every year. Unless we put our knowledge to use, the number of preventable accidents is bound to increase."

But it would be another twelve years before the NRC, Parks Canada, B.C. Highways, the ski resorts, the heli-ski industry and the Association of Canadian Mountain Guides would get together and create the Canadian Avalanche Association (CAA). In the meanwhile, the Canadian Parks Service felt confident enough to produce a small pamphlet titled "The Do's and Don'ts of Winter Travel" for the park visitor. By then the two new alpine specialists, Peter Fuhrmann and Willi Pfisterer, had begun giving lectures on the subject.

In the winter of 1970/71, a number of Canadians went down to Reno, Nevada, to attend the U.S. Forest Service's first National Avalanche School. Included in that group were Hans Gmoser and several of his ski guides from Canadian Mountain

79

Holidays (CMH). Peter Schaerer and Fred Schleiss were invited down as guest instructors, and in 1971, the first professional course took place at Rogers Pass. A second course was held in 1973 at Whistler, B.C., with 60 students attending.

By the winter of 1974/75 the interest was so great that several courses were needed each year to satisfy the demand. Instructors were now evolving out of the pool of keen and enthusiastic participants in the earlier courses. Administratively, it was getting far too demanding for Schaerer, Schleiss and Pfisterer to keep it up. It had reached the stage where a professional institution was needed to step forward and take over the responsibility of running these courses. The problem was solved in 1974 when the British Columbia Institute of Technology (BCIT) through its Continuing Studies Department took over the administrative responsibilities. New instructors grew out of the industry's budding talent pool while the National Research Council and Parks Canada continued to contribute teaching personnel.

In 1974, an avalanche accident on the west coast of B.C. further highlighted the need to provide avalanche information for those living, working or playing in the mountains. This tragedy led to establishing a task force charged with developing an extensive highway avalanche safety and control program in B.C. The task force designated over 70 areas on provincial highways in British Columbia that required avalanche forecasting and control.

The Ministry of Transportation's Snow and Avalanche Program grew into the largest avalanche safety program in Canada under the direction of Geoff Freer. Geoff picked up his credentials by working as Schaerer's assistant in Rogers Pass two years prior to the accident. He was one of the original task force members on the committee formed to look into the North Route Café accident but went on to run the new program. There was now a third player in the avalanche forecasting and control industry along with the Snow Research and Avalanche Warning Section op-

eration in Rogers Pass and the "Four Mountain Parks" avalanche control program in Jasper, Banff, Yoho and Kootenay national parks. They would be joined shortly by the heli-ski industry and the ski areas.

The technicians working for B.C. Highways would soon start to play a key role in avalanche rescue as well. Dave Smith, who worked in public safety in Kananaskis Country, joined B.C. Highways in the mid-eighties and brought with him considerable experience in mountain rescue. He reflects that it was a natural fit for the men working in avalanche control for Highways to respond to avalanche accidents when they occurred. More often than not, they were the only trained personnel in the more remote parts of the province available to attend. With the emergence of volunteer groups, however, they soon had help. They also found themselves working with the RCMP—particularly dog handlers—and ski guides from nearby heli-ski operations. One of the most significant contributions they brought to the rescue scenario was the training to evaluate the ongoing hazard to the rescuers and the ability to do something about it. Because snow stabilization was their bread and butter, they had access to bombs and helicopters and could quickly ensure safe working conditions for the searchers. It was a huge advantage in dangerous conditions.

WITH THE NEED FOR PUBLIC information and education on avalanche hazards becoming apparent, a small committee was formed in 1975 to address the problem. It was a three-member committee: Peter Schaerer with National Research Council, Ron Perla from Environment Canada and Geoff Freer with B.C. Highways. Ron Perla, an American, was an electrical engineer by profession, but had worked as a snow ranger for Ed La Chapelle in Alta, Utah. La Chapelle was a geophysicist (the counterpart of Peter Schaerer) who had been involved with snow research at Alta with the snow rangers. Ron moved to Canada in 1974 when he was offered a job with Environment

Canada's Glaciology Division. In 1976 Ron went on to write a major revision of the "Avalanche Handbook," the premier training manual on understanding avalanches in North America at the time.

This represented the first step toward Geisler's vision of a National Avalanche Centre. The original committee expanded to include other vested-interest groups (heli-ski guides, ski areas etc.) in the late 1970s. This led to the establishment of the Canadian Avalanche Association in 1981. When asked what led to the formation of the CAA, Freer was quoted as saying, "I think probably the need for an independent body to represent the field and move a bit away from individual organizations. Like Parks Canada had their own kind of approach, the [B.C.] Ministry of Transport's approach was basically the National Research Council's approach because Peter [Schaerer] and Paul [Anhorn] and I worked so closely together. Some people, and some organizations, needed an independent group. In other words, Parks [Canada] might not be able to do something from a political perspective, but if an independent organization like the Canadian Avalanche Association said, 'These are the standards for Canada,' then that put more pressure on Parks, the Ministry and the guiding companies to abide by those. I think that was really the other piece, having a unified voice for the industry to work with the federal government, provincial government and others. Also it got to the point that we [staff from Parks Canada, Ministry of Transportation and the National Research Council] were doing so many courses and training sessions that we really needed somebody to start taking it over." A number of different organizations now make up the Canadian Avalanche Association. Members include national and provincial parks in B.C. and Alberta, Parks Canada, the National Research Council, B.C. Highways, ski areas, mountain guides, backcountry lodges, heli-ski operations, cat-skiing operators and the mining industry, as well as the research and consulting businesses.

CONCERN ABOUT THE IMPACT of avalanches on human activity was initially aroused in the late fifties and sixties when structures like railway tracks, highways and dwellings were affected. There was not a great deal of emphasis on the welfare of individuals during the early years of avalanche research, simply because there was little ski-touring activity, and the loss of human life was isolated and sporadic. This began to change in the late sixties. Ski-touring grew popular out of a desire to ski virgin powder difficult to find in ski areas—though initially it was beyond the boundaries of ski areas where people found the untracked slopes. As people sought the ultimate experience in the sport, they travelled into more remote backcountry locations. The only way to reach this blissful heaven was to get there on skis, which greatly limited the number of turns a skier could get in a day after toiling to the top of a mountain. It usually meant only one run. Hans Gmoser solved this problem by introducing helicopter assisted skiing or "heli-skiing," which led him to found Canadian Mountain Holidays (CMH). This opened up a whole new landscape for the skiing industry. Suddenly people skiing together in large numbers were exposed to avalanche slopes when the extent of the hazard was not well understood.

When Hans first started heli-skiing in the Bugaboos in the late sixties, the snowpack was deep and stable and stayed that way for some years. But slowly the winters became milder, and the structure of the snowpack began to change. One of the things lost in heli-skiing is the opportunity to examine the snowpack. A person travelling on skis is in direct contact with the snow and can assess the hazard directly. The heli-ski guide, however, lands above the terrain and misses any direct feel for the stability of the snowpack.

Hans Gmoser himself said it so well in an interview; "I always felt in ski-touring you only do one at the most tour a day and on the way up you've got so much opportunity to really get a feel for the snow. I felt I could always pull one run out

81

of the hat and get everyone down safely. And you didn't have to spend a hell of a lot of time digging in the snow, because you have so much opportunity to observe. [With heli-skiing] we never thought of going out there and looking. We just went there and started skiing. And even if you spent a lot of time thinking about which would be the safest run today, one run wasn't enough. After one run you had to pull another run off. Now we do a lot of snow operations. All of a sudden, we began to realize, we were dealing with so many variables. You can dig all the snow profiles you want because you can dig a profile here and you go three metres over there and it's a totally different story. You go up, you go down, you change the exposure, so it's a lot of variables. What has really happened, and I've said it before, is that the heli-ski guides have gone through the same evolution as the bush pilot to the captain of a 747. At first it was the bush pilot by the seat of his pants, his judgment alone and with heli-skiing it's the same. You jump out, assess the situation and make your decision. Now before the guides go out skiing they've had so much input and they are actually programmed. They are part of the machine now. They know exactly which runs they are going to ski, they know exactly which line they are going to take, and they know exactly which runs not to ski. You can never eliminate the risk totally but you have to try."

For years the main competition for Canadian Mountain Holidays came from Mike Wiegele, a fellow Austrian who built the huge heli-skiing resort at Blue River, B.C. Mike studied the weather patterns of the different mountain ranges and felt the mountains west of Blue River held the most promise for great skiing. He was right. It took a while, but now the Blue River operation is one of the most successful heli-ski operations in Canada.

With the growing success of heli-ski operations, the business proliferated, spilling over into the development of multiple backcountry lodges and cat-skiing operations catering to the ski-tourer. But the sheer numbers of people exposed to steep ski terrain inevitably led to more accidents than had been seen before in a recreational sport.

For years there were no accidents within the industry, but this changed in 1974 when one skier was killed and two more injured at the CMH Cariboo operation. The numbers escalated even more in 1979 when the first of several big tragedies (now infamously known as the St. Valentine's Day avalanche) occurred on February 14th when seven people were killed. This was followed by the Thunder River avalanche near Blue River, B.C., eight years later in 1987 where seven more lost their lives. The worst to date, however, occurred in the Bugaboos in 1990, when nine people were killed on a run called Bay Street.

The government placed an ultimatum before the various businesses, saying, in effect, "Get your act together or be regulated by the government." Fortunately, the various operations were able to comply with this position and began to work seriously to minimize the risks.

One of the greatest aids to rescue operations came on the scene about this time. Rescue beacons first appeared in Canada in the late 1960s and by the beginning of the next decade, the Warden Service, the Association of Canadian Mountain Guides and the heli-skiing businesses were wearing them. The patterns used to find a buried victim were refined, and with better technology, detection became very rapid.

The ski guides also realized that they had to have a better system of recognizing existing avalanche hazard. By 1980, the ability to determine the avalanche hazard had improved, and with the development of the Canadian Avalanche Association, more sophisticated courses were available to pass on this information. The various heli-ski operations put significant effort into determining the hazard specific to their area; more important, they passed on the information. This effort paid off handsomely when the heli-ski industry was able to say they had had no casualties during the year 2003, which was a record-setting year for avalanche deaths due to a highly unstable snowpack.

4 Modernization: The Introduction of the Alpine Specialist

THE WORK DONE AT ROGERS PASS during the 1960s was quite important to the evolving public safety program in national parks. It resulted in more reliable forecasting, and skill in this field would become necessary for those to follow after Walter Perren's death in 1967. When the competition for the position was posted during the winter of 1968, two of the qualifying men, Willi Pfisterer and Fred Schleiss, had extensive training in avalanche work. It is revealing then, that Peter Fuhrmann, with his limited background in this field, had the confidence to apply for the job. The position was highly attractive in that it offered government security and a chance to develop a professional rescue organization. The wardens still had a long way to go before reaching the level of competence Walter had wanted to see, and the prospect of guiding them through the next phase would be challenging.

Willi had every reason to think he would get the job well before it came up for competition. When Walter died at the end of December, park managers realized they were facing a whole winter season with no one to lead the avalanche program. Willi was working for Fred Schleiss in Rogers Pass as avalanche observer and was asked to fill in. Walter had told Willi before he died that he had the qualifications and saw no problem with him succeeding. Clearly Walter felt that Willi had the greatest experience for the work ahead, but as Peter had noted, "Walter was not a political animal." Neither was Willi.

Willi Pfisterer grew up climbing and skiing in Mühlbach, a small village near Salzburg, Austria, under the influence of a dynamic grandfather who introduced him to both sports. As Willi says, "It was part of the family tradition." Though he became adept at both activities, he found the guiding quota for the village already filled. With no immediate future at home, he began to look for options. When the opportunity to go to Canada and possibly New Zealand arose, the young, bachelor thought "why not?" He arrived in Canada in 1954 with his friend Frank Stark, picking up what odd jobs were available—often not in the guiding field. Eventually he was able to work part-time as a ski instructor in Banff and finally as a horse guide for Bill Harrison, an outfitter in Edgewater, B.C.

Harrison sent Willi to his horse camp in Glacier National Park, where Willi made his first impressive climb in Canada: Mt. Sir Donald, solo on his day off. But it was an exciting pack trip back to Edgewater with a string of 28 horses that tipped the scales in favour of Willi staying in Canada. It took two weeks to cover the ground over the pass to the Beaver River through the wild, high country of Duncan Pass west of the Columbia River, on to the lush pastures at Edgewater. But it was one particular sight that caused Willi to stay. He talks quietly about the day "the front horses came out of the creek and up over a ridge and the wind was blowing in their manes and tails … and behind was the Great Glacier. And that was a real sight. That's when I decided I'm going to stay in Canada."

Shortly after, on the advice of friends, Willi went to Jasper where he opened a ski shop, married his wife Annie and started a family. It was here he began his skiing and guiding career in earnest. He obtained his guide's licence during this time along with Tony Messner, and was soon leading climbs up Mt. Robson and Mt. Edith Cavell. If he took clients up a new ascent, he charged a bit extra. Although Willi was struggling with English as a second language, his cutting sense of humour was very much in evidence. He and Tony Messner shared an easily climbed mountain as a reusable first ascent. They called it "Unnecessary Peak" because they made so many "first ascents." One day, Willi was taking up a new client when the man happened to spot a prune stone and wondered what it was doing on a virgin peak. Willi quickly scooped it up, and said it was his "moisturizer" and popped it into his mouth to demonstrate the usefulness of a prune stone when climbing a mountain. He thought ruefully to himself afterwards: "There I was on Unnecessary Peak, sucking on Tony's prune stone!"

In 1959, Willi accompanied Hans Gmoser on the second ascent of Mt. Logan, Canada's highest mountain. It was Willi's first time up north, and he loved the wildness and freedom of the country. Years later he would return as alpine specialist to initiate the much-needed rescue training for the wardens of the newly formed Kluane National Park. He added to his repertoire by making 60 ascents that summer, including climbs in the Bugaboos and Purcells. Many of these climbs were done with good friend Tony Messner from whom he learned a great deal—particularly in the more technical aspects of rock climbing and mountaineering.

Although Willi was busy with guiding and the ski shop, none of the work provided a reliable income—which was worrisome with a steadily growing family. He wanted "a position" with permanence and would say so every time Jasper Chief Park Warden Mickey McGuire asked him to help with warden training. In frustration he finally packed up the family and went down to the Big White ski area where he ran a ski school and ski shop. But failed promises of work with the government left Willi looking for work the following winter, and he wound up driving trucks and hauling house trailers from Chicago to Kamloops—a situation he found intolerable. As he described it: "You sit there in the truck and your legs die off and your belly grows bigger … and you drive by everybody."

The position with Parks Canada Willi was hoping for came first as an avalanche observer at Rogers Pass, where he worked until he moved to Banff to fill in for Walter. He had already established weather plots for Sunshine, Lake Louise and areas along the Banff/Jasper Highway and was well into a control program when the competition results came back. Willi was considerably shocked to find that Peter Fuhrmann had placed first, Fred second and that he, himself, had placed third on what should have been a shoe-in placement.

Peter's success was due to his achievements in the climbing world and an astute political savvy. He knew both qualities would be required to deal with park administrators who needed to be reminded daily why they had a public safety function. Peter's acumen and survival skills (political and physical) were honed through a particularly challenging childhood in East Germany, brought on by the rising tide of Nazi power leading up to the Second World War. Robert Sandford gives a brief but chilling synopsis of this period in *The Highest Calling:* "Peter saw the worst of what war can be and was very nearly destroyed by it. Separated from his parents when the tide turned against Germany, Peter fled with his grandparents to Dresden, where they experienced the worst fire bombing of the entire war. After the Russian invasion, Peter spent two-and-a-half years behind the Iron Curtain in a refugee camp. It was here that the Russians killed one of his uncles. Shortly after, his aunt took her own life. Conditions were so desperate that Peter nearly lost a leg to infection. He was so malnourished and sick by the time he was reunited with his parents in Nuremburg in 1947, he was immediately hospitalized."

Peter finished grade school, and he studied commerce for two years before taking a job with Shell Oil in Germany. It was during this time that his natural athletic abilities and exuberance for life led him into adventurous pursuits of skiing (compliments of Shell Oil), track and field, bicycling and motorcycle racing. The work with Shell Oil gave Peter a polish that would stand him in good stead over the years, but it was not what he wanted out of life. He was disillusioned with the highly structured oil company that was ruled by embittered former Nazi officers, and he jumped at the chance to immigrate to Canada with his new friend, Heinz Kahl, whom he met in a jazz bar in Munich.

The promised job with the oil company did not materialize in Edmonton, however, and as Heinz was eager to get to the mountains, they soon hitchhiked to Banff. Peter, who was never very enthralled with Edmonton, decided to take up climbing with Heinz as it was the only sport he could afford. Dutifully, they bought a small amount of climbing gear from Monod Sports in Banff, and were on their way to climb Cascade Mountain when they were picked up by the personnel manager of the Department of Public Works. He advised them to come into his office the following day to see what work was available. Peter did not get up Cascade, but he did get a job working as a draftsman and was on his

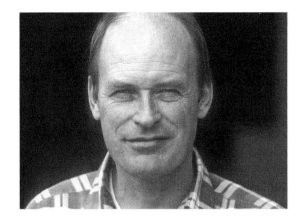

Peter Fuhrmann. BOB SANDFORD COLLECTION

way to a lifelong career in public service for the Government of Canada. What he did not realize was that the work would be in mountain rescue with the Warden Service. But that would not happen until he became adept as a climber. Peter had continued climbing with Heinz and others, but when Heinz announced he had received his guide's licence from Walter Perren, Peter reasoned that that goal was within his scope as well. He continued to climb diligently until he felt he was ready for his exam, and he made an appointment with Walter to take the test.

The test turned out to be very practical for the job Peter would eventually assume. Peter drove to meet Perren at the appointed time but was informed he had been called out to a couple of rescues. He headed for Mount Louis first, hoping to catch Walter there, but the team had moved on to Castle Mountain. It was a semi-comical episode that had brought the rescuers out to aid three climbers who had climbed the standard route on the tower but could not get down. The warden at the station had initially monitored their progress, saying they were on their way down, but when they hadn't returned after two nights, he realized they were in trouble.

When Peter arrived, he informed the warden that he was to meet Walter and was given the go-ahead to proceed up the route. Walter spotted him, and realizing that Peter was there for his test, immediately told him to come on up with his [Walter's] pack. Peter complied and was soon on the summit with Walter and the three stranded climbers. In the end, Walter went down the standard route with two of the climbers, while Peter took a more direct, exposed route with the third reluctant climber. At the bottom Walter said: "Well, that was your rock test." Later in the week, Peter took his snow and ice test, wrote the exam and became a Canadian mountain guide.

Peter began to guide for the Alpine Club, where he met Hans Schwartz. They became friends and eventually guided together at the Yukon Centennial Expedition, which led to a joint expedition to Huascaran in Peru the following year (1968). It was actually a guided trip that brought them some unexpected attention. Unfortunately, though they made the summit, problems with the descent and weather delayed their return to base camp. It was with some surprise, then, that Peter learned that the Canadian Ambassador was standing by with two fully equipped helicopters ready to fly to their aid, compliments of Catharine Whyte (benefactor of the Whyte Museum and wealthy, influential Banff resident), who "promised to pay whatever it took to find the missing Canadian climbers." He returned without help and intact in time to apply for the position.

Although Peter worked as a guide when he could, he had not given up his day job with the Department of Public Works. At the time he was working in the old customs building in Calgary only one floor above the Parks Canada office run by the Director General, Don Coombs. He actually met Coombs on a VIP trip to the Columbia Icefield (with Ottawa brass) where his mountaineering expertise was recognized. When Walter became ill, Coombs invited Peter for a coffee to discuss the future of the public safety program and mentioned that he should apply when the competition came up.

Peter was forthright during his interview and convinced the board he was the man for the job.

When asked by Bert Pittaway what the difference was between a vertical and a ring piton, he gave them the correct answer but immediately launched into what he felt they should be looking for instead of asking about pitons. He astutely predicted that increasing tourism would be the future problem for rescue work and pointed out the tremendous need for a "top-notch international rescue system." The idea that accidents were bound to increase was not startlingly new to the board, but the idea of an international-calibre rescue team probably was. Peter remembered, "I gave them a big spiel about what I thought the needs were and how it should be done. They all agreed and we had a good session after that." Willi had no chance against such rhetoric.

Fortunately for Willi, they needed more than one man for the coming work. Fred Schleiss, though qualified, found he was better suited to the work he was doing and was happy to go back to Rogers Pass. But before coming up with the compromise that would launch the modern era of rescue work, the board astounded Willi by asking him to help Peter with the avalanche work. Peter, despite having accolades as a climber, still had to gain Willi's level of knowledge in this field. They then expected Willi to return to his job as avalanche observer. Willi, however, had had enough of working for Fred in Glacier and had no intention of returning. He was heading out of town when he was asked to report to the Superintendent of Jasper National Park. Peter had realized that the job was more work than one man could handle and suggested that he split the position with Willi. Steve Kun had also come to this conclusion, and recommended that Willi take over in Jasper. Although all government jobs were locked up due to a hiring freeze imposed by Prime Minister Trudeau, the powers that be moved around this testy obstruction and had a job ready and waiting when Willi arrived in Jasper. It was one of the few occasions that a government employee found himself indispensable to the system.

In the end, Willi was responsible for Jasper, Waterton and Glacier/Revelstoke national parks, while Peter took on Banff, Yoho and Kootenay national parks. Eventually, Willi would also assume responsibility for the new northern parks of Nahanni and Kluane, and Peter would tuck Baffin Island under his wing. The two men with such divergent backgrounds and expertise would not only form the basis for a respected and successful international rescue operation, but would come to have a mutual respect and friendship few could have predicted. Willi with his sound operational skills, humour and rapport with the men was a perfect foil for the more worldly, silver-tongued Peter with his extravagant ideas and lofty goals. In recognition of the scope of work ahead they were given the new title "Alpine Specialist." In honour of this position, Willi always wore red knicker socks that he insisted only the specialist could wear. Woe betide the novice who showed up with socks even remotely red. Willi was likely to turn the spotlight on his ability for the whole trip—with not-too-kindly ribbing if they failed in any way.

The same year that Willi and Peter were hired, another significant event was unfolding that would affect the development of the burgeoning program. For a few years, there had been concern over the direction the Warden Service was headed. Until the mid-1960s, the warden's chief role was to look after a large backcountry district maintained throughout the year. But the tourist boom was being felt in the frontcountry, and problems with law enforcement, mountain rescue and wildlife conflict were increasing. Park management wanted to lead the men toward a modern idea of park management that did not support the district system. Though it was seen as an opportunity for advancement with a better salary, it was not popular. Ultimately it would lead to specialization in designated functions allowing the public safety function to flourish.

Suddenly all outlying facilities were centralized, and everyone reported to the main townsite office in the morning. The change was so abrupt that many wardens had nowhere to go and nothing to do. Centralization was a long-term project that was difficult to implement, as there was little immediate leadership for the new functions. It was into this void of general discontent—and personal loss—that Peter Fuhrmann and Willi Pfisterer stepped in to replace the beloved Walter Perren.

For as Peter later said: "It was very difficult for me to follow in his footsteps … even though I'd worked with the wardens … because everyone looked at him as the mountain God who walked on water, and I couldn't walk on water." Peter realized that one of his biggest challenges was to inspire the same confidence in his leadership that Walter had previously enjoyed. He astutely observed that Walter had a compassion for the older wardens "who were not really cut out to be mountaineers."

Both men set out to establish themselves by conducting local training programs in each park as well as holding joint regional schools. Willi, who had farther to go, was tireless in travelling to the parks under his jurisdiction, getting to know both the men and the country intimately. Peter had less travelling, but dealt with the heavier climbing traffic in the popular mountains of Lake Louise and Yoho, and the eastern slopes. To begin with, they taught the improvised rescue and simple cable-rescue system. Both felt that the equipment and personal-issue clothing the job required would have to be improved. Willi was particularly concerned with outfitting the men with proper clothing and boots so they would not show up in blue jeans and cowboy boots for a climbing school—or worse yet, a rescue. They also decided that the public safety function needed to be fully recognized and set about defining the objectives and organization in a "National Park Service Operational Policy Directive." This came out in 1969 and became the standard by which all parks operated. One of the key successes of the program was established early by standardizing the training, the equipment and the implementation of the program. Thus, if a warden from Yoho showed up in Waterton, he was totally in tune with the rescue gear and procedure for any scenario—be it a rescue or a training session.

The division of jurisdiction also conveniently suited both men in their preference for the type of travel and climbing they liked to do. Willi, early on, decided that the remote areas of Jasper and satellite parks were areas he liked to explore. One of his first goals was to visit every major icefield in the parks system, no matter how isolated. Peter, on the other hand, liked climbing close to home where he could hatch his ambitious ideas and stay connected to the pulse of the office.

While the bulk of the rescue work remained in the national parks, the Warden Service also liaised with other volunteer rescue groups that came into being in the early seventies. Willi and Peter were just getting started in reorganizing their joint approach to responsibilities, training and standardizations of equipment when a third mountaineering accident of significant proportion occurred—this time in the United States.

The accident, in December of 1969, occurred on Mount Cleveland, a massive 3,048-metre mountain on the border of the Waterton/Glacier International Peace Park. It involved four young climbers who were good friends at Missoula State University in Montana. They were all from divergent small towns around the state but shared a growing love of mountaineering that led them to attempt a first winter ascent on the remote north face. None of the party was old enough to have a great deal of experience, but they were fit and enthusiastic.

The weather had been unusually mild with no immediate change in the forecast in sight, so it was with light hearts that the five men hired a boat from the small town of Waterton, Alberta, now mostly shut down for the winter, and motored to the end of Waterton Lake to begin the climb. Since the boys had planned to be gone for six days, with a couple of spare days for unforeseen problems, they were not expected back until around the first

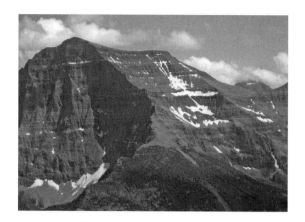

Mt. Cleveland. EDWIN KNOX COLLECTION

or second of January. Although District Ranger Robert Frauson was uneasy with their plans to climb the north face, the weather, aside from high winds, remained good. So it was not with any sense of trepidation that a brother of one of the boys decided to hire a light plane to check on the location of the four climbers. But what he found worried him. There was no trace of them except for what appeared to be their tracks leading into a fresh avalanche off the west face of the mountain. But there were a lot of goat tracks, and it was difficult to decide from the air if the tracks leading to the avalanche were human or not.

When the party had not turned up by January 2nd, the brother, now really alarmed, called Ruben Hart, Chief Park Ranger of Glacier National Park, telling him of his flight over the mountain. Hart immediately notified the Supervisory Park Ranger, who contacted the Warden Service in Waterton. Chief Park Warden Bud Armstrong set out with warden Jack Christiansen by boat for the remote U.S.-Waterton Ranger Station at the end of the lake before a message reached him, instructing him to wait for official support. What they found was not encouraging. The only signs of the missing party were some skis and snowshoes about two-and-a-half kilometres from the lakeshore and some tracks leading from the lakeshore toward the north face of the mountain.

Personnel in both parks now realized they might have a large search on their hands. And they were not wrong. The Mt. Cleveland search would be the first truly international emergency operation for the burgeoning Canadian rescue service. It would have far-reaching effects on the relationship between the two national parks. It would also be widely publicized, as the boys were well known in the climbing community, and finding them would become the concern of many well-known climbers.

Because the search was staged out of Waterton on Canadian soil, the leadership for the rescue was quickly assumed by the Warden Service, and Peter Fuhrmann was called in on the 3rd of January. Before he arrived, however, Glacier Superintendent Briggle arranged with the Montana Aeronautical Commission for another flight over the mountain using a fixed-wing aircraft. Again, there was no sign of the climbers, but the pilot reconfirmed the fresh avalanche on the west face and what appeared to be human tracks leading into it. A ground search party left early the morning of the 3rd to continue the search from the end of the lake while awaiting the arrival of Fuhrmann and the Banff wardens. They divided into two groups to scout the southwest ridge and check the tracks found by Christiansen and Armstrong. Ranger Colony, who had taken charge of immediate search organization, knew the limitations of a fixed-wing and arranged for a helicopter to be brought in. Thus began a series of less than successful efforts by the U.S. Air Force from the Malmstrom Air Force Base to deploy their Huey helicopter for rescue work.

Colony flew with the Huey on its first flight and found it unsuitable for this type of work. It had restricted vision, and communication between the pilot and observer was difficult as the dialogue had to be relayed through another crew member. In fact, several things hampered that first flight. The helicopter arrived an hour and a half late and was grounded soon after it took off when a small weather front moved in. After an

hour, the search was resumed, but the pilot was reluctant to work near the mountain with fog and flat light. Finally the Malmstrom Air Force Base ordered the helicopter to return to the Star Strip Base for the remainder of the day.

Meanwhile, Christiansen's group was having more luck. They found the climbers' main camp a half kilometre from the north face of Mt. Cleveland with the disturbing contents of climbing gear, sleeping bags and food for four meals. It was clear that the team had not been there for several days, indicating they could not travel or were not alive at all. Not far above that they found two small snow caves with tracks leading to the north col, which connected to the western portion of the north face via the northwest ridge. If anything, the puzzle deepened.

Fuhrmann decided to call in Willi Pfisterer from Jasper, who was technically responsible for all search-and-rescue efforts in Waterton Lakes National Park. Peter had come down from Banff at breakneck speed with wardens Bill Vroom and John Wackerle, hauling gear for every possible contingency: all the cable gear, rescue stretchers and avalanche equipment they could think of. Willi arrived the following day with Hans Fuhrer, Jim White and Mike Woledge. Ranger Colony, who still handled the Glacier National Park involvement, brought in a local support party and climbers from the Tetons.

Suddenly the weather turned cold, hampering boat transport over the iced-up lake. Further, the military pilot was getting more and more reluctant to be involved, finally saying he had orders restricting his landing in Canada. Perhaps it was just as well he withdrew, since the helicopter was not panning out at all. They considered using horses, but the opportunity to use snowmobiles became possible when five centimetres of new snow fell. Despite the difficulties, assignments were given out to co-ordinate a now major operation that was rapidly developing into a logistical nightmare. The weather bureau was even asked to step up their forecasts, but despite dire warnings of an impending front, the weather held till the 9th of January. After he was apprised of the situation, Pfisterer took charge of both the Canadian and United States rescue effort.

Supplies still plagued the planners, because the support groups had now gone down to the ranger station without the transportation problem being fully resolved. Despite the pressure, five search parties were formed and given their goals on the mountain. Fuhrman with Wackerle and Vroom headed to the north face to check the route; Hans Fuhrer's party went to investigate the tracks on the northwest ridge. Christiansen and Montana volunteer Pete Lev were sent to the west side of the mountain, and Doug Erskine and party established a spotting post on adjacent Goat Haunt Mountain to scan the north face with telescopes. Altogether, an impressive and comprehensive effort.

Pfisterer remained in base camp to coordinate the search and to struggle with the never-ending problem of using the military helicopter. Frauson had finally convinced the Malmstrom Air Force Base to commit a helicopter to the search, but they would not go until they were sure the weather was stable. This delayed the dispatch of the ground searchers and frustrated Willi no end. The helicopter, when it finally arrived at 11:30 a.m., was low on fuel with no service truck for refuelling. The military actually refused to allow the fuel truck to be based at Waterton townsite because it was on Canadian soil. This forced the helicopter to return to the Star Strip base to refuel, greatly reducing the search time. When the military aircraft finally did fly, they searched the Belly River, Stony Indian Pass and Waterton Trail, checking to see if the missing party had somehow got lost by taking an alternate route back. This did not pacify Pfisterer who was less than happy with the search pattern the Air Force pilot insisted on flying. The next to useless craft was finally let go when an alternate arrangement was made for a non-military machine to come from Missoula.

Despite the aggravation of the helicopter situation, the ground parties were making considerable progress. Fuhrmann all but ruled out evidence that the climbers had gone via the north face. More significant, Hans Fuhrer's party discovered tracks coming out of the northwest col and saw signs of milling around as if the boys were indecisive about where to go next. The tracks were made by only two men, who appeared to have climbed up to the col to reconnoitre a possible route up the north face. There was no sign that the party entered the west side of the mountain from this location—the tracks spotted previously from the air were found to have been made by goats.

The parties on the west side of the mountain, however, were not co-ordinated in their efforts to cover the ground. Christiansen's party was prevented from working the fresh avalanche on the west face because of the disturbing presence of Lev's group working above them on the mountain. They had found nothing so far, but were not happy about the thwarted effort to reach the slide. Lev's party moved too far toward the centre of the west side, and all efforts to turn them back failed. In the end they could not retreat before dark and spent a coolish night out on the mountain. The following day they went on to search the west face avalanche that had, up to then, been the secondary focus of the search.

By now the lake was frozen over, preventing the supply boat from reaching the ranger station at all and stalling the efforts of the Grand Tetons technical climbers who had arrived at their own expense to get on-site. On top of this, the helicopter was down again, because the pilot developed a severe head cold and could not fly. A relief pilot was sent for, but he still had to make his way from Great Falls. By this time, no one really held out any hope of finding the boys alive, and officials decided it was time to meet with the families and apprise them of the outlook. The long-predicted storm had still not arrived, but it was only a matter of time before the search would be shut down if nothing was soon found.

With this in mind, Superintendent Ross began to downsize the search.

On the 6th of January, a relief pilot arrived, and the teams began to make use of a magnetometer to find any sign of the climbers on the north avalanche. Using search dogs was discussed but then dismissed, because they would be superfluous. It is revealing that as late as 1968, the dogs were not yet appreciated for this type of work.

The mystery of the tracks up to the north col and the obvious interest the boys had shown in the north face plagued the searchers, especially when no indication of them having gone that way materialized. The chance they may have been buried by the west face avalanche was not excluded, but the tracks leading into it appeared to be made by goats. Things changed abruptly, however, when Lev's team found a pack near the toe of the west side avalanche. There was no doubt now that this is where the climbers went and all teams were committed to searching this area. The families were now certain that their sons had died, but although the teams continued to probe the west avalanche they found nothing. Finally they had to pull off the rescuers when the long-awaited front moved in depositing snow on the upper slopes, greatly increasing the avalanche hazard. They picked away at the north deposit, but finally one of the biggest searches in North America was over. Both Pfisterer and Fuhrmann knew the boys were buried in the west face avalanche deep below an icy snowpack that would entomb them for the winter. The storm hit early on the morning of the 9th and the search was stepped down permanently for the winter.

There would be a closure to the accident, but not until July of the following summer. The boys were eventually found roped together deep in the frozen avalanche debris of the west face slide. They had actually got above 2,500 metres, where the first articles were found, before the massive avalanche, probably triggered by their efforts, swept them over the broken ground. In the end, they had heeded the warning to stay away from the north face and had gone instead to the deadly, wind-loaded west face where they may have felt safer. The final Herculean efforts required to reach the boys in the frozen ice consisted of days of digging and tunnelling before the bodies could be freed and released to the families.

Though the loss was grievous to the American climbing community, the efforts made to find the missing climbers did yield some substantial gains. In the end, the search would not have saved one of them—they were long dead before anyone had any reason to look for them. However, both countries were enriched with the knowledge that they could work together on a rescue of that magnitude that had endless complications with jurisdiction and support requirements. The limitations with the helicopter were clearly illuminated and would be the principal area of improvement in the future. Ingenuity with solving problems had come to play, but more than this, personal contact had laid a foundation for future rescue efforts between the two countries.

ALTHOUGH THE WORK OF MOUNTAIN RESCUE in the parks was soon on track with the two new alpine specialists, Peter was frustrated by unnecessary deaths that occurred while transporting victims out from remote locations, or over technically difficult terrain. At the time it required many people to haul victims over cliffs, rivers, dense bush and crevassed glaciers. If the distance was too far or too rough or the weather totally unco-operative, the consequences for the injured were grim. With the enhanced interest in alpine sports, the number of people running into difficulty was rising sharply. It was with considerable interest, then, that Peter read a short article published in a German magazine—handed to him over the fence by a good friend and neighbour, Bruno Engler—about rescuers in the Alps using helicopters with a cable to reach stranded climbers. The instant Peter read the article he knew he had the answer to the rescue dilemma in the Rockies. He excitedly booked a

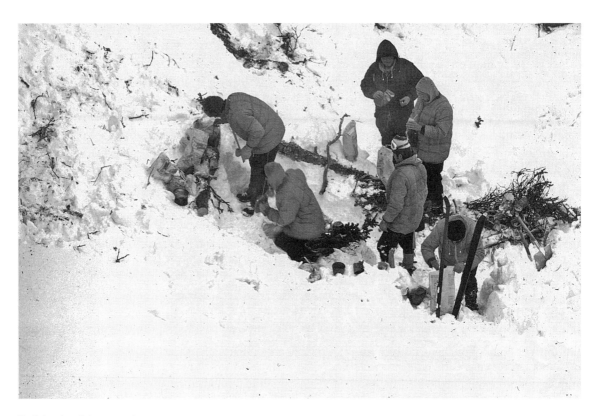

Training in winter camping. BANFF WARDEN ARCHIVES

trip to Europe to meet the man behind this new solution. Not surprisingly, the man was Ludwig Gramminger, who was already a legend in the field of mountain rescue.

It was actually Peter's holiday, and he had a good time. The two men were compatible from the start, and as Peter says: "We went to the opera, we drank beer and after that I knew what it was all about." He checked out the whole system but was concerned that their large, winch-equipped helicopters came from the air force. Their poor experience with the American air force on Mt. Cleveland with similarly large helicopters did not bode well for using a comparable system in Canada.

Another unexpected problem cropped up after an unusual accident on Yamnuska. During the early years of climbing, most climbers tied into the rope with a simple loop around the waist that provided poor support in the event of a fall.

Enterprising young sport equipment developers had since come up with a chest harness that kept the body upright when hanging by the rope. When a young climber took a leader fall on the steep Red Shirt Route of Yamnuska, he was only wearing a chest harness. Unfortunately he slipped out of the unsupported harness and fell to his death.

When Peter returned home saying that the wardens should fly under a helicopter from a long knotted rope sitting in a harness, the idea was not well received. He convinced them that the harness supplied by Gramminger was foolproof and perfectly safe to fly in, but it turned out he was wrong about that.

Before Peter could convince wardens to fly under helicopters, he first had to find a helicopter and a person willing to fly live cargo. Luckily, he found the perfect pilot close to home. Jim Davies, whose father was a park warden, was a

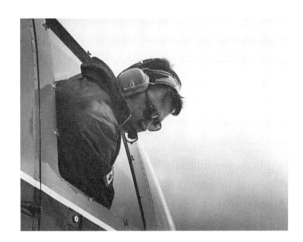

Jim Davies. JIM DAVIES COLLECTION

local resident of Banff, where he had grown up. His father eventually went into the construction business where Jim became acquainted with all sorts of equipment that led to a lifelong fascination with machinery. Jim felt this familiarity aided him in flying helicopters: "I was brought up on machinery: cats, trucks, tractors, everything ... so getting into helicopters was kind of a natural thing. It was just another piece of machinery."

Jim was also keen on the visual arts and enrolled in Fine Arts in SAIT in Calgary. But because he was always drawn to machinery, particularly aircraft, he started frequenting the Calgary airport. He was soon taking flying lessons, and he got his pilot's licence in 1959. This led to early exposure to helicopters, and he began flying them for Spartan Air Services. He flew in the Arctic, through the northern states and Newfoundland, and finally in New Zealand, where he really learned the scope of the versatile machine. The work of slinging culled deer from mountainsides was dangerous, but it taught him a lot about mountain flying. But, more important, he learned about vertical referencing, needed for long-line slinging. This was the key to his success as a rescue pilot.

In 1965, after flying with Hans Gmoser on a ski adventure in northern B.C., he became involved with Hans's fledgling Canadian Mountain Holidays enterprise in the Bugaboos. Once again he was flying exclusively in a mountain setting where he accumulated hours of experience with the tricky terrain and mountain weather patterns. So it was not strictly by chance that Peter asked Jim if he would be willing to come to Banff and fly men on a sling rope to small mountain ledges to pick up injured climbers.

Though Jim initially did not think it was feasible to fly wardens under the helicopter, he eventually became a master at it. But to truly understand the work, Jim accompanied Peter and Willi to Europe the following year to see the system firsthand. He also wanted to talk to the pilots to learn from their individual experiences. They concluded early that using a military helicopter was not feasible in the parks, where the small budget for fewer rescues was not sufficient to bring in the larger machines. In addition, the large machines were not appropriate for that type of work as the longer blades did not permit working close to steep mountainsides. They decided instead to adapt the small Bell helicopter Jim flew at the time to a fixed rope sling system.

The first big problem was how to attach a rope to the helicopter so it would not throw the pilot off once in the air. A swinging object attached to the skids was not the best solution, so Jim simply passed the rope through the belly of the aircraft. One thing that was not acceptable was attaching the rope to the cargo hook. It was too easy to hit the eject button and release the load, which in this case would be the rescuer and victim. Eventually they solved the problem by attaching two permanent hooks to the bottom of the helicopter. The hooks in turn attached to the rope with heavy-duty screw-gated carabiners. Peter devised the rescue line out of two strands of climbing rope knotted at four-foot intervals to keep it together in the air.

Finally on a windless day at the Banff airfield Peter explained the system to a crew of sceptical wardens. Peter recalls: "I said to Jim 'Look, why don't I sit in this marvellous seat and hook on with the knotted rope as per diagram—and you take off ten feet and put me back down.' And that's the first lift off we had." From there, it was magic. Jim flew the alternately terrified, thrilled or just plain excited wardens through space like Superman high above the tiny valley below. But soon Jim realized that if he had to fly the unweighted sling rope without a person on the end, it might fly up into the rotors. Jay Morton recalls that "Someone made a phone call to the garage and immediately somebody came roaring out with some bolts and plates from a guard rail, and they screwed them onto the end of the rope." He still has a picture of himself flying over the Banff traffic circle with "these goddamned guard rail weights hanging above my head."

Though it worked, the logistics of getting it accepted by both park administration and the Government of Canada proved daunting. The Ministry of Transport (MOT—later the Department of Transport), which controlled flight regulations in Canada, were a conservative lot, not given to strange new inventions that might jeopardize safety. Though slinging objects under helicopters was not new, flying human cargo on a nonreleasable attachment was. But first it had to be accepted by Parks Canada.

It did not help when Jim flew Jay Morton down the main street of Banff past the superintendent's office. As they flew by Jay waved happily at his boss, who was at that moment discussing why the airport should be shut down.

Superintendent Steve Kun was confidently explaining that the wardens would deal with any law enforcement problems that cropped up when one observant administrator replied, "and there goes one of them now!" Kun spun around in time to see a smiling Jay zoom by the window and disappear into the sunny skies. The next day Peter was called in to account for this unexplained phenomenon and to face some serious questions about the unborn program.

Steve Kun was not opposed to the idea of rescuing people by helicopter with this unorthodox method, but he needed much more documentation before presenting the program to the federal government. It was a Catch-22 situation where authorization could not be given till the system was proven, and that could not happen without authorization to use it. Fortunately, Peter was a bold man and willing to take risks for something he believed in. The axiom "forgiveness is easier to get than permission" was never truer than in this circumstance, and Peter did not pass up the chance to prove why this new approach to rescue was so important.

Peter went ahead with his training sessions and took the system to Jasper for Willi to introduce it to the wardens there. Peter recalls: "I drove to Jasper, and we had a very successful session up there. Quite a number of wardens flew under the machine with this system and things went very, very well." They had managed to commandeer a pilot who had long-line experience and was not afraid to sling the men around. The only thing that bothered both Peter and Willi was not having permission from MOT to fly with the unauthorized hookup.

On the return trip to Jasper, Peter got his first opportunity to prove the validity of the heli-sling rescue method. He overheard broken messages on the radio of a rescue problem involving a group of young people at Pinto Lake. One of them had apparently slipped on a steep ice slope near the top of the pass and had fallen about 150 metres into a narrow gulley. The young man was quite badly injured and failing by the time the rescue operation was underway. By the time the Warden Service was alerted, both the RCMP and the Alberta Forest Rangers were involved. Because the wardens had the greater experience in this arena, warden Jack Woledge found himself in charge.

Jay Morton remembers the rescue clearly: "We got called in so we're there, and it was going to be a horrendous operation. We had the Alberta Forest Service helicopter … and he started flying guys into really thick timber … with chainsaws to cut a landing pad so they could get this guy out.

Along comes Peter Fuhrmann on his way back from Jasper, and he had just been demonstrating the technique to the Jasper wardens. He comes up and asks 'What's going on?' so we told him."

The rescue went as Jay said, but not so simplistically. The pilot was young and capable and had already flown a number of rescuers to the top of the pass with the rescue mine basket when Peter arrived. The crew was working as rapidly as possible to build a rescue platform at the base of the gully to effect an evacuation by helicopter.

Woledge was more than relieved to see Peter with a better solution, as it was becoming apparent that they were quickly running out of time if they wished to save the boy's life. He was very hypothermic and beginning to pass in and out of consciousness. Peter immediately consulted with the pilot saying: "Have you ever done anything like this?" He replied "No," he'd never even heard of it. Peter quickly drew a diagram in the sand illustrating the principle and laid out the equipment. The pilot peered at the sketch, then with a quixotic look at Peter, said: "Well, sure. Why don't we try this?" Peter attached the long line and instructed the pilot to fly him around in the air a few times for practice before undertaking the far more difficult approach to the gully. The main problem facing the rescuers was how much the machine could lift at the higher elevation, with the downdraft in the gully. The early helicopters were notoriously underpowered, and were not able to sling more than a few hundred pounds. Despite reservations, Peter had the man convinced it was worth a try, and on the third flight they headed for the rescue site. On the way, Peter devised a plan.

The only communication between Peter and the pilot was through a large cumbersome lunch box radio he supported in his lap. He yelled: "I think the way to do this is to fly in nose first, as close as you can get to the site. You will probably have a downdraft, so hold the nose in and I'll unhook and you can get rid of me. Then go out and wait and see what happens." When Peter reached the boy he was unconscious, so he wasted no time attaching the rescue ropes to the mine basket they had him loaded in. He called the pilot back, directing him to point the nose downhill. They had hauled the stretcher out to the middle of the slope for greater tree clearance, which allowed the helicopter to fly straight down once he had the load, gaining much-needed air speed for lift. Even with this manoeuvre, the rescuers had to bodily lift the basket into the air and run with it to get it off the ground. The risks were enormous, as neither man was sure if the machine could lift both the victim and Peter. Suddenly, the unit was clear of the trees rushing dizzily downward toward Pinto Lake, from where they began a long arduous spiral flight back over the pass to the highway.

If Peter was relieved to not have crashed on takeoff, it was short-lived because the next message he got from the pilot was unnerving: "You know everything is going fine, but I don't think I can land you. I haven't enough power to come down and flare out without hitting the ground." The butterflies left Peter's stomach for his head as he rapidly absorbed this new information. In desperation, Peter got Woledge on the radio and instructed him to line up all the help he could find and face into the wind. He told the pilot to slow as much as possible when he reached the crowd. The ground crew could then catch the stretcher and run with it long enough to get the weight off the long line and detach the basket from the rescue carabiner. To great relief, they landed perfectly with only a few missed heartbeats. The victim was rushed to Peter's station wagon where he entered into the last and most perilous stage of his rescue: a drive at breakneck speed down the highway with Peter to the Mineral Springs Hospital in Banff.

The young man survived, and Peter now had the irrefutable evidence of a successful rescue to back him up. But before Peter took on obtaining the official stamp of approval from the Ministry of Transport or Parks to operate in the open, he was given another opportunity to save a life. Shortly after Peter returned from Jasper, a young corporal in the Canadian Army was hit on the head by rock fall while participating in a training climb on the east face of Mt. Edith just north of Banff townsite. The flimsy helmet the man wore was insufficient to prevent a massive brain haemorrhage, leaving him unconscious but alive. The leader quickly retreated, alerting the RCMP of the accident in remarkably good time. When Peter was given the details, he realized he must act fast, because head injuries require immediate attention. A ground team was out of the question if he were to save the man's life, so with little hesitation he called on Jim Davies to sling him in to the site.

Fortunately the winds were favourable, which helped Jim when he realized he would have to do some fancy flying to get Peter on-site. The steepness of the ground did not allow Jim to get close to the rock for fear of hitting the rotor blades. To get Peter to the stranded party, Jim was forced to rock the machine, setting up a pendulum motion on the long line that enabled him to swing Peter close to the face. After a couple of tries, Peter was able to pull himself in. It may have been at this moment that Jim became aware of the implicit trust he would have to have in the men he would work with. For at this moment Peter was briefly tied to the mountain and simultaneously clipped to the helicopter. Contrary to slinging an inert load that could be released, Jim had absolutely no control over this phase of the rescue. The machine was tethered to the rescuer until he unhooked. At that moment, a long thin line of trust quivered in the air establishing a silent dialogue between rescuer and pilot.

The unconscious man had been given little first aid and had only a triangular bandage around a big hole in the neck. The next difficulty was to sling in the large cumbersome mine basket to load the patient. It was a small exposed place to work in, but finally the young man was manoeuvred into the stretcher with Peter in place as attendant. Again, the same problem arose of dealing with an underpowered machine. Jim was not able to lift them vertically from the cliff. The solution was to have the men on the cliff face lift the stretcher skyward before attaching it to the rescue carabiner so that there was no weight on the machine. Then, while Jim hovered precariously close to the rock wall, they would push the stretcher into space followed by Peter who would jump with it. By leaping off the cliff, the weight would not come on the long line until they were in a steep dive toward the valley, allowing the machine to pick up sufficient forward speed necessary for rotor lift. At the count of three Peter and the oblivious victim hurtled off the edge into the exhilarating dive that levelled out once forward speed was achieved.

With more power on descending, Jim had the luxury of asking Peter where he would like to take the patient. Peter, who knew that immediate medical attention was required said: "Well let's land right in front of the hospital … radio ahead to tell them to have a stretcher ready on the front lawn." Jim contacted the authorities and within minutes the mine basket was lowered, with Peter attending, onto the waiting gurney parked at the front doors of the Banff Mineral Springs Hospital. From there the young corporal was quickly transported by ambulance to Calgary and the waiting neurosurgeon who was able to save his life. According to Peter, the sceptical superintendent, Steve Kun, saw the whole performance. For a moment Peter thought his whole career was over, but Kun was not blind to the potential of the helicopter in this service. All he wanted was to go through the right channels and get out of the "forgiveness" versus "permission" routine that was becoming all too common. An effusive letter from the attending doctors stating that the man would have died had he not received immediate medical attention, prepared the way for the permission Peter needed to use the helicopter sling for rescues.

The doors were open for Peter as far as the park was concerned, but this was just the beginning. Peter was well aware that he had been lucky on both rescues in having reasonable conditions to allow the helicopter to operate. But such operations were still dangerous with the limitations imposed by underpowered machines and clumsy radio communication. They needed better rescue equipment, trained pilots and effective liaisons with the ambulance service. They needed a whole lot of things, and trained rescuers were a big part of the program.

Fortunately for both Peter and Willi, they had a strong ally in the Regional Office. Every park function had a representative in this office, and at this time the ubiquitous Jim Sime had that role for the Warden Service. The Warden Service never had a better friend with more personal interest in the well-being of the service than Jim. Peter and Willi both worked directly for him, which suited them very well. Jim also controlled the purse strings for the newly developing function and was generous when expenditures were justified. And with the emphasis on helicopter rescue, expenses were necessary.

Although Peter now had the support of both Steve Kun and Jim Sime, they still needed to gain official approval at the federal level of the Canadian Parks Service in Ottawa. Peter was somewhat shocked at the degree of argument required to convince the upper powers that this was a life-saving tool that should not be ignored. Here he encountered the entrenched idea that people undertaking dangerous sports should be left to save themselves. The administration in Ottawa saw no reason to risk employees' lives (or money) to rescue these people. Peter quickly pointed out that leaving cadavers hanging around popular climbing routes or dangling above well-used hiking trails might not be the best image for Parks Canada. He also pointed out that without a second thought Ottawa was willing to spend millions of dollars to save pilots irresponsible enough to fly single-engine planes without filing a flight plan. All Peter wanted was a few thousand dollars to save accident victims, and he was able to argue that using the helicopter saved money. Slinging men into a rescue scene was very cost effective when compared to the expense of sending in a large ground party over several days to do the same job. And since the learned men in Ottawa were concerned with risking peoples lives to save climbers, Peter was quick to point out that the helicopter substantially reduced that risk by not exposing large numbers of rescuers to the hazards of the rescue. He was very aware of how much safer the rescue on Mt. Edith turned out to be when he considered the hazard the men would have been exposed to if they had had to climb to the victim. He then went on to a more "bucket of blood" approach, saying that the climbing era had arrived in the Canadian Rockies and that ground teams simply could not save lives like the helicopter could. Time alone prevented that. By eliminating the use of the helicopter, people would die needlessly, and it would lie at their door if that were to happen. The arguments were compelling and Peter soon had Ottawa's support.

It was probably just as well that Peter had to go to the lengths he did to convince Ottawa that helicopter sling rescue was necessary to bring Canada into the modern age of alpine rescue, because he had a much tougher sell with the Ministry of Transport. It certainly forced him to have the argument well thought out and practised before tackling this formidable arm of the government. Jim Sime was actually the principal negotiator with both with Ottawa and the Ministry of Transport, and he recalls that it took several months of delicate letter campaigning to elicit a positive response from this department.

The stumbling block was the attachment of the sling to the aircraft using a two-point contact flange on the bottom of the craft. Nothing like this had ever been approved by Ministry of Transport, mainly because of the danger to the helicopter and pilot. If the line could not be released, any entanglement with earthbound objects (such as trees or wires) jeopardized the survival of both machine and pilot. Wardens who later worked with this department point out that at the time helicopter regulations were relatively new in Canada and were adapted from

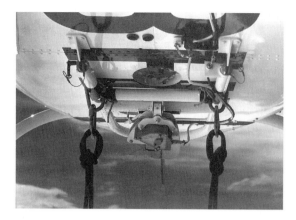

Original helicopter sling rope attachment. MARK
LEDWIDGE COLLECTION

the Federal Aviation Administration in the United States. These regulations stated that any load that extended below the side of the aircraft had to be jettisonable by the pilot. The regulations also prohibited suspending personnel outside the machine. The problem was that the record for accidents using the releasable load hook was unacceptable. The rescuers, on the other hand, felt much safer knowing they could not be jettisoned either by accident or by design. Both Jim and the men he would work with felt it was necessary to work as a team, with absolute commitment to each other, and to accept the joint risk.

After much negotiation, both departments finally settled on issuing a waiver for the new rescue technique that mollified but did not eradicate the unease the Ministry of Transport. The first stipulation was eminently suitable to Parks, as Ministry of Transport stated that because of the life-saving scope of the sling rescue, Parks could continue to use it, but it would be restricted to their use alone. No other agency or private company would be given permission to sling human cargo in such a manner. The second stipulation limited the rescue operation to areas not contaminated by overhead wires or other obstructions that could tangle the sling line. Since most rescues occur in open spaces, this was

doable, but the staging area had to be carefully regulated. In the end, permission to go ahead was granted, giving Peter and Willi the chance to bolster their success stories in case MOT reneged on helicopter rescue in the future.

BY 1972, WITH JIM PROVIDING the flying expertise, Peter and Willi had the public safety program in the starting gate. One of their first goals was to improve the equipment connected with the helicopter rescue system. Jim Davies had been working for Bow Helicopters up until that time but the potential rescue work gave him an opportunity to strike out on his own. Bow Helicopters was not interested in basing a machine in Banff, as they did not feel there would be enough hours to justify this commitment. Jim felt otherwise and approached Peter about taking on the contract himself. Peter, of course, was happy with the idea, so Jim arranged financing for the more suitable Jet Ranger. One of the things he required was a plastic bubble on the pilot's side so he could look down at the man on the end of the line. Prior to this, Jim had been removing the window to look down, which proved far too windy. Though there was static line slinging done in Europe, many of the pilots there had the luxury of having a winch system which lowered the rescuer to the accident site and did not require the pilot to look down to bring the person in. Because the line on the Banff helicopter was fixed, it was up to the pilot to spot the rescuer directly on-site, which meant looking down. This was a much more difficult manoeuvre for pilots and required several hours of training.

Very few of the wardens, who were at the pointy end of the line, questioned the ability of Jim to do his job. They had implicit faith that the pilot knew what he was doing, and if he could not go where he was asked, he would say so. The rescuer's job at the end of the rope was what the wardens concentrated on and became skilful at through rescues and training exercises. But initially, there was a lot to learn. What neither Peter nor Willi needed was a serious accident at this point. But despite taking care with the new system, incidents did occur. A lot of this had to do with refining the gear and its use.

Jay Morton recalls the day his "life flashed before [his] eyes" in understandable detail. "We assembled at the bottom of Mt. Rundle in the Spray Valley for a staging area, and we were going to have this exercise where we flew everybody up to the top of Rundle. We didn't have anything really finalized in those days. Like they didn't have the rope standardized, or packaged well, and we didn't have any helmets. Pretty basic. The last time I had done it, you just walked up and hooked your carabiner into the two strands of the rope." Peter also wanted to show the wardens how accurate Jim was in bringing the rope to the rescuer so he had Jay stand on top of a sign post. From this precarious position Jay tried to hook directly onto the looped rope at the end of the line while fighting the downdraft—ignoring the carabiner left in place. The sharp end of the open gate lodged onto the rope not allowing the carabiner to close. Before he knew it, Jay was in the air, eyes clamped to the open carabiner watching in horror as he flew to the top of Mt. Rundle. He had no radio and could not tell anyone of the problem. "I pretty well sat there and watched my life flash before me. It was a pretty horrible feeling … just as I took the strain off when my feet hit the ground, it clicked in."

The critique that day left a grim-faced Peter resolved to attach a solid steel ring to the loop at the end of the rope that could not come off the individual strands. It is now a permanent fixture of all rescue sling ropes. He also vowed to solve the problem of radio communication. Rapid advances in radio technology soon solved that problem with the advent of a small, harness-supported portable radio with detachable microphone. From then on, no one slung without a radio.

Because Sime had a substantial budget, Peter was able to bring over the latest stretcher innovation from Europe. It was a small lightweight cloth bag—called the Jenny Bag—that could be rolled up into a tight duffel for flight or backpacking. When spread out on the ground, it opened up to receive the victim who was then laced in place with a series of ropes and hooks. Once the victim was bound in place, the appearance was somewhat similar to a mummy. The trick, as it turned out, was to make sure the victim was properly secured.

Peter was called to a rescue for a young man passed out on the slopes of Mt. Rundle. Some hikers had spotted the comatose man near a small tarn well up on the mountain, but did not know it was the result of a drug overdose. They hurried down to the warden office to report the incident, conveying a sense of urgency. To save time, Jim slung Peter directly into the site, which was only a four-minute flight away, where Peter quickly popped the fellow into the Jenny Bag. Peter had enough first aid to know that vomiting is not uncommon if a person regains consciousness, and he left the man's head and torso accessible for immediate resuscitation. Halfway to the hospital, the victim suddenly woke up, but his drug-saturated, confused brain only registered a heavily bearded man looming over him, a sensation of rushing wind and above that, the ominous lettering "HEL." The bottom of the helicopter had large red lettering spelling out SHEL, but he only saw the last three letters. When he shrieked: "Who are you!" Peter answered as calmly as he could: "My name is Peter." This was too much. The man's wildest fears were confirmed, and in desperation he tried to escape—and almost succeeded with both hands free and with the energy of the demonically possessed. Jim glanced down to see Peter flailing away with both fists in an effort to subdue the madman before he leapt from the decreasing confines of the Jenny Bag. The waiting hospital staff watched in horror as they saw the helicopter approach with the struggling men, wondering what Peter was bringing to them this time.

The incident prompted a stern review of how to package unconscious people in the restricted bag, knowing that whatever the cost, they must be firmly laced up. Now victims are closely monitored so that they can be turned to a semi-prone position if vomiting begins.

Other problems continued to crop up with the sling harnesses. A near tragicomic incident took place near Elk Lake that resulted to another change in procedure. Again the lack of communication was a contributing problem. Joe Halstenson was the rescue warden in this case. It was a routine call requiring only one rescue person to pick up a man with an injured leg—or so it seemed. Joe attached the sling rope to the belly of the helicopter then stepped into the harness. He had a radio but did not set up a radio check before lifting off. The instant he was airborne, he flipped over backwards, and to his astonishment, found himself flying upside down. He had missed attaching the crotch strap that allows the person to sit vertically in the harness, and all he could do was hang on as best he could. The radio sputtered uselessly making it impossible to tell Jim to put him down before he fell out of the harness. He struggled like a worm on a hook hoping he did not have to fly too far in this dangerous position. Joe was somewhat disappointed, but not surprised at the reaction of his would-be victim. He spotted the two hikers on the trail from his skewed point of view, looking aghast at his approach. Upon finally landing in a virtual handstand, he unhooked with some effort, stood up and said congenially: "Hi!" They immediately replied: "What are you doing?" Joe said, "Well we got a report that one of you has a bad knee, so I've come to take you out." Joe recalls the man looked at him in astonishment and said: "There's no god-damned way I'm going out with you!" He tried to explain as they hobbled down the trail that he had had a little trouble hooking up but … From then on it was considered essential to send two people out at all times so that one man could check the harness, hookup and radio communication before anyone flew off to a rescue.

One of the main problems was the rate at which the rescues were escalating in relation

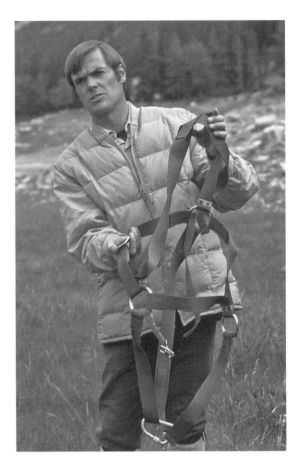

Bruce McKinnon demonstrating helicopter sling harness. JASPER WARDEN ARCHIVES

to the training the wardens were receiving. Everything was new and developing at a rapid rate. Novel equipment was being introduced at most regional schools as soon as Willi and Peter could buy it. With Sime's generous budget and Parks support for the public safety function, they were able to purchase many important pieces of equipment. One of the updated items was a sling harness just brought over from the Bavarian Red Cross. This confounded Hans Fuhrer and his partner Abe Loewen on a rescue they were called to on a sub peak near Mt. Edith Cavell in Jasper National Park.

A novice climber had fallen on a rather steep cliff and broken his leg, but the call didn't come in until late in the day. Nevertheless, Hans and Abe got there early enough to climb in to the site before the helicopter arrived from Valemount. Willi was at the base when the two men reached the victim and was able to sling in the stretcher. Once the man was out, Willi attached the new harnesses and slung them up to the waiting rescuers. Hans recalls the situation with some frustration: "It was starting to get dark when Willi said, 'Hans I'm going to fly in those two harnesses you're going to sling out with.' And I said 'What harnesses?' And he said 'Your harnesses. They are from the Bavarian Red Cross.'" Hans, however had never heard of them and was adamant he had never seen them on any training exercise. When they got them, neither man could make head nor tail out of the design and could not fathom how to put them on. The stress of the coming night and Willi's broken explanations over the radio did nothing to alleviate the frustration of deciphering the complicated webbing and carabiners. After many combinations were tried out unsatisfactorily, Hans decided to abandon the whole idea of slinging out and spend the night on the mountain. It would be no problem to down-climb the route the following morning in comparative safety. This did not sit well with Willi, who could not understand what the problem was, saying the harnesses were no different from the ones they had used before. Thereafter, all subsequent harnesses were manufactured with colour coding to distinguish the upper chest portion from the lower seat harness. Hans adds: "After that we had some serious training with those harnesses."

Concerns continued to crop up during training. At one point, the wardens realized that the rope strands had to be taped together, when one trainee's head got caught between the individual lines which spread apart when the rope became slack between the harness and the lead weight. The mistake was caught before the helicopter lifted the person up, but it was unnerving how close they came to a serious accident. Landings on steep slopes, delicate cliff faces or challenging snow and ice slopes had to be practised as well. Rescuers never knew exactly what the snow conditions might be like until they landed and got their footing. Winds also made for tricky landing. If it was really gusty, it could be difficult to detach in a safe manner and not be blown off the stance. The pilot had to hover above while the rescuer established a secure stance on the mountain. The time for this operation had to be kept to a minimum as this manoeuvre was very stressful on the engine in the early helicopters, and they quickly overheated. The teamwork between pilot and rescuer was critical at these times and good communication was essential.

There is no doubt that the helicopter was god's gift to mountain rescue, but it was not foolproof. During the late sixties and seventies in particular, the helicopter was "very unforgiving" and use was limited by weather and elevation. Not even the most brilliant pilot could fly during heavy storms, violent winds or poor visibility. Therefore, improvised rescue and cable training were never dropped from the syllabus of either regional or local climbing schools. Walter Perren had explored and refined most of the possibilities of improvised rescue but had only begun working with cable, and much was left to be developed in this field when Willi and Peter took over in 1968.

From the time the two men assumed the role of alpine specialists, they established concrete ties with the European rescue community and continued to be updated with advances made in the testing grounds of the Alps. All recent developments in cable-rescue equipment and technique were imported along with the latest climbing and survival gear. One of the biggest advances in cable rescue was the development of the winch. When Walter had had Bill Vroom go down to get the stranded men on Mt. Babel, all they could do was bring them up with a pulley system. It worked in that situation because there was plenty of room to work. The winch, however, was a small mechanical device which could be used in confined quarters, allowing greater control over the descent or ascent of the rescue team.

One of the first things that both men realized when they went to the international rescue conferences was that each country seemed to be trying to outdo the other in developing the latest gadget. As a result several different models of various equipment were on the market. But Canadians did not need to be restricted to one particular model because of affiliation to a particular country. As Willi said "We had no such scruples. We took whatever was best." And they certainly had choices. There was the German winch, the Swiss winch and the Austrian winch, all of which did the same job but operated slightly differently with different advantages. Peter observed that the one thing that was important, however, was to maintain uniformity so that the wardens could use them interchangeably among parks. Along with the winch came the cables, the cable connectors, the brake block, frogs and swivels. Eventually

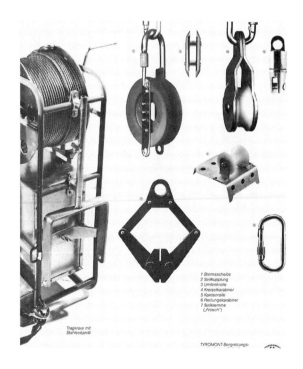

Original cable equipment. JASPER WARDEN ARCHIVES

plastic plates were added to the collection to keep the cable and connectors from digging into the rock or getting hung up on obstructions. There was also the spool that wound up the excess cable or let it out depending on the operation. All of this was becoming quite complicated, and it was apparent that a great deal of training was required to render the system usable in an efficient and safe manner. This soon became a principal focus of many of the rescue schools until Peter was able to say: "Many, many rescue and training sessions were done with the winch system, and we became quite fluent with it."

If Peter seemed like a kid in a toy store accumulating gadgets, Willi was equally passionate about seeing the wardens properly outfitted with suitable protective clothing and functional gear. He wanted the men to have skis that turned, boots that fit and bindings that did not break. They needed waterproof anoraks and pants, wool socks (grey not red), warm jackets and good tents and bags to sleep in. Although Sime had a sizable budget, it did have limits, and it was not possible to outfit every warden to the full extent. Willi did not have personal control over this either, as it was up to each individual park to provide adequate clothing and gear for the wardens they employed. It was particularly difficult to equip indeterminate seasonal staff who had to become quite clever in obtaining the coveted goods. Willi's best solution was to keep regional stores well stocked to supply the missing items.

Each park was also responsible for maintaining and equipping their own rescue room—which was usually quite a challenge for smaller parks with limited budgets. Both the chief park warden and the superintendent had other functions they had to provide money and equipment for, making acquisition of supplies a game of "scrounge" for the poor warden assigned to public safety. If either Peter or Willi descended on their assigned park and found gear in poor shape or missing, the warden in charge was immediately informed. If he was dealing with a particularly unsupportive CPW or Superintendent, the alpine specialist would likely go to bat for him. Because of the increasingly high profile of mountain rescue, however, it was not long before things began to shape up to the satisfaction of both alpine specialists.

In terms of training, neither Willi nor Peter were reticent in voicing their requirements. When they first took over, all the wardens were expected to participate in a rescue in some capacity. Most of the rescues still required substantial personnel and everyone was slotted into a training school at some point in their career. Willi recalls: "Once a year we had a big school for two weeks where wardens came from all over the place." But he soon realized that this was not enough. He explained: "We also needed the local knowledge, so we don't climb the same mountain in the same place every school. So we agreed we had to run local schools." Peter and Willi soon divided up the work to suit their natural talents. Willi remembers: "I was always the guy that did the field work and Fuhrmann did the paperwork and the selling. We really sort of complemented each other, because you have to sell your product to the guys above, you know."

Despite the politics and paperwork, Peter also ran his share of field schools and gradually the training programs took on the personalities of the two divergent men. The training schools were still divided up into novice, intermediate and advanced, but the scope of the training varied with the interests of the two men. Peter points out: "There were two different sorts of philosophies. Willi was always the one who wanted to go and explore new areas, whether on a novice, intermediate or advanced school. He wanted to go where nobody else had been. I stayed mainly in this area and concentrated more on the technical aspect, you know. I took them to Yamnuska and on a lot of rock climbs. But ice climbing became the fad, so I went up the Jasper highway and did all kinds of ice climbs in high visitor use areas."

Willi's main goal on his trips was to familiarize the wardens with the country and to instill the

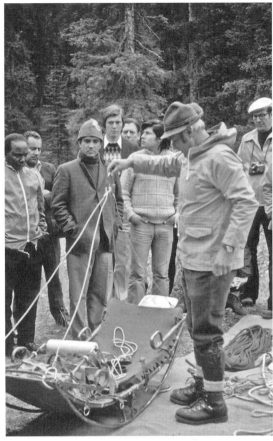

Willi Pfisterer demonstrating helicopter attachment system for slinging. JASPER WARDEN ARCHIVES

camaraderie of teamwork. Willi particularly liked getting "the attention of those guys for 24 hours." He could not go far enough to emphasize the fact that they were committed to each other for their very lives, and that the act of putting a rope on was part of that commitment.

One story he recalls had a humorous downside to it, but over the years it has become a fond memory for those involved, and it did get the point of commitment across. Willi very rarely finished a trip without throwing in a crevasse rescue practice to remind wardens about what they were ultimately training for. Toward the end of one particularly long trip on the icefields, Willi finally found the large crevasse that suited

103

his needs. But now he needed a victim, so Willi told the first man on the rope to jump in. The warden in the lead looked around in surprise and refused. Willi was incensed. He replied: "You mean you have been travelling on the rope with this guy for over a week, trusting him with your life, and now you don't think he's going to hold you?" Sheepishly, the young man looked back at his partner and understood the implication of his refusal to jump. He immediately threw himself into the crevasse. Willi laughs: "And he jumped but Johnnie didn't hold him! Johnnie almost went into the crevasse, too, but everybody else jumped on the rope to hold him." In the end they had a successful rescue practice, but one that clearly brought home the reliance they had to place in each other.

Peter and Willi set up rescue scenarios that mirrored actual situations they might be called upon to deal with. This meant training at night, starting late or going out under adverse weather conditions. Peter was particularly prone to start late, and his schools soon became nicknamed "Fuhrmann sanctions" after the harrowing movie *The Eiger Sanction* starring Clint Eastwood. The buzz around the office before one of these looming adventures took place was, "You going on the Fuhrmann Sanction?" Although some wardens objected to the onerous conditions they were required to survive, many felt they had achieved their objective and learned from the experience.

As WILLI AND PETER struggled to keep abreast of the climbing scene, other challenges were looming. Canoeing and kayaking rapidly became popular in the seventies, and the number of water rescues the wardens were being called to began to escalate. Tourists got into trouble everywhere: on trails, canyons, waterfalls, rivers and lakes. When accidents began to pile up, Peter realized that water rescue must become part of their repertoire. He remembers one incident at the end of a long demanding day after they had dealt with four mountain rescues. "It was a father and son caught on a log jam in the middle of the Bow River, and we didn't have a clue. We didn't know what to do." They managed to get a boat next to the log jam and bring the pair to shore, but it was a frightening experience. Peter knew there would be more to come and that some solution had to be found.

He tested their expertise with Jack Woledge, Bill Vroom and Joe Halstenson by experimenting with the only boat they had used for the log jam rescue. Peter recalls the boat "leaked like a sieve! We somehow stopped the leakage and got into the river with this thing, but it was a horror show. Unbelievable! I think we sank three times, then hit a log jam and nearly lost the boat."

Peter was pretty high on using the helicopter and turned his mind to adapting it to water rescue. Nothing on the market met the concept he had conjured up. He envisioned using some sort of metal cage that could be used to scoop people up and engaged the help of the mechanics at the Parks garage. He had a metal frame built with ropes for attachment to the helicopter, and was soon flying around in the thing, throwing inner tubes into the river to retrieve. The inner tubes were intended for the river victims, to keep them afloat until they could be dragged into the contraption. Jim soon found he had to fly downstream to keep track of the inner tubes. The opportunity to pick the tube up while flying against the current was too brief to be effective. The only concern Jim had was avoiding sweepers and low hanging branches that would entangle the contraption and put a quick end to that line of rescue work. Peter later found what he was looking for in a search and rescue magazine. It was called the Billy Pugh net and was quite similar to what he had dreamed up.

Jasper had more water-related accidents than Banff, because both the Athabasca and Sunwapta rivers are very attractive to boaters. Both rivers also have spectacular waterfalls that have been a death trap for the incautious, and despite protective railing, still account for a yearly loss of life.

Finding river victims was never easy, but on one occasion, the wardens came up with a different solution to locating the body of a dentist who had slipped over Athabasca Falls. They had searched for a week when Max Winkler came up with the idea of throwing a dead black bear into the river where the man went in, thinking it might wash up. They decorated the bear with colourful streamers of seismic tape for easy location as it floated along. It surfaced a few weeks later on a sand bar close to a tourist resort, where it attracted the attention of a rather large crowd. To their embarrassment, the wardens were at a loss to explain why the dead animal was all decked out in ribbons. Neither did it shed any light on the location of the missing body. The dentist continued to haunt the park for some time afterwards. It was not until two years later that the missing man finally gave up his bones, literally, in a backwash well below the Jasper townsite and miles from the falls where the accident occurred.

Although Peter and Willi incorporated water rescue into their scope of responsibility, it would be a while before jet boats and scuba diving became incorporated in the training. The technology had not advanced to that level in the early seventies, and Peter's innovations helped to span the interim.

ANOTHER RESPONSIBILITY that Peter and Willi inherited was avalanche control throughout the parks they were responsible for. Walter Perren had begun work in this area but had done little on any major road systems bisecting the parks. Both the Banff/Jasper Highway and the ski hills were seeing increased use but most control work consisted of closing the areas during periods of high hazard. As Willi often joked, the hazard sign at Marmot read: "High Avalanche Hazard: Closed Till Spring." Although this was an exaggeration, there was a serious element of truth in this early approach which was totally insufficient for the user public in the early seventies. When Willi moved to Jasper, warden Tony Klettl was in charge of avalanche control at the ski hill and headed the newly evolving public safety function.

Tony, like Willi, was from Austria, where he had a skiing background and had trained in mountaineering with the Austrian Army. He also volunteered with the Austrian Bergwacht (mountain watch) and was exposed to some rescue work both in the summer and winter. He came to Canada in 1952 and spent a year up north working on a new pipeline. He moved south looking for work in a more traditional environment and found Jasper more to his liking. He became established there and never left until he retired from Parks Canada and moved to Valemount, B.C. with his wife Shirley. During the mid-fifties his mountaineering and skiing background led him to join the ski patrol at the Jasper Ski Hill. This opened the door with the Warden Service and he never looked back. He ran the avalanche control and public safety function in Jasper for two decades while raising four children at the Cavell Warden Station near Jasper.

He started working at Marmot Basin when it opened in 1964. At that time the avalanche control work was limited to blasting cornices and ski cutting steeper slopes after a heavy snowfall. But as Tony recalls, it was "by guess and by golly" kind of work with no control of avalanche slopes. There was virtually no avalanche control along the Banff/Jasper Highway (now called the Icefield Parkway), which was closed during the winter. Much of this changed when Willi arrived in 1968.

Willi quickly realized that no formal control study had been put in place to monitor avalanche history or record necessary weather readings for forecasting. The task was not dissimilar to what he had dealt with in Banff, and with little fuss, he set about establishing an avalanche control program for the park. Besides obtaining the necessary equipment, he began training the wardens for the work ahead.

Exactly how to control the avalanches was initially up for debate. The blasting program in Rogers Pass worked well there, but it was not necessarily the answer for the other parks. The typical bureaucratic solution was to form a committee to come up with viable options applicable to each park. The committee was headed up by Chief Park Warden Andy Anderson who recalls: "I was the chairman, and they gave me Freddie Schleiss, Willi Pfisterer and Peter Fuhrmann. Now any two of those guys couldn't agree on anything." But they did agree that the snowpack in Alberta was entirely different from that in Rogers Pass. To keep the upper level of bureaucrats happy, Andy wrote up a series of reports that reflected his rather cutting sense of humour. He called the committee the "Avalanche Stabilization Study Team" and sent off his monthly summations to Calgary under the heading "ASS Team Report." But the irony of the name was beyond anyone at that level. It was never questioned, and as Andy recalls, "Nobody ever caught on."

Although they had several meetings with the Canadian army unit stationed at Suffield, Alberta, where they trained with artillery, it was some time before they developed a solution. They needed to find a safe way to deliver an explosive into the trigger zone, ideally during a storm cycle when the snow was building up. The howitzer was too powerful for the short range on the Sunshine road. The helicopter, which was Peter's solution to almost all public safety problems, was limited to flying in good weather and could not be relied upon to drop bombs in trigger zones during a storm.

In the end, Willi's solution for Jasper engaged the helicopter, a 106 mm recoilless rifle and a third gun called the avalauncher. The avalauncher was developed in the United States by Monty Atwater who modified it from a baseball pitching machine specifically for use in ski areas. It was mobile and operated using a compressed nitrogen cylinder set to deliver an explosive charge to a range of short targets within the ski area. Unfortunately early versions were very dangerous to operate. If the amount of nitrogen in the cylinder was undercalculated, the bomb could—and sometimes did—fall way short of the target and explode in unintended places. On a couple of occasions, it landed right in front of the gun. The only thing that saved the operators was the lack of delivery impact. The bomb merely flopped onto the snow softly enough that the detonator was not triggered. Now the unfortunate warden had to retrieve it and explode it in a safe location. Dealing with unexploded bombs is tricky work that has led to the death of more than one person working in avalanche control. Later versions of the machine corrected the initial faults, and it eventually became the workhorse in control work at ski hills.

The 106 mm recoilless rifle had many advantages over the howitzer, because it did not require a platoon of army personnel to operate and was able to reach targets along the highway that were out of range for the avalauncher. It was also affordable. Unlike the Snow Research and Avalanche Warning Section (SRAWS), who could spend $800 on ammunition without blinking an eye, Willi and Peter were happy to get the same amount of firepower for six dollars. Tony Klettl recalls that they had trouble getting the rifle at first, due to the unwillingness of the army to part with it, even though it was now surplus equipment. The first one, along with the shells, came from the United States; then it became available in Canada.

The helicopter was never a first choice for Willi. He did not like the combination of "two bad things: a helicopter flying in bad weather and dynamite." Klettl agreed with Willi after an unpleasant experience using the helicopter to drop bombs on avalanche slopes after a prolonged storm. He relates: "Oh, yah, on one trip I had a brand new down jacket, and there was a hundred-pound explosive right beside me. My goddamn jacket caught on fire when I ignited it! I guess one of the sparks hit me—actually, I had a whole bunch of little burns. The pilot said, 'I smell fire in here!' I looked down and there was burns on my jacket. So I figured that was not my cup of tea. That was one of the reasons in Jasper that we were pushing for a 106 mm recoilless." Using the helicopter, however, was often unavoidable. Many

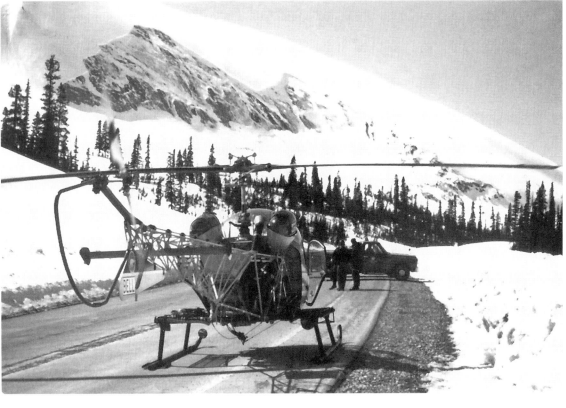

Bell B-1 used in 1970 for avalanche bombing at Parker's Ridge, Jasper. JIM DAVIES COLLECTION

of the targets were too high even for the recoilless rifle, whose use was also limited by the weather. Shooting avalanches down after the storm had passed, however, often gave limited results. After storms the weather often turned cold, leading to a tightening up of the snowpack and making it difficult to bring down the snow. If this continued, the resulting avalanche, when finally brought down, was often much bigger than the forecaster would have liked.

A more uncomfortable position the forecaster was often put in was the problem of reopening the highway after an unsuccessful, or partially successful shoot. But public highways could not be closed indefinitely and soon the pressure mounted to reopen the transportation corridor. Hans Fuhrer experienced a close call while acting as avalanche forecaster during the period he worked

at the Columbia Icefield over the notoriously dangerous winter of 1971–72. The hazard was high throughout the winter, but one particular storm came in suddenly, raising the hazard well beyond the acceptable limits, and Hans closed the highway. Unfortunately, two cars had slipped by the gates just before they were closed. One was heading to Jasper, the other to Banff. The sudden storm had passed quickly, leaving relatively clear weather and safe driving conditions, but that did not stop the two cars from colliding head on in the middle of one of the biggest slide paths in the area. Fortunately the people were unhurt and able to respond to Han's frantic effort to get them out of the cars and out of the slide path. Ten minutes later the avalanche released, covering both cars beneath tonnes of snow. Hans could only shake his head in recollection, still not sure how they had managed to collide on a clear road with no other cars in sight.

On another occasion, Hans called for the road to be closed after a large avalanche came down at Parker's Ridge south of the Columbia Icefield. He then drove down to the unmanned Banff end to close the gate. On the return trip, he encountered a bus full of hockey players on their way from Jasper to a tournament in Banff. Somehow, the bus had been allowed through after the road was closed. Chalking it up to administrative error, Hans turned around and escorted them through to Saskatchewan Crossing to let them through the gate. The bus driver had already encountered a minor slide he had been able to drive around. But Hans did not want to stay at Saskatchewan River Warden Station, which was closed, so he headed back to Sunwapta Warden Station. He had not gone far when he was engulfed in a dust cloud from a slide. Shaken, he continued on till he reached a solid wall of snow. A major avalanche had come down in the interim, and though he could go no farther, he did thank his maker that he had not been there at the time. Not knowing whether to curse the Jasper office for the foul-up, or thank them for keeping him from being in the wrong place at the wrong time, Hans returned to Saskatchewan Crossing where he settled in to make the best of what wasn't there. Three days later, having managed to keep warm and melt some water, he was finally rescued by helicopter.

Peter also had his hands full during these bad winters. He was responsible for the Trans-Canada Highway through Banff and Yoho national parks, as well as Lake Louise, Sunshine and Norquay, the three major ski areas. During the winter of 1970–71 when the mountains received some of the heaviest snowfall, Peter was on vacation in Mexico. When he returned in January he was aghast at the accumulation of snow. His vacation was decidedly at an end when he learned about the avalanche situation in Banff, Yoho and Kootenay national parks.

In 1970–71 there was still much to be learned about the ability of a large slab to propagate the release of huge quantities of snow from recessed gullies. Peter had had only two winters to establish a control program, and that gave very little indication of what he was dealing with in the unpredictable year of 1971. He was not alone, however, as it caught everyone off guard.

In those two years, Peter began experimenting with helicopter bombing, bypassing DOT regulations against taking primed high explosives into an aircraft by using nitrone, a blasting agent not classified as "high explosive," which was used in seismographic well exploration. Peter came across this little item over yet another lunch with the president of CIL, who had to get rid of the material now considered outdated in that industry. He was systematically blowing it up at considerable cost and was more than happy to give Peter two tonnes of the stuff to throw at all the mountains he wanted. Peter noted: "It wasn't normal Parks procedure, especially when delivered over lunch hour," but it did give him a "free" supply of explosives for several winters to come.

Peter started his campaign against the heavy snows at the Sunshine Ski Area parking lot. This was of great concern, because if the buildup of snow on the slopes above the parking lot or road resulted in a natural uncontrolled release, there would be no way to ensure the safety of anyone in the area. A dramatic change in the weather tipped the scales on taking action when a sudden warming trend made a natural slide likely to happen. Peter recalls: "We closed the parking lot, and didn't let anyone come down from [the ski hill at] Sunshine. We stopped everything. Then we flew up and threw a bomb into the Goat's Eye side path." The slide that came down was massive and indicative of things to come. When the dust cleared, Peter saw nothing but "utter chaos." The avalanche had buried 32 cars, pushed two busses across the lot and sent big fuel supply tanks shooting through the air "like torpedoes." It hit the Brewster information building and ticket booth, creating a pressure chamber effect that blew the whole roof off. But nobody was killed or injured. Peter remembers: "We were all aghast. The parking lot was destroyed."

Subsequent bombing along the paths above the road left slide deposits six to nine metres deep, requiring a major cleanup just to reopen the place. Any skiers caught up at the hill had to hoof it out over the snow and timber debris of the now very wide slide paths. There were no immediate repercussions, even though Assistant Superintendent Guy Myers, who was new to the mountains, was a bit unstrung about whether the correct action had been taken or not. It was new to everyone else as well. But it was hard to argue with saving lives and very difficult to second-guess if leaving a slide to nature would not have resulted in loss of life, so the program continued.

The next concern was the Banff-Windermere Highway, but the road was little used at that time, and no one complained about the several days it took to clean up the massive slides released by Peter's nitrone bomb. But Mt. Bosworth was a different story.

Although Peter had not included the snow collection basins on Mt. Bosworth at Wapta Lodge above the Trans-Canada Highway in his control program, he had eyed it nervously from the beginning of his tenure as alpine specialist. He had "advised the superintendent a number of times" that Mt. Bosworth posed a critical threat to the highway, and under the prevalent conditions, Peter was convinced it was a disaster waiting to happen. All hesitation was removed when a small avalanche scudded across the highway, obscuring a car from the view of a trailing vehicle that reported the incident. Although the first car had scooted through safely without realizing an avalanche had come down, no one knew this and it led to a tense search of the debris that night.

Peter has no trouble recalling the conditions the day they flew up to stabilize the slope: "It was drizzling on the summit of Mt. Bosworth—terrible high hazard conditions. I threw the bomb out of the helicopter, and the moment it hit the snow, the slide started. The explosion hadn't even happened yet. I could have thrown a rock into the slide, and it would have accomplished the same thing." As they flared away from the slope, they could see the fracture line of deep instability snake through the surface of the thick slab, spreading across the slope in both directions, releasing tonnes of dense snow that began to move slowly down, the slide growing larger as it descended. The awesome inertia of potential energy converted instantly to working weight when the bomb went off, hurtling the solid blocks downward, ripping out huge hundred-year-old stands of timber in its rush to the highway and the CPR tracks below. Neither man had ever seen anything like it in their lives.

Neither had Andy Anderson, who was now chief park warden in Yoho National Park and knowledgeable about avalanches himself. He had worked in ski areas in the avalanche control program with Walter Perren and knew quite a bit about explosives and avalanches—but this scared the pants off him. And for good reason. He was part of the observation team below and could not see if he was clear of the slide through the fogged-up windows of his truck. Haste never hurt under those circumstances, and he quickly threw the truck into reverse, hurtling backwards to avoid the oncoming avalanche. From a relatively safe position, the men watched the massive slide roar across the road, over the lake below and on up to the CPR tracks on the far side of the valley. Chunks of timber flew into air the out of a dark cloud of snow and debris air like thin black reeds. The slide had taken everything out right to the ground. It had also widened the previously unconnected narrow chutes into one huge slide path.

If there had been no immediate repercussion over the Sunshine parking lot (except for impending lawsuits), that was not the case this time. Much of it had to do with the freight train that was on the track when the slide hit. Although it was not derailed, it resulted in a panicked call to Anderson from Superintendent Harley Webb to

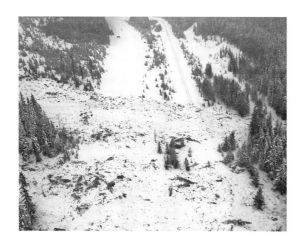

Mt. Bosworth slide 2003. MARK LEDWIDGE COLLECTION

stop all bombing immediately. Not that there was any need to drop another bomb. Still in alarm mode, Harley then called Jim Raby, the regional director in Calgary, who contacted Assistant Superintendent Guy Myers in Banff to sort it out. Myers sorted it out by shutting Peter's program down altogether. The situation was only temporary, however, when Jim Raby, the director of Western Region, supported Peter's initial decision to bomb the slope and instructed him to "get back and do what was best." Undoubtedly there was some fallout over having not notified the CPR of the control actions, but no one had thought the slide would go that far.

There was one concern remaining for Peter in the wake of destruction left by the Bosworth Slide Path. A second major slide path near the small town of Field also threatened the Trans-Canada Highway, as was evident from some old aerial photographs Andy had unearthed while looking into the avalanche history of the park. The photographs clearly showed a slide had come down from the upper reaches of Mt. Burgess and crossed the highway some years earlier. The town lay directly below this path, and if anything of the magnitude of the Bosworth slide came down, Field would be wiped out. The advice of other avalanche experts such as Peter Schaerer and Fred

Schleiss was to pass on this bombing exercise and spare the town. Fortunately for those facing sleepless nights, the weather grew cold shortly after, tightening up the snowpack and reducing the hazard. The major events of the 1970–71 winter were over, but a succession of heavy snow years would follow. The year had brought a much greater understanding of the power of avalanches and control programs were modified accordingly.

As Canada blossomed in the 1970s, so did the public's awareness of the value of national parks, and soon new ones were being created. The ones that affected Peter and Willi were two new parks in the north and three more in the east. Kluane (22,000 square kilometres) and Nahanni in the north came under Willi's jurisdiction while Cape Breton, Gros Morne and Auyuittuq (Baffin Island) were handed over to Peter. While the development of mountain rescue in Western Canada was not affected by the eastern parks, the same could not be said for the northern parks, Kluane in particular. Though Nahanni had some significant mountains that posed a challenge to serious climbers, the major attraction in the park was the Nahanni River. The higher mountains offering extreme climbing conditions are in Kluane (home to Mt. Logan, the highest mountain in Canada).

Willi's first mandate was to write a public safety plan for Kluane, but to do this he first had to determine who could be called upon for emergency rescues. The initial staff certainly weren't brought there for their climbing ability. He did not find any such resources in the community either. He soon realized that any rescue capability had to come from the south, so he and Peter assembled a team of wardens to climb Mt. Logan—just to let them know what they would have to deal with if called upon to effect a rescue in this remote park.

Peter was anxious because the high altitude required the wardens to become acclimatized. It did not help that Haines Junction, the park headquarters, was located at an altitude of only 610 metres. Before they left, however, Peter arranged for a high-altitude check at the ambulatory care centre in Calgary, where the men were subjected to a battery of tests. The nine men selected went to climb the mountain in 1973 and faced some of the severest weather and altitude conditions the wardens had yet encountered.

Both Peter and Willi were along as joint leaders of the expedition with a group of men ranging from their late thirties to the youngest, Clair Israelson, at age 22. For some, the experience was a nightmare of personal survival, carrying brutish loads through severe storms and plunging minus 40 degree Celsius temperatures. Despite the disappointment of not making the summit, they came together as a team. Both Willi and Peter were happy with how the men and equipment worked and felt much more confident about the inherent problems of the park. From that time on, Willi regularly went north, training the local wardens as well as bringing others from the south to climb several of the high peaks in the park. Extending the wardens' capacity to respond to rescue situations beyond park boundaries was considered an essential part of the mountain rescue program.

During this period of experimentation and development of the public safety program, the rescues continued unabated. Though Willi and Peter were in charge of establishing the program, running the training sessions and overseeing the implementation of equipment, the final goal was to have the wardens run the rescues. To this end, both specialists let the wardens conduct rescues where possible. To begin with, Willi often called in more experienced guides, which caused some initial resentment, but that only lasted until the wardens were capable of effecting rescues on difficult terrain without outside help.

This was seriously tested on the 3–3½ couloir, a very demanding new ice route in the Valley of the Ten Peaks at Moraine Lake near Lake Louise.

The two men from Salt Lake City in Utah, U.S., were experienced climbers who set off early in the morning of August 13th to climb the route. Despite the early start to avoid rock fall, the leader was hit on the head when the team reached one of the steepest parts of the climb. It was only 10:00 a.m., but the climbing was severe enough that his partner was slow returning and did not get help until 6:00 p.m. Before he left, however, he pulled the seriously concussed man off to the side under the protection of overhanging rock and covered him with a light sleeping bag.

Despite the lateness of the day, Bill Vroom flew in with Jim Davies and the survivor to locate the man and assess the difficulty of the terrain. It was not hard to locate him, but it was a forbidding place so steep that Jim was concerned about hitting the rocks with the rotor blades. Finally Bill saw an outcrop of rock not far from the injured man that Jim could reach with the long line and that provided some sort of stance to get in an ice anchor.

His backup partner on this occasion was warden Monty Rose, who was not that experienced in high-angle rescue. Before they went in, Bill had to show him how to attach the sling line to the Jenny Bag, which he did from a nearby airy staging perch high on the mountain. Then, with some trepidation, Bill went in alone to set up the anchor for Monty and the rescue gear. Though it was midsummer, with calm warm conditions and good flying weather, it meant the rock fall hazard remained high. The tricky part for both of them was the time it took to set up the anchor. Bill needed the security of being attached to the sling line while he put in the ice screws, because a second rock could easily take him off the mountain. Bill's curt description describes the balancing act they both had to maintain: "Jim slung me in until I touched the ice, then with some of the expert flying we have come to expect as routine from this pilot, he held me almost perfectly still while I sank the toe spikes of my crampons into the ice to steady myself." The helicopter was also in jeopardy from rock fall while Bill completed this

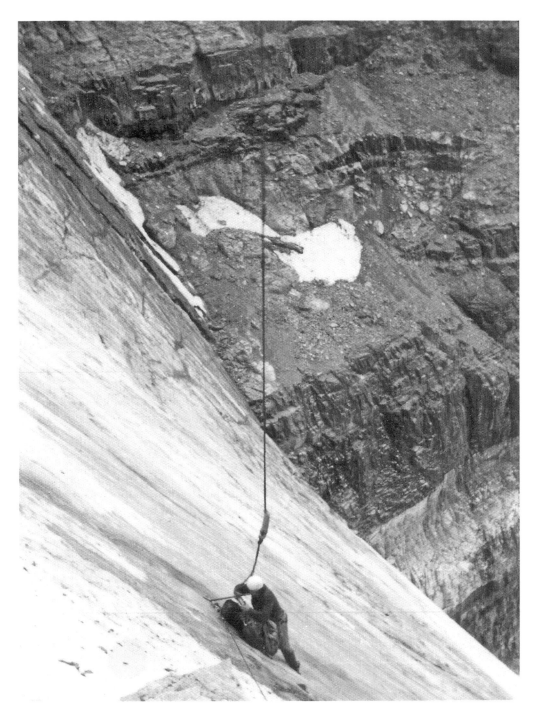

Bill Vroom at ice anchor. JIM DAVIES COLLECTION

manoeuvre. With great relief, Bill signalled him off to bring in Monty and the rest of the rescue gear, and soon the two made their way to the climber and the shelter of the overhanging rocks.

Monty finally got a good look at what he had let himself in for and was horrified. The stark verticality of the place was emphasized by the dark blue ice runnels in the chute that rattled with rocks that zinged out from the skyline far above. On top of this, a storm was coming in. Any thought of getting the man off under the rushed conditions of high winds, rain and coming darkness soon faded.

Bill quickly realized they would have to spend the night out and radioed Jim to see if he could sneak in some bivouac gear before the storm hit. His rescue report states: "Jim came up very quickly with a pack slung on the helicopter rope. When he approached the ice chute he had his landing light on and light rain was falling. He slung the pack in to Monty who was anchored out in the ice chute." The full force of the storm hit just as Monty reached their protected stance, and Bill knew he had made the right decision.

The one item they had not been able to bring into the shelter was the rescue basket left out in the ice chute and tied to ice screws. Bill wrote vividly about watching the basket being pummelled by rock fall when illuminated by brilliant flashes of lightning through the dark, heavy rain. As he watched the basket swaying on its lone ice anchor, Bill suddenly thought that the victim would be far more comfortable if they could retrieve it and have him lie prone on the comfort of the foam pads lining the bottom. Though it was risky, Bill decided to take a chance with the rock fall, and he brought the stretcher back to the shelter of the rocks. Within minutes the victim was comfortable in the stretcher now hanging securely from ice screws. When daylight came at 6:00 a.m. they manoeuvred the victim and stretcher with some difficulty over to the rock outcrop in the chute. The continuous rock fall hampered everything, making any action in the open exceedingly

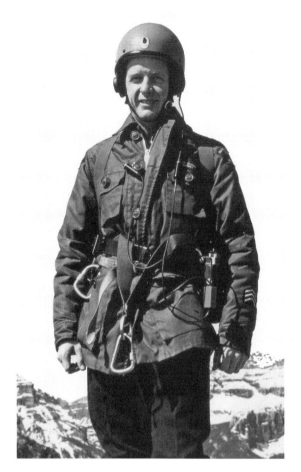

Bill Vroom. BANFF WARDEN ARCHIVES

hazardous. When Bill finally had the victim and stretcher secured to the anchor, Jim was already overhead ready to retrieve the load. Again there was the short, dangerous point of transferring the weight of the basket to the sling line while still hanging on the ice anchors. Bill writes: "Jim lifted the helicopter slightly and took the weight of the basket on the sling rope … I then quickly took out my knife and cut the two sling ropes that the basket was hung to the fixed line by. The basket swung clear from the mountain on the helicopter sling rope, and Jim swung the helicopter out from the mountain and proceeded directly to the Moraine Lake Road." Monty was next to go with a load of gear, but Bill remembers that just before lifting off, two large rocks went sailing by, barely missing him. Jim was back quickly to pick up Bill and conclude an extremely demanding rescue.

This rescue plus another technically demanding rescue on Cascade Mountain that summer prompted Peter to direct a memorandum to Banff Chief Park Warden Andy Anderson on the necessity for the Warden Service to maintain a highly trained public safety staff on call at all times. In this instance a disoriented climber had rappelled into the steep east face—possibly trying to take a direct line down—and become stranded after losing all his gear while setting up the next rappel. Here he was stopped by an overhanging cliff which was impossible to descend without the rope. Again, the helicopter was used to swing the rescuers in on a 15-metre line, but this time they were assisted in landing by the climber, who was able to reach out to them and secure them to the fixed protection. Getting off was quite another problem. Jim was again flying the mission and now had to pendulum the free line into both the climber and the rescuer, who was also technically stranded with the climber. Jim was getting quite proficient at this rather tense action so close to the rock face and was able to manoeuvre the line in. Peter states: "This is technically a most important moment as in this case the changeover must be made simultaneously as otherwise either the rescuer falls off or the aircraft could be forced into a crash."

It was the intention of both alpine specialists to upgrade the wardens' rescue profile and bring it as close to the European standard as they could, but as Willi admits, it was Peter who kept the ideas and connections flowing. One of Peter's early achievements was to introduce basic medical training for the wardens, qualifying as many as possible with an EMT (Emergency Medical Technician) certificate. This was a rigorous two-week course that allowed the wardens to administer basic first aid in the field with some degree of confidence.

Another major step forward was Peter's insistence on joining IKAR, the International Commission for Alpine Rescue. This European rescue association was instrumental in presenting and reviewing all the latest rescue equipment brought to the market by innovative companies. As Peter reflected: "One of the big things during Perren's time was that equipment was always slow to come to Canada because it was developed in Europe." Peter realized that both he and Willi had the advantage of speaking German as well as a European background to fit in with such an organization. Joining IKAR meant Canada could fully participate in an international exchange of both equipment and ideas. Canada was accepted, and thereafter both men enjoyed attending the annual conference. It also gave rise to one of Willi's insights into his partner's personality and exceptional gift for the gab.

On one of their earlier trips to the annual conference, Willi found himself with Peter at the Calgary International Airport preparing to board their flight to Europe when Peter discovered he didn't have his passport. Willi was fully prepared to see Pete attempt a mad dash back to Canmore at breakneck speed to recover the delinquent document but was more surprised by Peter's unflappable demeanour when he coolly said he had no intention of driving back. When Willi asked what he was going to do, Peter calmly replied he would just explain to the authorities about the error and carry on with their plans. Willi ruefully recalled that Peter did just that: "He talked his way through it all!"

Through the years of their greatest influence, the two men found a way to balance their strengths, eccentricities and talents to bring the Warden Service to a high standard of mountain rescue.

5   Rescue Dogs

When a new industry reaches a period of exponential growth, it often does so on more than one front. This was certainly true of the public safety function during the early seventies. While Peter Fuhrmann was introducing sling rescue and modern cable equipment, Willi Pfisterer and Jim Sime were pursuing the use of dogs for avalanche search and rescue. Willi was familiar with dog use in avalanche searches in Europe and saw a need for them in Canada. But it would be an uphill battle before they were fully established as part of the rescue team.

The first modern-day reference to avalanche dogs was in Switzerland during the winter of 1937–38, when a dog located the last victim, who could not be found by probing. By happenstance one of the rescuers had brought his dog Moritzli along. Suddenly one of the searchers noticed that the dog kept returning to one spot that had already been coarsely probed. They started to fine probe, getting a hit within minutes. This was most fortunate for the young skier, who was still alive.

The "Moritzli Incident" as it was later referred to, caught the attention of a dog expert in Berne, Switzerland. Ferdinand Schmutz postulated that dogs could be trained to find people buried under snow using their sense of smell. When he mentioned it to the Swiss Army, they agreed and four dogs were duly trained. After the war when recreational skiing returned in earnest, the Swiss Alpine Club began acquiring their own avalanche dogs. Soon other countries like France, Italy, Austria and Germany got involved and the program grew from there.

Dog use in Canada actually started in Alberta with tracking dogs when a Lethbridge police constable used his bloodhound to track a man who had killed a Royal Northwest Mounted Police constable in southern Alberta in 1908. Their use was expanded and was eventually taken up by the RCMP in 1932.

What made the RCMP important in the evolution of search-and-rescue dogs in Canada was the broad base of expertise accumulated over several decades. Their dog teams are stationed in rural as well as urban locations and are trained in a multi-faceted program that combines search-and-rescue with law enforcement. The RCMP developed a sophisticated understanding of working dogs and a well-rounded comprehension of how scent works in different situations.

In the United States, interest in avalanche search dog capabilities grew out of existing volunteer search-and-rescue organizations. The late 1950s and early 1960s saw the number of avalanche fatalities begin to rise and avalanche dogs starting to be used in the Western United States. This new post-Second-World-War wave of interest in skiing soon caught on in Canada. With that came a gradual increase in recreational avalanche accidents across North America. The need for trained dogs got its start when they were used with some success at the Granduc avalanche disaster. Despite this early success, it did not lead to the immediate deployment of dogs. During the search for four missing men on Mt. Cleveland, avalanche dogs from Washington State were briefly considered but were ultimately not used.

The second recorded incident where a dog was used in the recovery of an avalanche victim in North America did not occur until March of 1969 on Mt. Ranier in the U.S. The incident involved a man who had failed to return from a solo ski-touring outing. Though his vehicle was located, his whereabouts could only be guessed at. Still, there were a couple of areas he could have wandered into that had recently avalanched. One of these areas had already been checked by park rangers who found neither ski tracks nor articles. With no realistic hope of finding the person alive or even certainty of his location, rescuers brought in four avalanche dogs twenty four hours after the man had been reported missing. Initial results were not encouraging, as the dogs, from the German Shepherd Search and Rescue Dog Association in Seattle, Washington, found nothing that first day.

The following morning, one of the dogs indicated the victim under 60 centimetres of snow. Rescuers found no ice mask around the man's mouth and nose, so death had come quickly. The dog handlers had good cause to feel vindicated in their efforts, and the rescue established confidence in the dogs' search capabilities. Though it was a good start it was followed by a ten-year hiatus in the United States without a recorded success using dogs. In the meantime things were starting to happen in Canada.

Some of the RCMP dog handlers were getting involved in avalanche searches simply because the RCMP were the officially designated search-and-rescue authority in many parts of the country. There were a number of different RCMP dog teams scattered throughout B.C. that could be called on in an emergency, but unfortunately many handlers were not trained to meet the mountaineering challenge that many searches presented. Few had skiing abilities, let alone mountaineering skills to augment the noses of their well-trained dogs. They did not get that kind of training at the police academy—but they still shouldered the weighty responsibilities of being first responders no matter what the problem.

One RCMP dog handler who broke the mould was Dale Marino, who had picked up winter mountaineering and avalanche awareness skills while employed as a park warden in Glacier/Revelstoke National Park.

Marino had become interested because of the rash of avalanche accidents which gave the dog more opportunity for work. Marino could also see that there was a future for the RCMP in avalanche searching if they received the proper training. He brought this to the attention of his superiors but, initially, received little support. They didn't understand that specific training was needed for both dog and man. This attitude left some handlers trying to operate in unfamiliar terrain where they were more a liability than an asset.

Despite the unenthusiastic support of superiors, one RCMP dog handler got a chance to use his dog on an avalanche in 1971, bringing about the second use of a dog for avalanche recovery in Canada—but it happened more as an afterthought, when all other means had failed. A few days before Christmas, three men were heading out for the festivities from a bush camp in the Flathead Valley near Fernie, B.C. They were travelling in two vehicles and were stopped by an avalanche blocking their path. All three men got out, leaving their vehicles running and climbed up onto the deposit to assess its size and the seriousness of their situation. Suddenly, they were hit by another avalanche which swept them away. When they had not returned by Christmas Day, a search team was sent out. They soon found the vehicles empty of fuel, with the ignition switches left on, on the far side of a huge avalanche deposit. The team assumed the men had been buried in the avalanche and the RCMP took control of the search. It was an extensive area, and bulldozers were brought in for snow removal while searchers dug through the debris with shovels. The first body wasn't found until December 29th; it was not till January 3rd that a dog was called to the site.

The dog quickly located the second body lying in water and buried under two metres of hard snow. The third body was uncovered by a bulldozer soon after. The bodies were all located in close proximity to one another, indicating the men were in a group when hit by the fast-moving avalanche. The dog proved to be the superior search tool, and that fuelled the notion that "any search dog is better than no avalanche dog."

If the RCMP were slow to recognize the need to train dog handlers to work in the mountains, it was not the case with Parks Canada. Willi Pfisterer, recognizing that the handler had to be a good skier as well as knowledgeable about avalanches, thought the dog profile would fit well with the Warden Service. The first professional avalanche dog handler in North America was Alfred Burstrom with his dog, Ginger. It was August 1969, a time when Burstrom was searching for a new role in a changing Warden Service. Over the years he had shown a keen aptitude toward animals, and when Ginger came along it gave him a chance to put his name in the hat for the dog position.

Ginger started out life behind the eight ball, being the runt of a litter of 11 pups belonging to fellow warden, Gordon McClain. McClain gave the last remaining pup to one of Alfie's children, thinking it would be good for the kids. Burstrom soon realized the dog showed great potential as a search dog and approached his chief park warden about using him in this capacity.

A meeting was held in Jasper in 1969 with Chief Park Warden Mickey McGuire, Jim Sime and Willi Pfisterer to discuss the possibility of using dogs. The program soon had a green light at the regional level; all they needed were some candidates. They considered several park wardens but chose Burstrom because of his mountaineering training, superior travelling skills on both skis and snowshoes, and his ability to relate to animals.

Early in 1970, Sime got approval from Ottawa to establish the dog training program, and he approached the RCMP training facilities at Innisfail. In the meantime, while visiting in Europe, Pfisterer brought back a copy of the Swiss avalanche dog training standards. Staff Sergeant Terry Kehoe was the head trainer at the Innisfail training kennels and Sime sat down with him to discuss developing the program within the existing RCMP training curriculum. Kehoe had a course for potential dog handlers coming up that spring. It was an occasion when potential and existing RCMP dog handlers from across the country were brought in and evaluated by the training staff. When the Staff Sergeant offered Parks Canada a place on the course, Sime volunteered Burstrom's name. Sime and Pfisterer were gambling on Burstrom and his dog, knowing that the future of the program depended on the team's success.

After Burstrom qualified, it was Ginger's turn to be assessed. Before he even got started, he had three strikes against him: First, he was relatively small for a police working dog, second, only one out of 80 dogs statistically made the cut and third, Ginger's heritage was in question. His breeding remained controversial even after he graduated from the RCMP training kennels months later. His pedigree simply wasn't in keeping with the RCMP's penchant for training purebred German shepherds. Coyotes were not considered. Kehoe was up front with Sime when they sat down to discuss Ginger a few days after the training course. "Where in the hell did this dog come from?" he boomed. Jim, defensive and subdued at

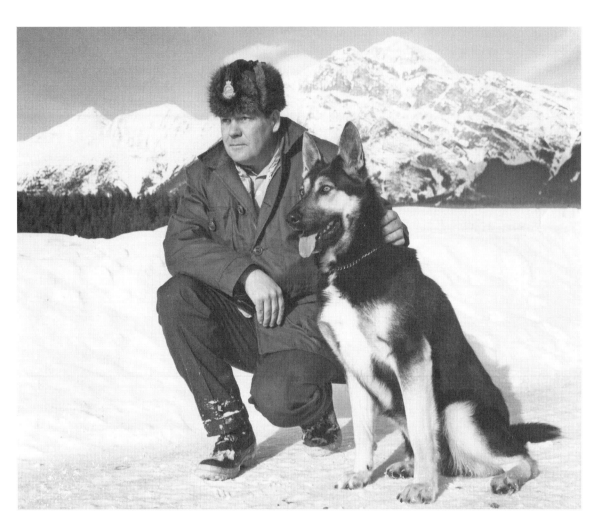

Alfie Burstrom and Ginger. ALFIE BURSTROM COLLECTION

Kehoe's brusque manner, began to relate Ginger's history. "Well his father was a big German shepherd, but his mom was half coyote. I know that's controversial around here, but I don't think it matters." Despite the unorthodoxy of the dog's breeding, he was accepted in the program. If the handler had been an RCMP officer, however, the coy/dog probably would have been refused.

As far as Kehoe was concerned, though, there were many unanswered questions. Coyotes were viewed as sneaky animals of prey who did not display traditional signs of courage. They were not considered life companions—how dependable would Ginger be in the wilderness? It was quite likely the dog would develop an "animal hang-up" and be distracted by animal tracks. But Kehoe's fears proved groundless. Ginger was so good that the staff sergeant wanted more dogs with some coyote in them (something Burstrom took to heart in a future breeding program). Ginger and Alfie went into training in September, 1970, for four months and graduated in January, 1971, as the first certified professional avalanche search dog team in North America. In keeping with Parks Canada's wishes, the team was trained in all RCMP dog profiles except attack work.

Pfisterer had originally looked at three European avalanche dog training standards: the German, the Swiss and the Italian. He and Fuhrmann chose the Swiss standard, and Fuhrmann translated it into English and then submitted it to the RCMP, who incorporated into their training manual. Pfisterer provided a much-needed training standard for the handlers so that they could be comfortably and safely employed in avalanche search situations with requisite mountaineering skills.

Once they started working in the field, Burstrom and Ginger blossomed into an effective unit, though it took a while for some within the Warden Service to accept the usefulness of the dog. The idea of using a dog on search-and-rescue operations, poaching cases or for looking for lost kids in campgrounds was new to everyone. The nearby RCMP detachments had no such doubts. From the beginning, Burstrom and the dog were in demand, getting a large share of RCMP calls from communities surrounding Jasper. The closest RCMP dog was at Stony Plain near Edmonton, 300 kilometres away. As Burstrom said, "They had me chasing god knows who. They were used to a working dog." Burstrom and Ginger were the first of a long line of Parks Canada dog handlers who fostered a unique relationship with their counterparts in the RCMP.

ON FEBRUARY 20TH, 1972, Alfie Burstrom finally got the call he was trained and waiting for. For Shirley Klettl, wife of veteran public safety warden Tony Klettl, it had been a quiet morning. It was just past noon, the kids were in school, her husband was at work in town, and she looked forward to some quiet time to read before the kids came home. Sudden the solitude was broken by a loud rapping at the back door. A haggard and exhausted man with a broken arm stood outside. His tale of surviving an avalanche on Mt. Edith Cavell and travelling on foot without skis throughout the night astounded her. He had struggled along a 15-kilometre snow-choked road

to report the accident, hoping to save his friends. At one point he had lost the road and struggled for hours in waist-deep snow before regaining the road. When he had left the accident site, one of his buddies was still alive on the surface, but there was no sign of the other two. After spending an hour looking for the missing climbers without success, he had returned to his friend, making him as comfortable as possible before going for help.

Willi Pfisterer was at Marmot Basin Ski Area supervising some avalanche control work when he got the call and left immediately to interview the survivor. Wardens were called in from all points of the park and by 1:15 p.m. there were 12 men including Burstrom and his dog, Ginger, and one RCMP member at the start of the Cavell Road waiting for the helicopter.

With one man known to be alive, time was everything, so Pfisterer had the reporting person brought to the staging area for the interview, recalling: "He was really bashed up with a broken arm, and I asked him some questions, and he precisely answered them. He gave clear answers and I knew exactly what had happened and where it was on the mountain. So the thing to do was to get there as fast as possible—because of the light."

The story unfolded, telling a tale of tragedy for well-known members of the Edmonton section of the Alpine Club. On February 19th, the party of four had registered out in Jasper to attempt the first winter ascent of the east ridge of Mt. Edith Cavell, using the standard summer route.

By four that afternoon the weather turned cloudy and warm so they decided to dig a snow cave for the night at the top of the steep gully. The survivor was inside the snow cave putting on the finishing touches when he heard a crack, and the roof collapsed on top of him. The other three were outside in varying degrees of unpacking, when they and the survivor were carried down the mountain with the mass of avalanching snow. After sliding, tumbling and free falling over numerous cliffs, they came to rest near the saddle at the base of the mountain, 600 metres below.

119

Amazed to be alive, the survivor found himself near a big rock clear of the avalanche deposit. When he tried to get to his feet, he realized one arm was broken near the elbow. Only one other person lay on top of the wide avalanche deposit. He looked hastily around for the other two, but saw nothing but camp debris on the surface. He returned to his friend and splinted his broken leg to his sound one and made him as comfortable as possible. He left for help at 8:00 p.m. knowing it was going to be a long night.

Back at the staging area, one group of wardens left by snow machine up the unplowed road for the base of the mountain while the rest waited for the helicopter. Willi Pfisterer flew in first with Max Winkler and immediately spotted one person on the surface of the snow. Pfisterer and Winkler quickly reached the victim, but he had died, apparently from internal injuries rather than exposure. They did a hasty search of the slide but came up with nothing but camp debris. The helicopter, now flying Burstrom, Staff Sergeant Al Moore and the dog, continued to be delayed by snow squalls, and did not reach the site until 4:00 p.m. Three more men came up on the next flight while the bulk of the team set up a rescue base at the tea house.

Burstrom soon had the dog at the edge of the deposit and gave the search command. Before Alfie could direct the dog, however, Ginger was distracted by the body on the surface and immediately went to check it out. Unfortunately, one of the searchers was preparing it for evacuation when the dog suddenly arrived. Annoyed at the intrusion, the rescuer yelled, "Get this goddamn dog out of here." Burstrom's anger quickly flashed to the surface and was controlled only by the need to get the dog searching again. Ginger, however, had never encountered a body and lingered around the area before returning to search the deposit under Burstrom's direction. The search was also complicated by all the human scented articles on the surface. Soon though, the dog started to ignore articles and concentrate on what was under the snow.

Pfisterer had his own concerns, because daylight was running out. In an hour or so they would have to either fly a camp to the site or return the next morning, weather permitting. He decided to give the dog an hour before taking action. Ten minutes after starting the search, the dog found the first body buried under 20 centimetres (eight inches) of snow. It wasn't hard to recognize the dog's frantic attempt to uncover the body as the snow flew from his digging effort. Not surprisingly, the person was deceased. Ginger located the second body 50 minutes later, just as the issue of flying a camp in was being addressed. All efforts now went into getting the bodies and rescuers down from the mountain. The evacuation was completed by 8:30 p.m.

The dog was the reason for the success, and Pfisterer recognized how important it was to have the dog team on the first flight on future incidents. Burstrom realized that articles on the surface can be a major distraction for dogs, and he would incorporate it in future avalanche dog training. The helicopter was another distraction that would need to be addressed on future avalanche accidents. What pleased Alfie most of all, however, was that Ginger worked so well despite the distractions. The dog actually found a dime on the surface of the snow, proving how well the dog concentrated under the conditions.

Burstrom saw a significant increase in dog calls after this success. Wardens took new interest, and many volunteered to act as quarries in training scenarios. Alfie still has the 1964 10-cent piece in his scrap book to this day.

THOUGH DALE MARINO had championed the benefits of avalanche dogs, the RCMP were not convinced about the avalanche profile until 1972. After Alfie and Ginger completed training in 1971, their principal obligation was to Parks Canada; they responded to incidents beyond these borders only if there was no emergency in the park. But other teams would soon be needed, and the RCMP was the obvious agency to fulfil that need. What changed their thinking was a search for four lost skiers at Whistler, B.C., in April of 1972.

A man and woman out skiing for the day were declared missing when they failed to pick up their infant child at the ski resort's babysitting service. The RCMP were notified and shortly thereafter another couple was also reported missing. It was soon ascertained that the two couples knew each other, indicating they were probably skiing together. The ski patrol conducted a night search but found nothing. The next morning numerous aerial and ground searches were conducted throughout the area. By noon new information came forward that the missing skiers were last seen heading toward the Back Bowl and not the West Bowl where the original couple had been spotted.

By daybreak the following day, the RCMP had three helicopters involved in the search as well as two (uncertified) RCMP dog teams. The first dog team went to the Burnstew Basin area where a couple of avalanche deposits had been located. Dale Marino and his dog Rocky were put on an avalanche deposit in the Back Bowl area close to where the skiers were last seen. The team worked the slide deposit from the top down, but much of the old avalanche was disguised by new snow, and search personnel had difficulty defining the avalanche boundaries. The search was further hampered by deteriorating weather and a mounting avalanche hazard prompting the removal of the probe team. That left Marino and Rocky on their own to work the deposit. It was unnerving work, but to Dale's relief, two ski patrollers were established as spotters, one to watch for any new avalanches from above and the other to keep an eye on the two in relation to where they were on the deposit. Marino also had his escape route picked out if a warning was sounded.

After a couple of hours of searching, Rocky found the first victim, and then in the short span of a half hour, the other three were found in the same general area by probers called in to do a hasty search. This was a big success for an avalanche dog, for it came at a time when the worth of dogs was being evaluated. Although Dale and Rocky were unofficial in their capacity as a avalanche search team, they were rapidly becoming seasoned veterans.

Finally, with the avalanche profile established at the Innisfail Dog Training Kennels, Marino was able to convince his supervisors that he and his dog should be trained in this field. The program would be administered through the RCMP but conducted under Pfisterer's direction in Jasper. They decided to train not one, but two dog teams in the new profile, and Doug Wiebe, a promising handler stationed in Prince George, B.C., attended with Marino. The course was taught by Bernie Johnson, the RCMP dog trainer from Innisfail, and Willi Pfisterer, the Jasper alpine specialist. It was a success and it established a precedent for the future. During the winter of 1972/73, Marino and Wiebe became the first two RCMP dog teams in the avalanche program.

While Jasper is the largest national park in the Canadian Rockies, Banff is the busiest and the one with the highest profile. With Burstrom and Ginger's growing successes, it became apparent that Banff needed to catch up, and so in the summer of 1973 Banff selected two wardens with sufficient mountaineering background to be considered good candidates for training. Both were sent off for evaluation by the RCMP. That fall, Earl Skjonsberg and Jack Woledge went into training and graduated four months later. The early winter 1973–74 saw the second annual RCMP avalanche dog training course, with six teams attending, including Skjonsberg and Woledge from Parks Canada. Helping out with the instructing was Alfie Burstrom, assisted by Ginger, who demonstrated how it should be done.

A week after the dog course, a skier went missing at Bow Summit. It was later discovered he had gone skiing on the 9th of December, but it was not until the evening of the 17th that he was reported missing. The man had not registered

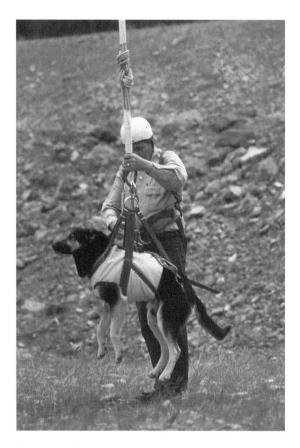

Ginger in helicopter sling harness. JASPER WARDEN
ARCHIVES

Burstrom quickly saw an opportunity for Skjonsberg and Woledge to have their dogs exposed to a corpse and called them over on the radio. Before they attracted any attention, the two dog handlers had their dogs satisfy their curiosity about the unsettling presence of a dead body. Alfie came to know the importance of exposing a dog to a body after his experiences on Mt. Edith Cavell. The handlers considered this manoeuvre, viewed as macabre by some, necessary because working dogs have been known to be traumatized by the experience.

Banff's first success with the new dogs came just outside the boundary of Sunshine Ski Resort near Lookout Mountain. A skier had gone missing, and a search of the area that night had come up with nothing. The search narrowed the next morning after two new slide deposits were located near the boundary close to Delirium Dive ski run. The two Banff dog teams were flown to the site in the early afternoon. Though one of the dogs immediately located a ski pole, they found nothing further that day. The next morning the dogs resumed searching, and a couple of hours later, Faro, Skjonsberg's dog, found the missing man.

AVALANCHES DON'T ALWAYS RESULT in death. Knowledge of proper procedures and right action are important in saving lives. At an accident at Parker's Ridge, skiers did follow procedure, but in the end, inattention resulted in a death. The Parker's Ridge area near the Columbia Icefield is very popular with ski-tourers. It provides good ski terrain close to vehicle access, but is plagued with an abundance of avalanche terrain that has accounted for numerous fatalities. Many of these accidents occur in small, localized pockets that are terrain traps. One nasty little spot at Parker's Ridge near the Hilda Creek Youth Hostel has claimed the lives of more than one person over the years.

In February, 1976, seven people were returning from a day of skiing when an advance group of four came upon this small, infamous slope.

out, and there was little to indicate where he had gone other than the fact that his car was parked at the Peyto Lake parking lot. When no clues were found, the search was quickly broadened.

On the 19th, a helicopter survey found an old avalanche deposit above Peyto Lake. Conditions were so dicey that one of the dogs triggered a full-depth avalanche that cleaned out the entire basin despite earlier stabilization efforts. Fortunately no one was in the way of the avalanche, and the dog managed to scamper clear. On the 22nd the search area moved west of the parking lot. After two hours of searching, Ginger found the missing skier in an old avalanche deposit 40 to 70 centimetres (16 to 28 inches) below the new snow.

They showed evidence of having some avalanche awareness, however, when the leader assigned one of the group to watch while he crossed the slope to establish a last seen point in case a slide occurred. But for whatever reason, the observer was distracted by the group and failed to see the man disappear beneath the slide he immediately triggered. All the observer heard was a noise as the slope released; he did not see his friend in the fresh avalanche deposit of the small slide.

One skier was quickly sent for help while the others frantically searched for the missing person. Other skiers arrived from the youth hostel to lend a hand. By 4:35 p.m. the Warden Service had been notified, and a first party consisting of three wardens and a dog was on its way. At this point, the group's lack of training became evident. Rather than use what tools they had (skis and ski poles) to probe the small deposit for the victim, they had randomly dug where they *thought* he might be, digging up a considerable area to no avail. Once the rescuers arrived, everyone was quickly removed from the deposit, and Burstrom put Ginger to work, immediately finding the body buried 10 metres from where the group had been digging.

EACH AVALANCHE EXPERIENCE adds to the list of dos and don'ts that dog handlers and rescue leaders use to determine how best to deploy dogs. Because there was a lot to learn in the early years about the strength and limitations of the dog team, not all rescues were successful. This was hard on the handler, because it cast aspersions on the dog's ability.

Sometimes search conditions compromised the dog's skills. One such situation developed in 1979 on an avalanche in the Stanley Glacier Basin of Kootenay National Park. It involved four cross-country skiers who were caught in an avalanche they had triggered when putting in a few turns on the open slope after returning from a day's outing. All four skiers were caught and carried 300 metres down the mountain.

When the avalanche came to rest, one young woman found herself buried to her chest in an upright position. Once free she helped a second partially buried woman before the snow set. There was no sign of the remaining two skiers. A group of ascending skiers in a different party quickly came to their aid. Again, lack of training was a factor—rescuers realized that though the party carried avalanche beacons, none of them were turned on. Twenty minutes later the first victim was found under his pack, lying on the surface at the upper end of the deposit. While they continued to search for the fourth person, another skier went to report the accident.

The accident had happened at 4:00 p.m. and by 5:30 p.m. Jack Woledge and Earl Skjonsberg were on-site with their dogs. Shortly after arriving, Woledge's dog uncovered a woollen headband at the lower end of the slide, but the probe team found nothing else there. Meanwhile the two dogs and their handlers tried to work amongst the distractions of the helicopter taking off and landing nearby and the activity of the twelve people on the probe line.

The dogs were having no success in the area they were working and began to lose interest despite the pressure to continue. As night drew on, wind and heavy snow scattered surface scent, further exacerbating their efforts. The densely falling snow was also increasing the avalanche hazard, and the rescue was reluctantly called off at 10:00 p.m. By then the dogs were exhausted.

Earl Skjonsberg had no problem recollecting the events surrounding that search 24 years later. "I remember the Stanley Glacier in Kootenay. Old Alfie was out there with us too. That was the time I just about wrecked my dog. I worked him so much that he just quit. He wouldn't do anything anymore. He never found anything on the search. If he had found something it would have given him some incentive. In the end he just wouldn't do anything anymore. I took him home and later I took him out to play and he just said the heck with you. He wouldn't look for anything. So I put him in his kennel and left him there for three of four days. I thought, 'Holy smokes, I've wrecked him.' But he finally came out of it."

The next day the control of the rescue was handed over to Hans Fuhrer from Kootenay National Park. It had snowed heavily overnight and the avalanche hazard was extreme. He wisely called off the search until the area stabilized. The storm quit two days later, but a large avalanche crossed the initial avalanche, increasing both the search area and the depth of the deposit. Finally the park wardens were able to safely return to the scene. Despite having four dog teams now on-site, success continued to elude them, though they found more articles.

Frustrated dog handlers began to think the body was buried too deep for the scent to reach the surface and when it did it was being scattered by the wind. The probe teams were instructed to screw two standard size probes together to add length. They finally located the victim under six metres of snow. But now, rescuers were wondering why the dogs, who were very experienced, hadn't found the victim.

Obviously the depth of the burial and the strong winds hindered the dogs, but the helicopter (which can be controlled) was a major distraction. The proximity of the probe line to the dogs was also a distraction. Human scent was everywhere, confusing the dogs who had to sort out it all out. In the end, the analysis of the search was invaluable in setting up criteria for future avalanche searches with dogs. But the perception that the dogs had failed shook the confidence of the search team.

The handlers realized they needed to train the dogs to work around these problems and to be assertive in how best to deploy dogs. They decided they needed a code of practice to give the dogs every chance for success. For example, during the Delirium Dive search, the helicopter had used the avalanche deposit as a heli-pad, contaminating the slide with spilled hydraulic fluid and scattering human scent from the surface of the slide.

Rescuers had to learn to take articles off the slide once they were found, leaving a wand instead to mark the location. They had to forbid smoking, eating or urinating—surprisingly common occurrences—near the deposit.

But learning all of this was a slow process for both the dog teams and the public safety wardens, and it would be a few years before many vital lessons were incorporated into avalanche search protocol.

In March 1980, a group of 14 skiers had been transported by Sno-cat to a meadow just above timberline on Mount Mackenzie near Revelstoke, B.C. Their plan was to ski the West Bowl rather than the Northwest Bowl, which had claimed an avalanche victim the year before. But for whatever reason, one of the group hung back, then plunged down the untracked Northwest Bowl despite being warned to avoid it. The action triggered the release of a massive slide 200 metres above, sweeping the reckless powder enthusiast down the mountainside.

The rest of the group waited at the bottom for this last fellow, but when he didn't arrive, a few of them skied over to the edge and saw a fresh avalanche deposit in the Northwest Bowl. Immediately they headed to the deposit. Having only their skis and poles for probes, they searched for twenty minutes before sending a small group off to report the accident.

The local RCMP coordinated the rescue effort and flew a dog team in from Vernon, B.C. The local Provincial Emergency Program group, as well as ski patrol, private heli-skiing groups and park wardens from Glacier/Revelstoke National Park were also called in. A Parks Canada group, composed of Willi Pfisterer, Alfie Burstrom and his dog Ginger from Jasper, and Earl Skjonsberg with his dog Faro from Banff were flown immediately to the site by helicopter. Here they found the RCMP dog team searching the upper reaches of the deposit where the body was least likely to be found, while a probe team worked the bottom of the deposit. Unfortunately, the dog handler had never been exposed to an avalanche search and had no reason to question the deployment of either the dog or the probe line. The inexperienced dog handler assumed the search leader was familiar with how to deploy resources in a situation like this and followed instructions.

When Pfisterer arrived, he took over as the rescue leader and immediately sent the RCMP dog team to search the bottom of the slide. Once the RCMP team got there, the dog immediately found the victim under 30 centimetres of snow, two metres from where the probe line had quit searching.

Willi also learned over time that a dog handler would sometimes go off and work with his dog away from the attention of others to avoid the spotlight. It was a chance for the dog to work without distractions, but it also meant being able to work without critical scrutiny. Often dog handlers felt intense pressure to achieve success, but working with all eyes focussed on the team was intimidating. It was important that the dog work where success was most likely, even if it was at centre stage.

Though the learning process was often slow it was sped up in Banff during the winter of 1981. During one weekend, wardens were to confront three accidents in less than 24 hours. By February, after a prolonged cold snap, a significant layer of old surface hoar was covered by new snow at higher elevations, leading to a serious avalanche hazard. But the construction of these layers would ultimately teach the dog handlers (and search masters) a lot more about the complexities of some avalanche searches.

The nightmarish weekend started in Yoho National Park in the Waterfall Valley above Twin

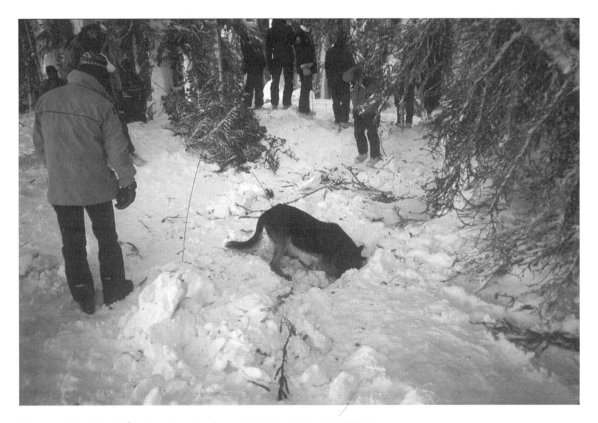

Dog searching Healy Creek avalanche deposit. DALE PORTMAN COLLECTION

Falls on February 21st, when a group of four back-country skiers were caught in the first slide. They were following a creek down a small alpine valley when they encountered a narrow gully with steep banks on either side. It was a terrible little terrain trap that demanded respect even under good conditions. With the hazard being as high as it was, it was deadly. Though the skiers were spaced out according to safe travel procedure while passing through the steep little section, they missed seeing the event. The leader had just made it through the gully when he heard a noise behind him that sounded like a call. Looking back he saw that a small slab avalanche had fractured from the top of the steep slope and that the person behind him was missing. The two remaining skiers immediately turned their rescue beacons on to receive, but they couldn't detect a signal from the victim. They marked the last seen point then dug three or four holes about two metres deep hoping to uncover him. Finding nothing, the party skied to Twin Fall Tea House from where the leader continued on, taking seven hours to reach the highway and report the accident.

The Warden Service organized a search party and a helicopter for departure in the morning. This included two avalanche dog teams: Alfie and Ginger from Jasper and an RCMP team, Chris Banham and his dog, from Cochrane. Alfie and Ginger went in first with the rescue team.

Rescuers randomly probed the area while the dog went to work on the deposit, immediately showing interest near the creek. Probing revealed nothing, and the dog was moved to another area of the deposit. After some searching, the dog returned to indicate at the first location. Again probing turned up nothing. Clair Israelson, the rescue leader, understood the dog's role but felt his indication was weak and not a confirmation of the body location.

Burstrom knew his dog, and he was sure there was something there, especially with the dog repeatedly returning to the same location despite the weak indication. Finally a lone rescuer screwed

an extra length onto his probe and after probing around, hit something well down in the snowpack. He left the probe in place and started digging. Another searcher, who also had faith in the dog, joined the shovelling while the rest watched with interest "though slightly sceptical" as Alfie remembers. The second searcher was well down in the hole shovelling when the bottom suddenly collapsed, dropping him into the creek and onto the body of the victim. An hour and a half after the dog had started searching, they located the body six metres below the surface of the snow in the water. Alfie was quietly pleased with Ginger, whose ability was approaching legend. The dog's indication was impressive, considering the depth of the burial and the fact the body was submerged in water. It also explained why the ski party could not get a signal from the victim's rescue beacon, for it had shorted out in the water.

The recovery had just wrapped up when another accident began to unfold near Bourgeau Lake in Banff National Park. Two skiers had been climbing up a steep creek bed toward a large alpine cirque west of Bourgeau Lake when they triggered an avalanche. The lower skier saw the snow cracking above him and then suddenly found himself moving down the slope. Using a swimming motion, he was able to keep his head above the snow, eventually coming to rest only partially buried, five metres from the edge of the deposit. He dug himself out and went looking for his friend, who was completely buried above him somewhere. After searching for twenty-five minutes, he skied out to the highway on his one remaining ski and reported the avalanche around 4:30 p.m.

A three-man search party was on-site at 5:10 p.m. and immediately started a hasty search of the deposit. A dog team (Skjonsberg and Faro) arrived on the second flight and began working the lower end of the deposit. A strong wind, however, was pushing the scent uphill, preventing the dog from developing a wide search pattern, and the dog covered the area faster than Skjonsberg would have liked. Within the span of a few short minutes the team had worked into a secondary search area well above the toe of the deposit. The dog became distracted by the other searchers and the buzzing helicopter. At one point the dog ran over to investigate a collection of packs left on the deposit, and Skjonsberg called him back.

By 6:00 p.m. the dog search was deemed unsuccessful, and a ten-man probe line moved onto the middle of the deposit and started coarse probing. The dog continued to search, but the probe line was now upwind of the dog, compromising his ability to use the wind for searching. It also meant they did not search the toe of the deposit where the packs were located. One-and-a-half hours after the probe line was formed they found the body located under a metre of snow right on the extreme lower edge of the deposit near where the packs had been.

The weekend was not yet over. Though some wardens were now uncertain about how well dogs worked on avalanches, much of this was put to rest on the next call that came hot on the heels of the Bourgeau slide. Once again, Alfie's mongrel proved how well he could work, given the chance. Ginger, now 12 years old, was near retirement and practically deaf. But the seasoned dog could still get around, and he didn't need much direction from his handler. He had served Parks Canada well, often carrying the program through tough years. Now it was time to give it one last shot on Mount Thompson.

When three mountain climbers set out on skis from the Peyto Hut to climb Mount Thompson, one member of the party travelled slightly ahead of the other two. His route took him onto the northwest ridge and to the summit, where he intended to join the others. The other two went east from the hut into a steep bowl punctuated with broken cliffs to the ridge that would take them to the rendezvous site. They never made it and were last seen at 10:30 climbing up the snow slopes.

The survivor waited on top for some time and then headed down the mountain, following the route the other two had ascended. Halfway down he was caught in an avalanche and carried 160 metres farther down the mountain. He was fortunate to be on the surface and managed to dig himself out. At that point he observed two other avalanches in the same bowl, which had not been there when he had last seen his two friends. He returned to the Peyto Hut, but when his companions had not returned by 4:00 p.m., he skied out to the highway arriving there at 8:30 p.m. He quickly flagged down a passing car and got a ride to Lake Louise.

The second team that assembled the following morning at Lake Louise now included Gord Peyto, a new Parks Canada dog handler, as well as the seasoned dog handler Chris Banham, from the Cochrane RCMP detachment.

Burstrom was pumped for this search and wasted no time getting to the deposit ahead of the others. With a poor weather forecast, he wanted this to be a quick recovery. After a short ski, the team approached the toe of the first deposit and saw a ski pole high up on the avalanche. Ginger found the first person buried under a metre of snow, nine metres out from the toe of the avalanche. Alfie put him back to work immediately, and seven metres away Ginger found the second body. It was all over in less than five minutes even before the other handlers had a chance to get to the search site.

Though Alfie worked well with Ginger, Earl's dog was often unreliable around other people because of his aggressive nature, and Jack's dog had health problems that sometimes affected his working capabilities. The uneven success of the dog program prompted a review of procedures to determine where improvements could be made.

The review recognized that a dog could cover an avalanche deposit 30–50 times faster than a probe line. With the spotty use of avalanche beacons in the seventies and early eighties, dogs were still the most efficient search tool available. Everyone agreed that the dog should be on scene first and be given a chance to work without the distractions of a probe line or unnecessary helicopter activity. The question of contamination was addressed. Most important of all, the review recognized that dog handlers must know how to use the dog properly and insist they be given the chance to do so. In other words, they must be more assertive in the field. This also meant being fully trained in avalanche behaviour. The dogs must be trained to ignore unanticipated distractions, though it was recognized that like people, they had good and bad days when it came to focus, concentration and energy levels.

With many of these nagging questions addressed, the dog program moved forward into a new phase. Earl and Jack had pioneered dog work in Banff National Park and had had success in elevating the dog program. With their retirement came the desire to hire younger dog handlers with broader skiing and mountaineering skills.

Jack had one last success while searching for two climbers who went missing on Mount Stephen near Field, B.C. A helicopter search was initiated, but falling snow and poor visibility hampered progress. Eventually tracks were found entering the starting zone of a recent avalanche, and a short time later the helicopter spotted one victim on the surface. Once the body was removed, Woledge and the dog were slung into the site, and after a short search the dog found the second body. With that, the team took pleasure on being able to retire on a positive note.

When Woledge retired in 1981, Parks selected two wardens, Gord Peyto and Dale Portman, to be in place when Skjonsberg would retire in a few years. Peyto started training in the fall of 1980 and graduated with his dog Saxon in January, 1981. Portman started to train in September of that year and was out in the field with Chip in January, 1982. Portman was stationed in Lake Louise, Alberta, while Peyto worked out of Glacier/ Revelstoke National Park in British Columbia. Alfie Burstrom was working with a new dog and went into training at the same time as Portman. But Parks Canada actually created another dog position during the expansive years of the eighties

and brought Scott Ward in as Earl Skjonsberg's replacement in Banff. Scott graduated from Innisfail, Alberta, in 1984 with Gypsy, a female, and joined the boys in the field.

Ward, Peyto and Portman were about the same age and had grown up together in the outfit. They found it easy to set up mutual training sessions. This camaraderie kept their enthusiasm up, and soon their dogs were performing at very high standards.

ONE OF THE ADVANTAGES the warden dog handlers had over the RCMP was being part of an experienced rescue team. By contrast, the RCMP dog handlers, who responded to incidents outside of national parks, often found themselves the only experienced person on-site working with volunteers who had only basic avalanche rescue training. The RCMP dog handlers realized their mountain rescue training had to expand to include avalanche behaviour and search management. Parks Canada stepped up its mountain rescue training for the RCMP, placing more emphasis on these skills.

The dual role of the RCMP dog handler was emphasized on two avalanche accidents involving snowmobiles in 1984. Recreational snowmobiling was rapidly becoming the new "fun sport" that appealed to people who had no familiarity with mountains or mountain hazards. Many of them came from cities—avalanches were as foreign to them as tidal waves to the desert dweller. The practice of driving to the highest point on an avalanche slope meant heading into the trigger zone, which often led to the release of a major avalanche. Because snowmobilers didn't understand avalanches, they were generally not equipped with proper survival gear (except for shovels needed to dig out a bogged-down machine).

The first of a rash of accidents occurred in the Flathead Pass, just west of the continental divide. Three snowmobilers on a day trip were trying to drive successively higher on a fairly large avalanche path using the previous track

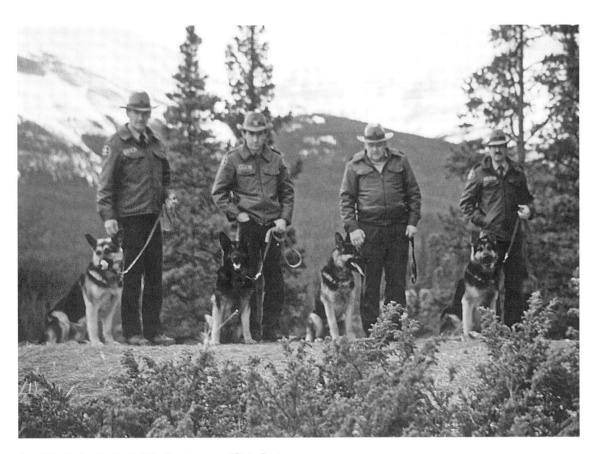

Gord Peyto, Scott Ward, Alfie Burstrom and Dale Portman. DALE PORTMAN COLLECTION

as a runway to launch themselves upward at maximum speed.

While two of them parked in the middle of the avalanche runout zone, adjusting the carburettors on their machines, the third madman made another run up the track. He was heading down for another try when the huge slope released, quickly gobbling up both him and the machine. When the two snowmobilers below saw what was coming there was little they could do. One fellow with a spark plug in his hand ducked behind his snowmobile while the other jumped on his machine and tried to outrun the wave of snow but to no avail. It was now two o'clock in the afternoon.

Fortunately another group of snowmobilers were playing in the area and were able to render assistance. The fellow who had started the avalanche found himself with a fractured hip, partially buried in the run-out zone. The second victim was completely buried, 30 centimetres down with internal injuries. There was no sign of the third man or his dismantled machine. Totally unprepared for such an event, the remaining snowmobilers tried to use branches as improvised probes to search while two others went for help.

Four hours later, the first party of rescuers arrived. Under the direction of a Provincial Emergency Program coordinator, the probe lines began working the deposit. Three quarters of an hour later, Gord Burns, an RCMP dog handler from Cranbrook, B.C., arrived with his dog Griz. He immediately assessed the hazard and then requested floodlights be brought in for the searchers. But he was dismayed to find the site was almost impossible for the dog to work because of all the contamination. A helicopter had landed on the part of the deposit that had the highest probability of search potential. The entire surface was littered with food and paper from lunch remains; people had urinated on the deposit; and pieces of snowmobile lay scattered about. Rescuers cleaned up the site as much as possible before sending the dog in.

In addition to this, Burns was unable to establish the last seen point of the missing man. Nevertheless, the dog soon found the buried snowmobile and other articles, allowing probers to move in and search more thoroughly. They soon found the third victim buried under two metres of snow, close to his snowmobile. In the official report on the accident, Corporal Burns commented, "Snowmobilers seem to be attracted by open smooth slopes. This was the case on the day of the accident, when tracks could be seen on several avalanche paths." He goes on further to say, "The party was aware of avalanches and the associated hazard, and the survivor stated that he had not wanted to push his luck and therefore stayed at the bottom." They may have been aware of avalanches but clearly knew nothing about trigger zones.

The second accident took place at remote Redfern Lake, 120 kilometres west of the Alaska Highway on the eastern slopes of the Rocky Mountains. Winter access to the area was only by snow machine or by helicopter at the time. On February 11th, 1984, five snowmobilers left a trapper's cabin for an outing in the mountains. By noon they had driven 40 kilometres and had stopped below a large knoll in the middle of an avalanche path. One member left with his machine to do some exploring, followed shortly by another, leaving three men sitting below the knoll. The men below the protecting outcrop suddenly heard a sound like an explosion and seconds later saw a rider coming full speed down a gully toward them. He was only slightly ahead of a huge avalanche cloud that soon overtook him, swallowing him from sight. The three men below were saved by the knoll.

They could see one partially buried machine when the dust settled, but there was no trace of the two riders or the second snow machine. The three survivors searched for two hours before one of the men drove 30 kilometres away to a cabin where he could call for help by radio phone. The closest available avalanche dog was 650 kilometres away and could not reach the site till the next day. In the meantime, the two other men had returned to the scene and managed to locate the second machine by probing with oars from a boat, before darkness forced them to quit.

The first help to arrive the next morning were volunteers with proper probes from the Provincial Emergency Program. RCMP dog handler Jim Brewin arrived on-site at 1:00 p.m. and immediately saw that several holes had been dug near the snowmobiles and that people were scattered about the deposit randomly probing. Jim, who had sufficient training to recognize the avalanche hazard, first established an avalanche spotter and an escape route in case of further avalanches. He directed the searchers where to probe, and they found the first body a half hour later.

The dog indicated a spot near the second machine, but probing turned up nothing. Though the dog searched elsewhere, he returned to the same spot again and strongly indicated. Brewin continued to probe the site without success. But the dog returned to the spot a third time, pushing people aside and again digging with his paws. After more digging and probing, the body was discovered 2.1 metres down in an upright position. His helmet had a few probe marks on it; it had felt like a layer of ice to the probers.

The snowmobiler who had driven like hell ahead of the billowing mass of airborne snow had finally run out of luck. He was found five metres from the edge of the deposit, mere seconds from climbing to safety up the other side of the small valley.

It was becoming evident that volunteer groups like the Provincial Emergency Program needed better instruction in avalanche search management and safety. Parks Canada and the RCMP, in conjunction with their dog handlers, started to provide instruction to local Provincial Emergency Program groups and began to include them in future training scenarios.

TEACHING DOGS TO TRACK FUGITIVES was a big part of the RCMP training program, and Parks Canada quickly adapted the dogs' ability to find missing people. Though it was less common to use dogs as the primary search tool in ground searches and water rescues, they saved many lives. The United States began using dogs to search rivers and lakes in the mid-1980s. In Canada, their use came about more or less by accident.

Early in Burstrom's career with Ginger, he was called to search the Maligne River for a missing girl who had fallen into Maligne Canyon, a popular tourist attraction in Jasper. Burstrom was initially brought in to check deep holes in the canyon, because he was adept at rappelling into dangerous places. But he felt that was a waste of his expertise, and he insisted he be allowed to search the riverbank with Ginger instead. The search master thought this was a waste of time, but to save arguing, he sent Alfie to walk the lower reaches of the river with Ginger as company, if that's what made him happy.

It was not long before Ginger pulled yet another trick out of the hat. The dog soon indicated a point where the river was deeply undercut. Burstrom couldn't see anything in the dark water, however, so he continued his walk along the bank. But Ginger knew what he was there for and returned to the same spot, peering into the water again. The dog was working a scent that was obviously reaching him on the riverbank. The wind was blowing lightly from the west, assisting him as they worked the east bank.

Warden Dale Portman was there that morning and remembers seeing Burstrom peering into the swiftly running water. He remembers that "[Alfie] called over warden Max Winkler and myself to look as well. You could see something waxy like, maybe a hand, waving in the current, but we had to look hard to see it. We put a rope around Max's waist and I held him while he crawled into the river. The current was strong, and I remember this big man bracing himself submerged up to his chest. Sure enough he felt clothing and then a hand, and it was a bit of a struggle to get her free, but he did and we pulled her up onto shore."

Though it was a body recovery, the dog's success was the talk of the town for several days afterward. The ability of dogs to detect bodies in rivers soon led trainers to see if dogs would have similar success in still waters such as lakes. Some of the RCMP dog handlers in B.C. were now training their dogs to specifically search lakes and rivers. A U.S. training video had recently surfaced on how to train dogs to search rivers and lakes from the bow of a boat. The Parks Canada dog handlers were eager to extend their training into this profile and found themselves getting together in Jasper, one fine summer morning in 1990, for their first Water Rescue Dog Course. It went over well using training aids and methods recommended in the American training video. The RCMP, who had taken the lead in developing this capability in Canada, were happy to pass this expertise to Parks Canada dog teams.

In the summer of 1991, Gord Peyto and his new working dog, Baron, had the first success in a national park using this new method of searching. Since Ginger's success in 1971, Parks Canada dogs had only found drowned people who were washed ashore. That was about to change. Two men had gone canoeing in Hector Lake near Lake Louise when their canoe capsized, and both men ended up swimming for shore. Only one man made it, and the wardens in Banff initiated a search for the second person. Peyto and Baron were searching from the shore of the lake when the dog winded something out in the lake. The

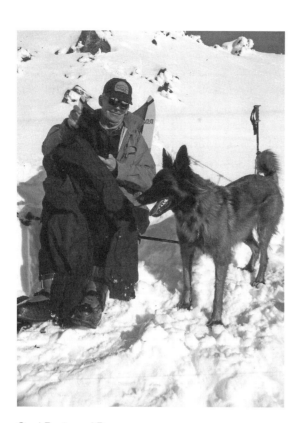

Gord Peyto and Baron. HANS FUHRER COLLECTION

recovered; technically the dog could not be credited with finding a submerged body. But because rescuers had seen the body from the air, everyone realized the importance of the dog's indication. It unofficially confirmed that the training was not wasted.

Dogs were also becoming useful in ground search and rescue. However, when dogs are required to look for lost climbers in mountaineering situations, they are often limited by steep terrain. But dogs have other heightened senses besides smell. On two occasions Parks dogs turned around a search that would otherwise have resulted in the deaths of the missing people.

In a late afternoon in July of 1987, the weather held good promise as two staff members working at Sunwapta Falls Bungalows went off to hike up a mountain just across the valley from the lodge. It was a popular retreat for staff, and they were last seen sitting on top of a rock outcrop in the early evening. When they hadn't returned the next morning, the lodge notified the Warden Service in Jasper. It was decided that because there was a known last seen point, a dog would be useful in determining which way they had gone.

Portman and his dog Sam picked up a spotty track which they followed to a minor timbered ridge where the track petered out. They were accompanied by Art Lawrenson. It had been drizzling all morning, but by noon the team was overtaken by a wet snowstorm. They located a promising footprint, and so the trio continued to climb, but the dog was finding little scent to work with. The wet snow was accumulating on the flat slab rocks above treeline, covering scent and becoming treacherous and slippery for all—particularly for the dog, who was having trouble maintaining his purchase on the slippery rocks. They carried on climbing until Portman decided it was too dangerous for the dog to continue.

If the couple had come this way, they were going to be in serious trouble, because they had set out with only light blazers and had no spare warm clothing or food. As a last resort Portman

dog ran back and forth along the shore feathering the wind, trying to zero in on the scent. Finally the dog jumped into the lake and swam out for some distance. To Peyto's astonishment, Baron then started to swim in a tight circle in one spot. Peyto quickly jumped into a canoe and paddled out to the dog, who was now swimming in even tighter circles and poking his head into the water. Peyto threw out a buoy to mark the spot and retrieved his remarkable dog.

Because the lake water was so silty it was hard to see much from the boat. Thinking it would be easier to spot a figure from the air, he sent for the helicopter. Sure enough the wardens could see a body in the murky water, two or three metres below the surface. It took a few hours to get a dive team to search the lake; unfortunately the visibility was so poor they could not find the body. To this day the body has never been gave out a couple of yells then listened for an answer over the wind. They heard nothing and turned to start down. But on a whim Portman decided to give one more call before retreating. "I gave a couple of yells, then listened for an answer. When none came, I turned to start climbing down—until I noticed Sam. He was looking up the mountain, ears cocked, while slowly angling his head back and forth. He seemed to hear something we couldn't. I pointed this out to Art, who looked at Sam with both puzzlement and hope. It was enough to convince me to continue."

Sam was left tied to a rock while Portman and Lawrenson climbed farther. He goes on to say, "Art and I pushed over the slick rock. After about 15 minutes, we stopped and yelled again. We were going to have to turn around soon, as we were getting into terrain where we would need a climbing rope to continue … Finally over the sound of the wind, we detected a faint echo. Someone was calling for help. We had found them."

The couple were still a considerable way up, however, and so a climbing team was called in. Portman was concerned that the dog might break free from his tether and try to join them, so he returned to the dog. Lawrenson continued on and eventually got within 15 metres of the couple but could go no farther without a rope. It became too steep above and too exposed below. It took the rescue team, who had slung in with a break in the weather, another two hours to get to the couple with directions provided by Portman and Lawrenson over the radio. The weather was making things very treacherous for everyone. The severely hypothermic couple had to be lowered very carefully down through the rocks before they arrived at a spot where the helicopter could sling them out. In hindsight, if the dog hadn't heard them and if Portman had missed the indication, they would have perished.

In the second case, Scott Ward and his dog Smokey were called out to what was reported as calls for help on Sulphur Mountain in Banff National Park. It was March 1989, and it had been a mild winter with little snow around the townsite. When Ward investigated, the staff thought it was probably some kids fooling around above the hot springs. There wasn't much to go on, and when he yelled up the mountain, he got nothing in return. He decided he would try to pick up a track behind the hot springs with the dog. The dog quickly picked up a track, but lots of people frequented the area so Ward wasn't too excited about it.

The dog tracked up the mountain in a zigzag fashion through the trees and small cliff bands. It was tiring even for a long distance runner like Ward, and he had to make the dog wait on a few occasions while he caught his breath. Eventually they arrived at the base of an area covered by interlocking cliffs where the dog struggled to keep his footing. If the track continued upward it would eventually lead to a gradual climb to the summit and the top station of the gondola lift.

The dog now started to track laterally toward a snow-choked ravine when his head swivelled to the right, and he started clawing his way up a steep slope toward a man perched on a small rock shelf. The man had broken his leg while scrambling over a cliff and had given up on anyone hearing his cries for help. Nightfall was quickly approaching, and he had little clothing to protect himself from the sub-zero temperature that would ensue.

He had started the day hoping to gain the ridge and have an easy stroll to the top of the mountain and the gondola terminal. From there he planned to take the gondola down and celebrate by taking a dip in the Sulphur Hot Springs. It is doubtful he would have survived long that high up on the mountain in March, especially with the light clothing he had on. He was soon packaged up and slung off the mountain in the diminishing light of the day.

Because dogs are able to cover avalanche ground much more quickly than rescuers can, they are often used instead of a large rescue team to recover bodies when conditions are dangerous. But sometimes recovering a body is just not worth the risk—a conclusion Portman came to after being called to search on a route called Slipstream, an ice climb on The Snow Dome in the Columbia Icefield. It was April 4th, 1989, and two separate parties were climbing the route. The two Americans in the first group had reached the top and were looking for the descent gulley, which was difficult to spot from the corniced edge of the rounded mountaintop. At about the fourth or fifth vertical gully to the south, one of them decided to probe his way cautiously to the edge and peer over for a better look. Not being roped to his partner, he promptly disappeared from view when the piece of cornice that he was standing on broke away. With no protection, his partner was not able to safely approach the edge to ascertain his fate.

When the second party got to the top of the climb a couple of hours later, they met the survivor at the start of the descent route and assisted him down. But this American was just not having a good day. On the descent, a member of the second party fell into the bergschrund. Because they were now roped up, they were able to bring him up unharmed but not without consequence. While assisting him out of the crevasse, his partner suffered a dislocated shoulder. He was left behind in a tent at the base camp while the other two walked out to the highway to report the accident. It was now well into the night when they arrived at the warden's door at 2:00 a.m.

Darro Stinson, the rescue leader, assessed the situation early the next morning and determined that the main objective was to evacuate the injured climber and then concentrate on searching for the American who had fallen. The rescue party was in place at 7:30 a.m., waiting for the helicopter to arrive from Valemount, B.C. In the meantime a party of two were sent in on skis to the base camp. When the helicopter arrived at 9:10 a.m. they quickly evacuated the victim at the tent site, and he was out by 9:30 a.m. Now Darro hoped for a similarly quick recovery of the missing climber.

A helicopter reconnaissance showed a probable accident site where a metre-long section of cornice was missing. It was directly above the four or five chutes on the east face just south of the ice climb. The rescuers determined that if the victim had not got hung up on the face of the mountain or come to rest on the fan, he would have continued down into some large crevasses below where recovery would be very difficult.

Scott Ward, the dog handler from Banff, was called in, and he viewed the search area from the air. Spindrift avalanches had been falling on the site throughout the day, and Ward declared the present conditions too unstable to put the team in the area to search. Due to the continuing avalanche and weather conditions, the operation was suspended for the day. The next day, April 5, produced even worse conditions, with 20 centimetres of new snow overnight and poor visibility. It wasn't until the 8th that the weather lifted sufficiently for the helicopter to access the site. Even so the area was shrouded in clouds until mid-afternoon when things started to clear up. At 4:00 p.m. the helicopter finally lifted off with Dale Portman and his dog Sam, from Jasper, and Frank Staples. On the flight to the search site, they were entertained by the collapse of a monstrous ice fall that bellowed down the mountain, obscuring any view of the search area for five minutes.

The helicopter returned to the staging area, because it was too dangerous to search until a bombing run could stabilize the place. Three sets of three charges were dropped in the gullies south of the slipstream above the search area with good results. Lookouts were then strategically placed with panoramic views of the entire east face of Snow Dome. Again Portman, Staples and the dog flew to the site. The two men and the dog roped up to cross the glacial terrain in a gradual ascent to the site. Once there, the group unroped and the dog began searching the avalanche fan below the 4th and 5th gullies. Below lay a giant crevasse that would easily consume any avalanche debris that reached it. While the team searched, Staples dug a pit. As Portman said later, "I looked below and saw the gaping chasm of a huge crevasse waiting for us. Frank stood by the pit he had just finished

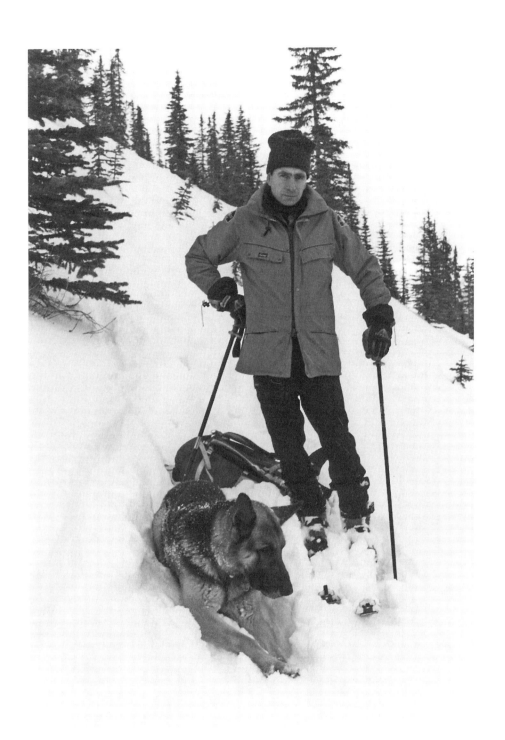

Scott Ward and Dana. KANANASKIS COUNTRY PUBLIC SAFETY ARCHIVES digging. It was about 1.5 metres deep and just big enough for the three of us to fit into if necessary. We had 8 to 10 seconds to reach the hole if or when the next avalanche came. If the ice broke above, the lookout in the valley would sound the alarm over the radio and we would sprint." If they had been hit by even a light avalanche they would most likely have been swept off the steep slope into the crevasse below. After working the area for a couple of hours with no result, daylight was running out and the search was suspended.

With two areas still to be searched, it was decided that Ward would be called up again from Banff to help out. The next morning, warden Murray Hindle accompanied Portman and Sam on the first flight. They were unnerved to see the area they had landed on yesterday covered in huge blocks of ice from a fresh icefall overnight. They were able to land nearby. As Portman, Hindle and the dog proceeded to rope up, an avalanche swept down and covered the entire search area; it would have swept them into the crevasse below had they arrived five minutes earlier. A lively discussion ensued among Stinson, Hindle and Portman, and it was decided that conditions were far too dangerous to continue searching for the missing climber. They felt they had been seriously tempting fate. The victim was obviously dead and there was no need to add to the body collection.

This situation repeated itself a few years later when two climbers fell off Slipstream without a trace. The base of the climb is a fan that gets rapidly steeper with the approach turning quickly to ice. It is not a place to spend time loitering about and is certainly only searched using the dog after careful consideration. The two climbers that fell that day were found later that summer in the large crevasse at the base of the fan.

DALE PORTMAN RETIRED from dog work in 1992 after 12 years as a dog handler. In that period he saw the dog program evolve into the multi-profile capability the current dog teams enjoy in Parks Canada. Prior to leaving this part of the job,

however, he was happy to have the chance along with Scott Ward and Gord Peyto to participate in updating Parks Canada's dog training standards to correspond with the update done by the RCMP in their new manual.

When Dale Portman retired as a dog handler, he helped pick his successor, Will Devlin, who took over the Jasper position in 1995. Scott notes that Devlin's avalanche forecasting background allowed him to bring "RCMP and Parks avalanche dog training [courses and validation] to a higher level." It also meant they moved on to more challenging scenarios and terrain. Gord Peyto retired from the Warden Service in 1997, and Scott Ward retired from his dog position in 2001. Devlin spent six years as a dog handler in Jasper and took over running the public safety program there as well. By the end of the decade, Devlin concentrated fully on running the program, and the dog handler position was filled by Darien Sillence. Mike Henderson and Attila competed successfully for Scott Ward's vacant position, which now completed the full complement of Parks Canada's dog teams. Gord Peyto's position in Glacier/Revelstoke was cancelled due to government downsizing in the late 1990s, and was not refilled.

The dog program in Parks Canada was uncommonly lucky in having Alfie Burstrom and his remarkable dog Ginger to set the standard and prove the value of the dog. But one successful team does not ensure the acceptance of those that follow, and each successive dog handler had to prove again that the dog was worth the kibble the parks were paying for his upkeep. Each success and failure was felt keenly by every man who took on the job—the pressure never let up. Both Darien and Mike often felt like they were proving for the first time that their dog could do the job. And this did not change—each new mission was like the first. Ultimately, the dog man is alone in the field with all eyes on him. But the opportunity to work with dogs and to rise to the challenges of the job seem worth the risk as the competition is fierce when the positions become available.

6 The Climbing Generation: Camelot Years

EVEN BEFORE WALTER PERREN took on the daunting task of forming the first professional mountain rescue program in Canada, the frontiers of climbing were being pushed by young aggressive men fresh from Europe who had already exceeded anything dreamt of in these uncultivated Alps. This new wave of aggressive young climbers were soon ticking off the formidable routes on the north faces of the higher peaks in the Rockies.

Ironically, much of the push in climbing came from the men who had founded the Guides Association under Walter Perren's direction. Hans Gmoser—now a good friend of Walter's—and Leo Grillmair both became guides, as did Brian Greenwood and Don Vockeroth, the excellent young Canadian climber who went on to establish some of the hardest routes on Yamnuska. Unfortunately, the veteran wardens were far behind these new climbing standards. This same group of climbers were also taking their expertise into the national parks and pioneering audacious new routes on the big mountains such as Mt. Alberta and Mt. Temple. Some of these climbs led to rescues such as the one on Mt. Babel.

Then there were the Americans who were attracted to the grotty, dangerous north faces of the Rockies described by Chic Scott, author of *Pushing the Limits,* as "cold and wet and raked by rock fall … enough to frighten the bravest climber." Usually found in the remoter parts of the country and often beset with bad weather, they presented some of the greatest mountaineering challenges of the day. But the wardens didn't worry as much about men like Chris Jones or the Lowe brothers as they did about those who would follow.

Daunting challenges were opening up on other fronts as well. The new sport of ice climbing on frozen waterfalls was being invented right at their back door. Bugs McKeith, a naturalized Canadian from Scotland, joined up with British climber Dick Howe to climb some truly scary routes. The whole sport was revolutionized by the invention of the pterodactyl, a cunningly restructured ice axe with a head that is bent sharply downwards with serrated teeth on the undershaft to provide bite in the ice. A climber could actually swing the instrument overhead, imbedding it into vertical ice, allowing him to pull himself up. That, and the newly reconstructed front 12-point crampon which eliminated the need to cut steps and increased the angle of ice that could be climbed.

There were other developments in both skiing and in river sports as well. The latest development in the skiing world was the use of light cross-country skis from Norway. The principal proponent of their use was Don Gardner, one of Canada's leading climbers and cross-country ski racers in the sixties. He loved to engage in long-distance winter ski trips in the mountains, made possible by travelling on light gear. If the wardens thought that abandoning snowshoes for downhill ski gear was a stretch, the move to "misery sticks" was beyond them. News of Don's proposal to ski from Jasper to Lake Louise via the Great Divide on cross-country skis left them baffled. Although they did not refuse to register the trip, someone mentioned the men should not expect a rescue at the end of the thirty-five day trip if they didn't return. Rescue was not something any of the men expected, but the success of their trip did open the door to travel of this nature on all the big icefields.

In the summer, the rivers were now being scouted for the burgeoning new sport of kayaking. Whitewater challenges were accelerated to higher grades, almost to the point of going over waterfalls. In fact, the Germans, who seemed to be particularly advanced in this sport, did undertake paddling over smaller falls if they thought they'd survive. Rafting through rapids was also gaining in popularity, and it was not long before rafting companies sprang up to tap into a whole new tourist adventure.

What was pushing this bold front in all realms of mountain activity was the emergence of a new class of citizen with an open-minded approach to life … the Baby Boomers. The Boomers had missed the depravation of the Second World War and the hardships of the depression. Perhaps it was the predictability of the world that led them to adopt radical changes in thought and action. They rebelled against pedantic security in a chaotic celebration of freedom that was often risky. They sought out new experiences and did so explosively in numbers that staggered the resources of the national mountain parks, which had to deal with the swarm of neophyte adventurers.

WHEN PETER AND WILLI took over from Walter Perren, they inherited an aging generation of wardens who had valiantly taken on the mantle of public safety because it was part of a job they loved. But engaging in risky sports was never a way of life for them, which limited them from reaching the top of the profession. Both Willi and Peter knew a younger generation of wardens were needed to fill this role.

Unfortunately, when both specialists took over in 1968, Prime Minister Trudeau had slapped a hiring freeze on government staffing, preventing the recruitment of any new wardens. Willi, himself, had only managed to get on through a reclassification procedure in Jasper, which still baffles him to this day. One young warden, Bob Haney, who hired on as seasonal in 1965, slipped under the wire of this freeze only to find himself a youngster amongst the older veterans. He was well aware that mountain rescue was part of the job and realized that doors would open if he improved his skills. The hiring freeze was actually to his advantage when a job came up in Rogers Pass, as he was one of the few wardens on staff available for the work.

Bob was not totally a neophyte when it came to skiing; he had received some rudimentary training while working at the ski hill in Lake Louise. But he recognized that he had a lot to learn in skiing and in avalanche research and that these would be the requirements of the coming age. He leapt at the chance to work in this environment and learn from those who were setting the standards of the day. He was not wrong. Rogers Pass would prove to be a valuable stepping stone for many a young warden with aspirations for the field of public safety and the jobs that lay beyond.

Gordon Peyto had also started in Waterton and had taken the same wise course of working at the pass during 1969–70. Gord, however, was a very good skier. He was the grandnephew of one of the original wardens, Bill Peyto, and had grown up in Banff where he learned to ski at an early age. He was young, fit and strong, so adapting to the rigours of deep powder skiing at the pass was not a big stretch. He soon played an integral part in the public safety program in Glacier National Park, which eventually led to his becoming a dog handler.

While Willi saw the recruitment of Gord and Bob as a beginning and worked vigorously to encourage them to come into the public safety program, he knew this was not enough. Another young Waterton warden, Duane Martin, also recognized that the older men were limited in the role of mountain rescue. He reflects: "The guys in those days did not relate to the climbers … they saw climbers as risk takers and always questioned the sensibility of those who undertook the activity." Duane was not about to start climbing and soon found himself seeking a better future in other areas. But the seventies wrought unexpected changes, and within five years he returned to take up the sport and to play a vital role in public safety in Jasper National Park.

Indeed, the whole warden way of life at the end of the sixties needed the infusion of younger people, which began when the hiring ban was lifted in the early 1970s. The wave of young men and women would soon generate these changes. The earliest and one of the most dynamic of these was a very youthful Tim Auger.

Like many of the gifted young climbers on Canada's west coast, Tim evinced a predilection for climbing at an early age. He was actually raised in Winnipeg, Manitoba, so his inspiration did not come from visions of beckoning heights, but rather from telephone poles, houses, fences … anything vertical. Fortunately for Tim, his parents moved to Vancouver when he was 12, and sensing a growing interest in the sport, his mother brought home one of the classic books of mountaineering, *The White Spider* by Heinrich Harrer. The mountain setting and the inspiration of the book set Tim on a course he never deviated from. By his late teens he was headed for where "the real action was" … a mountain called The Chief at the nearby town of Squamish. The Squamish Chief had a major geological feature called The Grand Wall which was exactly what it sounded like. A huge soaring vertical wall of solid granite rock that challenged climbers to leave their signature and dare others to follow.

Tim was inspired by the climbers who established first ascents on this daunting ground. His own first ascent of University Wall established him as a leading Canadian climber at a fairly young age. Though Tim thought he had found his true calling, he also pursued a degree in fine arts at the University of British Columbia in Vancouver. Tim longed to chase his climbing dreams to Yosemite and other rock meccas in the States, but he needed to earn money if he wished to stay in school and keep climbing. But he wanted to remain in the mountains at least, so he was particularly attentive when two other young men "cut from the same cloth" showed up on his doorstep and mentioned the possibility of working on trail crew in the parks. Chic Scott was making a name for himself as a climber in the Calgary area, but it was Jerry Walsh who sparked Tim's attention when he mentioned he had the trail crew job in Yoho National Park. What could be more ideal? Work in the summer in the heart of the Rockies and climb in the off-season down in the States while finishing a degree in the winter … great planning! Tim's previous summer jobs in "fishing-camp country, swatting mosquitoes" paled by comparison.

Inspired, he sent off an application to the park and was hired on in the summer of 1967. While there, he became acquainted with the Warden Service, and though he had no intention of following this line of work, the wheels were set in motion. Tim was not disappointed in his first summer at Yoho. He met up with other climbers of great calibre like Fred Becky and Galen Rowell with whom he was able to undertake some good climbs—one of them a difficult new route on Mt. Louis near Banff. But possibly more significant, he was introduced to the intoxicating mountain world of Lake O'Hara. Before setting foot in the place, he had heard all about it from the family of a climbing buddy in Vancouver. He was not disappointed and soon became enchanted with the peaks surrounding the small alpine lake. He didn't know it then, but Lake O'Hara nestled in his heart, laying the spell that would cement his future decisions and a career in public safety with the wardens.

Rescuing people for a living was not something that occurred to Tim either at the time, but he thought it something a responsible climber should be familiar with. He spent time in the Vancouver area training with the local MRG (Mountain Rescue Group), learning improvised rescue and extending his knowledge of rope work.

This came in handy during that first summer when he convinced Sid Marty, the local Lake O'Hara warden, to climb Grassi Ridge—one of the great classic rock climbs in the area. Tim can't help but remember it was one of those fine fall days that blesses the lake and surrounding peaks with jewel-clear air and balmy temperatures. They were surprised by the unusual presence of two parties ahead of them. This meant they were just below when a member of the first party dislodged a large rock which landed on the foot of the second party leader. Peter Spear, the injured man, happily accepted the aid of the warden and his assistant, Tim—who engineered the rescue.

As Tim says, he knew a little bit about improvised rescue: "We had the ingredients because I had heard about the split coil carry … a coil of rope is split in a certain way so you can put the patient's legs through [the loops] and basically pick them up like a pack and piggyback them down." He added "The second ingredient was having Sid. Sid is big and quite strong, so he was the obvious one to actually pick Peter up." The two of them were able to lower the injured man straight down a gully system to the Lake O'Hara Fire Road without undue complication. Although they were "a way up off the ground," Tim was quite comfortable with what he had to do and was quite pleased with the outcome. It was the

beginning of what he would spend the rest of his life doing for a living.

Tim returned to Lake O'Hara as the local warden in a seasonal position after writing to ask if the job was available. Ironically, he got a letter of acceptance from the park just as he was rolling into a big climbing year at Yosemite, which put him in a momentary quandary. But "there was this gnawing thing … you know, it was the beauty of Lake O'Hara that made me think: you've got to go back there. That place is like heaven … and there are *mountains!*" Truly hooked, he was in his element, and despite mouth-watering postcards from friends in Yosemite, climbing everything he had hoped to get up, he immersed himself in the new job.

The other wardens, too, were happy to have him. Gordon Rutherford, a senior warden who was his boss, remembers those years fondly. And Tim was quite happy to extend his talents to other wardens or anyone else who wanted to get out and climb. In those days there was not an overabundance of willing partners, though he could still count on Sid Marty to show up. Gord Rutherford was of the same mind and truly enjoyed getting out with Tim in his district. When management abandoned the district system and swung into the function system, Rutherford was put into the public safety role and so continued to climb with Tim for the years he remained in the park.

BY THE LATE SIXTIES, even before Walter Perren died, Tim realized park managers were "actively looking for guys who could travel well in the mountains and had a good potential for learning to climb." When the hiring freeze was lifted, there was a spate of applications from young men who were attracted to the Warden Service, even if they didn't come equipped with the skills. One who would have a lasting influence on the development of the public safety program was Clair Israelson.

Clair was actually hired through a very active recruiting program in 1971 while attending BCIT studying, appropriately, park planning. He recalls

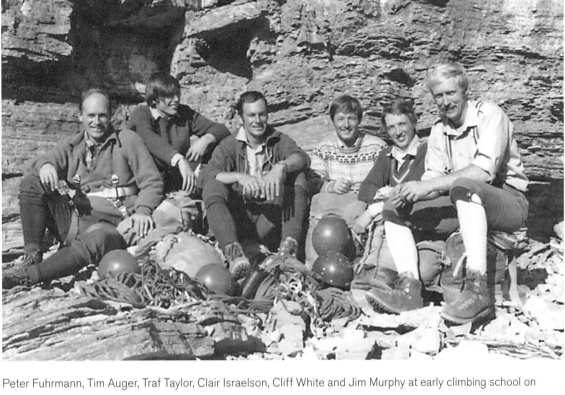

Peter Fuhrmann, Tim Auger, Traf Taylor, Clair Israelson, Cliff White and Jim Murphy at early climbing school on Castle Mountain. BANFF WARDEN ARCHIVES

that national parks came through looking for potential candidates and invited many for an interview. Clair was intrigued. Obviously the recruiters made the job sound pretty attractive to Clair, as he was just the material they were looking for. Not only did he have the right academic credentials, he also looked like he could do the work. Relatively tall with an athletic frame and squinty eyes that could be disconcertingly direct, he impressed the board enough to hire him. Though "it sounded like a fun thing to do for the summer," he had no intention of staying on full time. But after his first summer as a seasonal park warden in Waterton Lakes National Park, he changed his mind. As he puts it he "had a wonderful time and stayed for 26 years."

Though he had not taken up climbing to the degree that Tim had before becoming a warden, he knew he "had a huge interest in the mountains." In fact, running off to the mountains almost jeopardized high school through playing hooky, but that was where he wanted to be. This led to involvement with the outdoor club at school and ski trips on the north shore mountains of Vancouver. He was introduced to basic climbing and certainly did plenty of scrambling in his forays from school, but his real development as a climber began once he joined the Warden Service.

The potential for doing exciting work became evident to Clair shortly after he arrived in Waterton for the summer and was exposed to "all kinds of different training opportunities." Once again, the older wardens were happy to send the young guys out on schools they were rapidly losing interest in, which was no problem for Clair. "I couldn't believe it! … I mean, here I was … they were paying me to come to work, and then they'd send me off to climbing or skiing schools. I'm going to complain about that?"

One of the most important events of the summer was meeting Willi Pfisterer, who would become a teacher, mentor and lifelong friend. Willi set by example, and no greater impression could be made on a young man at a turning point of his life. Willi, of course, knew the importance of nurturing the future fodder for the rescue program he was entrusted with developing. He encouraged Clair to come to the schools, made sure he even had the equipment he needed and in general pushed him into public safety. Once Clair realized that this was what he was being groomed for—and what he wanted to do—he embraced the program with a vengeance.

After his summer in Waterton, he was offered a choice of two term positions for the winter: one in Rogers Pass and the other in Yoho National Park. He chose Yoho because he felt he would get the greatest exposure to a winter training environment there rather than Rogers Pass. He was rewarded by being sent on yet more schools, this time touring in the "wild places in the Rockies." Although he had the basics of skiing on groomed slopes, this was a whole new dimension of the sport that required good travel as well as skiing skills. Gord Rutherford, still in charge of public safety in Yoho recalls Clair returning from one school on the Wapta Icefield with very badly blistered feet. So bad, in fact, that he went to work in slippers until his feet healed. But Clair learned fast and never had to wear slippers to work again.

During that winter he was also introduced to avalanche control. It was the year following the huge avalanches of the 1970–71 season when the disastrous buildup of snow resulted in damage to roads, railroad tracks and parking lots. No one wanted that to happen again, so helicopter bombing was pursued throughout the winter. Bombing from a helicopter was very much in its infancy, with several of the older hands from Banff taking a lead role. He recalls John Wackerle,

in particular, as being very involved and capable, both in knowledge and experience in avalanche control. In fact, there was a lot of overlap between the younger, inexperienced wardens coming on strength and the seasoned veterans.

But the younger generation was eager for the responsibilities of rescue work, and as Clair's enthusiasm for the job escalated, so did the training opportunities. He was still shaking his head over how much Parks was prepared to invest in him, and he responded by applying himself to learn as much as possible. It paid off when he was invited to be the youngest member on the first warden team sent to climb Mt. Logan in the spring of 1973. Clair never looked back. He spent the next summer in Waterton, but things were moving fast, and that winter he was offered a full-time position in Banff. With characteristic independence and astuteness, he immediately asked to be sent to Lake Louise.

Clair initially went to Lake Louise as a "generalist" warden; he was assigned to the Lake Louise ski hill in the winter, but spent most of the summer in the backcountry. During front-country shifts, he was assigned to general duties (campground patrols, bears, jams, law enforcement problems, highway accidents), which included rescue work when required. At the time, Monty Rose was responsible for the public safety program and was also in charge of the ski hill operation. Though Monty had seen his fair share of rescues, climbing was not a natural vocation for him, and by the mid-seventies, he was happy to see the younger men take over. As soon as Clair learned to read a thermometer, he was given a green light to take up most of the duties at the hill. But this set him back a bit, because he did not feel he was ready for the responsibility. Nevertheless, he took the work very seriously and set a high standard for himself. This early mantle of responsibility set the tone for Clair that never let up during his tenure with Parks, and anyone who came to work for him knew early on it meant working hard under a baleful eye.

During the years when Clair first arrived, the ski area was undergoing review for expansion. In the 1960s Lake Louise put a bid in for the 1968 Winter Olympics but was turned down because of the controversy over allowing this activity in a national park. This was followed immediately by a proposal from Imperial Oil to build an international ski development not unlike the Imperial Ski Village in Aspen, Colorado. This unlikely development was thwarted at the last minute by an aggressive lobby group called the National Parks Association of Canada under the direction of Steve Herrero, a young biologist at the University of Calgary concerned about the welfare of the local grizzly bear population. But since the government had shown some initial leniency toward development, the various ski hill operations tenaciously dug in and lobbied for boundary definitions and expansion within their domain. The action prompted a review of all ski hill expansion, dragging in the ever-present issue of avalanche control. Clair was thrust into this controversial political atmosphere where he actually thrived.

It was a heady time to work at the hill in Lake Louise. Clair recalls: "We had a challenging atmosphere, we were all learning and we liked to be learning. And we had people who were motivated." The hill provided winter employment for many young seasonal wardens as well as opportunities to learn to ski and pick up the basics of avalanche control. Everyone seemed to have the constitution of an ox when it came to celebrating at the end of a long work shift. They still showed up the next morning as though they had slept peacefully all night. But they had to be alert to throw hand charges off wind-blown ridges, cut steep snow-loaded slopes, load and fire the ava-launcher at tricky targets and, if the weather was good, get a series of bombs off with the helicopter. It was demanding and physically exhausting work but with rarely a dull moment.

By 1975 the explosion of public safety incidents was beginning to overwhelm the wardens assigned to the work on a semi-casual basis. Up until then, the wardens had been on a rotating schedule of two weeks in the backcountry and two weeks in the frontcountry. But it was rapidly becoming apparent that this part-time approach wasn't sufficient to keep on top of the rescue demands. In Lake Louise, Clair found himself now heading up the public safety program full time under area manager Jack Woledge. Jack was trying to be an effective dog handler at the same time and was happy to let Clair run the public safety shop. With carte blanche to go ahead, Clair revamped the rescue room, updated the equipment, set up training schedules for the warden staff and in general took command. As the rescue load increased, he became even more acutely aware of his responsibility not only toward potential victims but also to the wardens themselves. He was determined to make it his business that nobody was hurt on his watch. Clair realized that training for mountain rescue must be a total commitment excluding any other work-related activity—for himself and any other warden wishing to play an active role in public safety.

One early episode brought home to Clair just how seriously the Warden Service was behind the standard of the day. When Clair mentioned he was going to climb the Greenwood Route on the Tower of Babel, he received a rather shocked silence. He felt the senior people in public safety thought he was going beyond his limits by foolishly undertaking such a drastic climb. In reality, it was not a difficult route by the standards of the day; in fact, Clair had some serious training ahead of him to bring himself up to the level of climbers setting new routes. Clair realized he had to set his standards with the Association of Canadian Mountain Guides.

SIMILAR CHANGES WERE OCCURRING in other national parks. The parks under Willi's jurisdiction were also seeing a much-needed influx of young wardens eager to be involved in public safety or any other exciting aspect of the Warden

Service. In Jasper, a young Brian Wallace was hired immediately after the hiring freeze was lifted in 1970. The other two wardens, Al Stendie and Abe Loewen, were targeted by Willi for as much public safety training as possible. Within the next two years a spate of others followed. Dale Portman transferred in from Lake Louise, while Duane Martin and Marv Millar came aboard in the early seventies. Murray Hindle joined the Warden Service in 1972 and immediately launched himself into the public safety program, signing up for every available training course. Because he was very slim and wiry, he appeared smaller than many of the others and always seemed to find himself at the bottom of a crevasse whenever these rescues popped up. Willi appreciated him, particularly after he discovered Murray had a slightly rebellious, independent streak. Willi liked war-

dens who argued a bit. It showed they cared and were thinking about what they were doing. What impressed everyone else, almost to the point of annoyance, was Murray's on-the-spot readiness for any rescue that came along. He travelled with his radio on and his knickers in the truck.

During this period, Tony Klettl was the senior warden assigned to the Marmot Ski Hill, which had opened in 1964. From this he also took over the role as the warden responsible for public safety in Jasper National Park. Again, the ski hill provided both winter work and the opportunity to learn the skills of the job for the young seasonal wardens. Although Marmot did not undergo any of the expansionist struggles of the ski areas to the south, they did move into some tricky avalanche terrain that needed control work, and a program similar to Lake Louise evolved at this hill. The

144

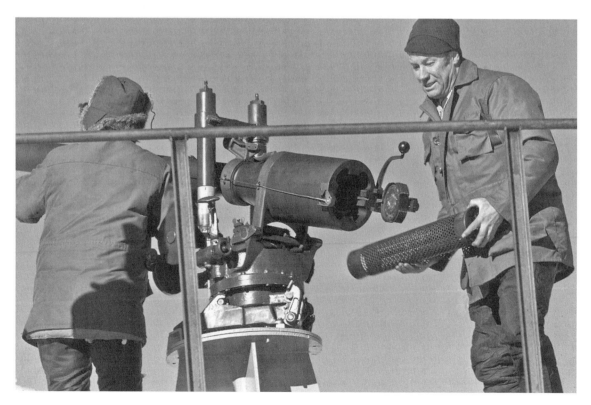

Tony Klettl and unknown warden firing a 105 mm recoilless rifle at Marmot Basin in the early 1970s. JASPER WARDEN ARCHIVES

same exciting atmosphere prevailed here as well. Everyone lived at an elevated level during the work day, trailing off to weekend parties or just an evening bar scene that slowed no one down.

They were working with marginally safe equipment that always added spice to the day. A new piece of equipment that would become invaluable (once it was refined) was the avalauncher. In 1965, Marmot acquired the first avalauncher from Rogers Pass, where it had proved ineffective. It simply did not have the range to reach the lofty trigger zones at the pass, but Tony felt it could be of use at Jasper, both along the highway and at the ski hill.

Though Tony swore by it, the Lake Louise boys in Banff considered the avalauncher a joke as well as a very dangerous piece of equipment and would have nothing to do with it. Tony always thought the objection to the temperamental machine was its mundane appearance rather than problems with safety. He was finally able to show the fundamental usefulness of the gun when they acquired a safer one in the early seventies. With rumours of much improved performance, Clair asked Tony to bring the gun to Lake Louise for a demonstration. The gun performed very well in that environment and was soon the instrument of use at Lake Louise as well.

Although Willi and Peter tried to keep a commonality of operation in public safety, each park had a unique environment to be considered. Jasper was much bigger than Banff both in the size of its wilderness areas and the scale of its mountains. While it was possible for operational pairs to rotate in and out of Banff's smaller backcountry areas, this was impractical in Jasper. The backcountry districts were far too large to shift people in and out of quickly, so it was just the wardens assigned to operations on the highway who handled most of the rescues. During the late 1960s and very early seventies, the principal wardens Willi turned to were old hands like Max Winkler, Hans Fuhrer and Tony Klettl. Some younger wardens had taken up residence at Sunwapta Warden Station, which was also a front-line resource, doubly so since most of the rescues occurred at the Columbia Icefield. During this period, Willi was quite happy to have these experienced men to span the interim training period of the young recruits.

Certainly a very young Dale Portman was glad of this expertise when he and Max Winkler responded to a strange rescue on Pyramid Mountain, which looms over the town of Jasper. The rescue occurred in 1973, just when the mountains were losing the last remnant of snow. The two young men on the hike had nothing in common other than camping in the local townsite "free" campground. On reaching the summit, the younger man could see the town directly below him and decided it was much quicker to go directly down on what appeared to be easy ground. The second man did not want to leave the known route and opted to go back the way they had come. There they parted company and never saw each other again.

The descent proved to be much more technical than the first man realized, and he became trapped on one of the lower cliff bands. Pyramid Mountain, however, has a radio tower on the summit, and one of the service men happened to be riding the cable car that accessed the station when he heard a vague shout in the afternoon gloom. In the deteriorating weather, the wind buffeted the sound around the steep gullies and crannies of the open face, making it difficult to hear. But the conscientious man reported the imagined or real shouts to the Jasper Warden Service anyway.

There was no option but to check it out. Max Winkler was one of the more experienced climbers in Jasper, and he had no hesitation about going directly up the face of Pyramid to confirm the report. Dale Portman, who had now joined the Warden Service after working in Rogers Pass, went with him.

They proceeded up the face rather blindly, hoping to locate the source of the shout somewhere in that broken face. Some metres up, Portman was in the lead, struggling with a short, steep section when he hauled himself over a shelf and came face to face with the missing man. He was so startled he almost lost his hold. Both men were shocked at this close eyeball encounter, and for a moment they just stared at one another. Finally Portman asked, "Why didn't you yell out when we hollered up the cliff?" The terrified man replied, "I didn't hear nothing! I've been too scared to move." As was the case. He had lowered himself to the point of no return. Only no one knew he was there. His erstwhile companion had simply presumed he had found his own way down. By sheer luck the man in the cable car had chosen that day to check the tower and had heard the feeble cry. Were it not for that, it is unlikely he would have survived the night. It was a situation that would become very common during the seventies but not always with the same happy outcome.

It must have seemed that everything was packed into those first few years in Jasper for Dale, for no sooner had he arrived than he was introduced to heli-slinging, which for a cowboy seemed a bit questionable. He watched as several of the young wardens donned the complicated harness and flew off as if getting on a ride at the fair. It seemed even more serious to him when the pilot was not really sure of what he was doing. And, in fact, that was the case initially in Jasper. They were with a pilot who was not used to delicate flying, which resulted in one unsettling ride. Duane Martin was present when Willi and Clair were flown up to land on the side of a mountain near the Jasper Airfield for a practice session. From the ground, it seemed there was a tense moment when the pair appeared to be snagged against the rock. This was followed by a hard landing that left them questioning the pilot's ability.

Portman soon realized that darkness and bad weather also limits helicopter use when he found himself on another rescue with Max. Two inexperienced young tourists were making their way up a dry rock-pounded avalanche gully well above the Beaver/Medicine Lake trail in Jasper National Park, when the leader was struck on the head by a rock. It was dark by the time Portman found himself tossed about in the cab of a warden truck that Alfie Burstrom was driving along the fire road leading to the gully. When they got there, the man was being carried down by the first party of rescuers who were happy to see the fresh reinforcements. They found it taxing bringing the victim down in the stretcher. The drive back to town finally unnerved one unseasoned warden who could no longer stand the moaning and thrashing of the unconscious man. Without thought, he began to yell back, "Shut up, for god's sake!" as if the man could hear him.

The tense band of rescuers rushed the man into the hospital where they were requested to stay until the doctor completed his initial assessment. In the early seventies Jasper had a small contingent of capable but unspecialized doctors with minimal staff to deal with emergencies of this nature. The doctor, suspecting the seriousness of the injury, quickly consulted a neurologist in Edmonton by phone. In the end, the wardens had to hold the severely agitated victim down while the doctor relieved a haematoma on the brain with a hand-held drill. It is unlikely that the patient was aware that an anaesthetic could not be administered for the operation, as consciousness never did return. The young man died on the way to Edmonton.

The fact that the man died after he had left the care of the rescuers, though disheartening enough, was of some relief to Portman, who had not been around a rescue that entailed death before. He felt it would have been worse if he had died in the stretcher. The unfortunate rescue soon picked up the chilling title "The Black and Decker Rescue" in reference to the Black and Decker hand drill that was new on the market for Christmas that year.

Death was a fact of mountain rescue that would sooner or later affect anyone who remained to do the work. The warden who was unnerved by the head-injured victim knew immediately it was not for him and soon left the Warden Service. But other wardens did stay to deal with the darker side of mountain rescue. This also meant dealing with the death of people known in the small community of Jasper. Because Jasper did not have a reliable pilot or a readily available machine that could respond immediately, the wardens remained versatile with both improvised rope rescue and cable rescue. At that time it was also more economical, as the helicopter was an hour's flying time away from either Hinton or Valemount.

It was with considerable ingenuity then, that the wardens recovered the body of a telecommunications officer who serviced the CN communications tower on the top of Pyramid Mountain behind the town of Jasper. The well-known man was a good skier and outdoorsman, who sometimes kept up his conditioning by running down from the top instead of using the tram that serviced the buildings on top. On one late day in June, he decided to walk down but soon encountered more late spring snow than he probably expected. He overcame this by riding a snow shovel, instead of struggling through the thigh-deep snow. Within minutes he was out of control and plummeted over a series of broken cliffs into a deep gully. He was subsequently reported missing, and a small search party was sent out in the morning. The body was actually found by warden Tom Davidson, who had been training his dog in elementary search and tracking.

Though Duane Martin was called in to act as rescue leader, it was Brian Wallace who learned a lot about the limitations of the cable. Wallace remembers that the tram car was used to bring up the rescuers and heavy cable gear. Because it was manoeuvrable, they were able to position the car directly above the gully that the victim had fallen into. They rigged the winch and cable drum right on the car, so that they could lower the line and rescuer directly to the accident site. The day was cloudy and snowy as the boys lowered Brian into the void. He recalls it being a weird sensation to go off the tram before contacting familiar rock, one made more so by the swirling snow.

Once he was down, he decided to detach from the cable. This was met with protest from above, and he was told to "keep the cable on." The problem was, he actually had to traverse over to the body. Tom Davidson had scrambled up to the body and was waiting for him to help prepare the victim for removal. But Brian was having problems with the traverse. As he proceeded, he asked for more slack cable until he reached one big boulder he could not get around. Suddenly the cable tightened up, jerking him off his feet. He was pulled back off his stance only to pendulum wildly back across the face into a pile of rocks. Fortunately for him, he had positioned his pack in front of his body, which protected him from the impact.

That did it. He was over the steep part of the descent, so he took the cable off and scrambled back to Tom, holding the cable in his hand. In short order, they bundled up the body, attached it to the cable and worked the body back to where it could be raised and ultimately taken down by the tram. Though disgruntled with his fling across the face, Brian felt they had learned something about avoiding traversing across broken faces at the end of a cable. It was a lesson taken to heart by the rescue team as well. In future, diagonal traverses were avoided or protected if possible.

OTHER PARKS THAT WILLI was responsible for mirrored the same shift to a younger Warden Service, though at a slower pace. Rogers Pass in Glacier National Park was fortunate in acquiring Gord Peyto in the early years, not so much for his climbing ability as his remarkable skiing talents. Again, Willi was dealing with a park quite different from Jasper or Banff. Glacier is a park with very steep terrain and demanding glaciers, where the principal danger comes from crevasses and avalanches. When Gord arrived in Glacier as a permanent warden in 1972, he had already come to know Willi Pfisterer through his years in Waterton. One of Willi's first objectives was to get the park staff trained for helicopter rescue. When Peter and Willi had first decided to use the helicopter for slinging rescuers, the only option had been to ask the pilots if they were willing to do the work. If they agreed, then training proceeded. It was a risky way to find out if the pilot was any good at the work, but up to now, no testing procedure had been established. When Peter first asked Jim Davies if it could be done, Jim had replied that he didn't think it was possible.

When Willi arrived in Glacier with the sling gear, he simply asked Fred Baird if he was willing to sling wardens onto the side of the mountains, then showed him the sling rope. Fred was dubious at first but agreed to give it a try. Gord Peyto was also dubious when he saw the four little ropes but went anyway when Willi volunteered him as the first candidate. He tensed up as soon as he was off the ground, clutching both the rope and the awkward lunch box radio cradled on his lap. When Willi saw him clinging to the sling rope he radioed up saying: "Let go of the rope, lean back and relax." Ever mindful of Willi's instructions, Gord did just that only to have the harness slip suddenly down around his legs, giving him a heart-jolting shock. Fred flew him around long enough that he eventually calmed down and became comfortable with the rig.

Gord later felt that it was good timing, because only a few days later, he was called to a rescue on Mt. Sir Donald. A young climber, thrilled at having reached the top, celebrated with a bottle of wine, only to lose his balance and fall 915 metres to a bergschrund on the Uto Glacier. Typically, the report came in late in the day, and Gord saw it as a good opportunity to try out this slick new rescue solution. Fred slung him to within two metres of the body and within a short time, Gord had him placed in the stretcher ready to be flown out. This first recovery was technically fairly challenging, as Gord was slung onto a steep snow slope that required a good ice axe belay. When he placed the axe in for an anchor, however, it broke through

into empty space below. He quickly relocated, discovering at once the dangers of slinging onto unknown ground on glaciers. The operation was over in 20 minutes, which convinced the pilot that this was a very expedient way to do rescues. Gord calculated they saved two days' of work and avoided using a minimum of 12 men, all who would have been exposed to the dangers of travel over the broken glacier. Fred Baird went on to be a fine pilot for the park in this field for several years after.

Despite growing expertise with the helicopter, each rescue scenario had its own individual complications that made it unique. It was not always possible to rely on past experience as a blueprint. Gord Peyto recalls that "One of the worst rescues [he] was ever on," was the heart-rending effort to save co-worker and friend Jim Tutt. Jim was a popular young worker with the snow research crowd at the pass who loved to get out on a good trip any time of the year. When Peyto said that "everything that could go wrong did go wrong" he was largely referring to having no break from the continuous bad weather that plagued the attempt to save the man's life.

Jim and his colleague Doug Orn were ski touring well back from the highway on Youngs Peak near the top of the Illecillewaet Glacier when the accident occurred. They were moving upwards along the crest of the peak when they changed leads for breaking trail. They were not roped, and when Jim moved aside to let Doug pass, he fell into a snow-concealed cornice crack that was several feet deep. He fell to the bottom, nearly a metre from the top of the cornice. Because they did not have a rope, Doug was loathe to go down for fear of not being able to get either himself or Jim back out. He heard no verbal response, so he took the next course of action and skied out for help before daylight was gone.

Doug was a good skier, and he made it back to the pass in time to mobilize both Peyto and the helicopter that day. With good luck they would be able to land close by and get him out of the hole before night closed in. Peyto was ready immediately with the rescue gear. But by then it was getting dark and the weather had turned stormy. By the time they got to Lookout Mountain, close to Youngs Peak, the winds were howling. They searched under deteriorating conditions for a place to land but realized the best the pilot could do was hover close to a small ledge long enough for Peyto to gain his footing there. In classic understatement, Gord laconically recalls that "it was not a nice place." The moment he was out the door, the helicopter was jolted by a violent blast of wind that sent the tail rotor flying by his head—then it disappeared from sight. With sudden panic, he realized that he was left with nothing—no pack, no skis, no radio and no warm clothing. He settled down on the miserable ledge, wrapping his thin jacket about himself, wondering "what next?" as the storm rolled in for the night.

Much to his relief—and the pilot's relief to see him alive—the helicopter returned in a moment of clear weather. (The pilot was sure he had taken Gord's head off with the sudden manoeuvre.) This time, he was able to land long enough to let Doug disembark with the gear, including the precious skis. But by then there was no chance to get to the accident site, and both rescuers settled down to a long cold night that left little hope for the survival of their friend.

A second party was able to fly in early the following morning to meet the boys on the ridge. From there, in continuing stormy conditions, they proceeded to "a small hole" where they found Jim about 10 metres down the fissure. When they brought him up they were amazed to find him still alive, but he was very hypothermic. It was small consolation that he died in the arms of his friends, but it is not uncommon for people to hang on only to succumb in the presence of their rescuers.

WATERTON LAKE NATIONAL PARK was also very different from Jasper. This small beautiful park was highlighted by spectacular mountains composed of exceptionally crumbly rock and attracted very little mountaineering activity. It was popular, however, with hikers and large youth groups who frequently underestimated the dangers of mountain travel.

One seasonal warden who graduated from this park to become active in public safety was Tom Davidson, who was actually from Waterton. Tom's introduction into this field was not so pleasant. It was sudden and dramatic, underscoring the power of water and the need for quick action. The incident occurred at Cameron Falls, a very beautiful waterfall on the edge of Waterton townsite, which is consequently very popular with the tourists.

Tom was on duty in town when a cry for help went out from the falls. When he arrived, all he could see was a young boy being carried to the surface then submerged again by the strong back-eddy in the pool beneath the falls. It was the first accident he had been to, and all he could think to do was keep his eye on the boy. Fortunately, Max Winkler, the newly appointed CPW from Jasper, had been notified almost at the same time. He had just moved into park housing close to the falls and was at home when the call came in. When he arrived, he saw Tom standing on shore pointing to the small pale figure as it rose again to the surface. Without a thought, Max stripped to his shorts and dove in. He brought the boy to shore with one mighty heave and tried to resuscitate him.

Tom was astounded. He could not believe the assurance that Max had displayed in retrieving the young boy. Max, however, was a powerful man who also happened to be an excellent swimmer. Unfortunately Max did not know CPR (a recent innovation not yet taught in standard medical training) and could not save the boy. It is difficult to say if it would have helped, as the child had been in the water over five minutes before he was retrieved, but Max always wondered if knowing CPR might have saved his life.

The other young warden who arrived in Waterton to work in the public safety field and stay was Derek Tilson. He had actually started in Kootenay National Park in 1973, where he received all the benefits of being a young eager seasonal warden in a park full of aging wardens who did not want to either climb or ski.

Kootenay was a quiet park in the seventies, with little climbing activity, and park management saw no need for a public safety function. Derek was keen, however, and felt a warden should represent the park on the school whenever possible. He asked to go and was sent. There was little money for equipment or clothing and Derek had to be creative in getting properly geared up. He relied heavily on regional stores and supplemented that with his own gear and what he could borrow from others.

Derek did not come to the Warden Service as a climber or skier, but he took it up eagerly and found that he had a natural aptitude that he developed quickly on the schools. He had a strong slim build well suited to climbing, which might have led him to more technical climbing had he moved to a full-time position in Banff the following year. Before, he accepted, however, Max Winkler, whom he had met briefly in Jasper, asked him to come and look at Waterton as an alternate choice. Derek went and never looked back. Just as Tim had been captured by Lake O'Hara, so the infinite variety of the jewel-like park put its hold on Derek. Though it did not offer the extreme climbing opportunities to the north, it suited him. He would remain the backbone of the public safety program in the park well into the eighties, much to Max's great satisfaction.

THE PARK WAS RUN BY THRIFTY MEN who did not care to spend much money on helicopters and who tended to rely more on improvised rescue. The park was plagued with high winds and very poor visibility that limited flying opportunities. Willi did not mind, feeling that it was important to keep things simple and basic. He felt Banff sometimes used the helicopter too much. Derek often heard the comment "they use a helicopter if someone stubs his toe in Banff." When Waterton did need a helicopter, they usually brought in

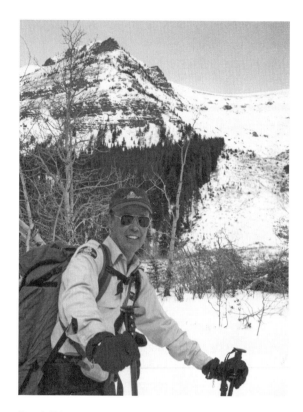

Derek Tilson. EDWIN KNOX COLLECTION

an Okanagan Helicopter from Cranbrook or Fernie. They stayed in the loop, however, with developments, always trained religiously and kept the gear in good order, ready for use.

Derek early on became acquainted with the nemesis of the park: the poorly equipped youth group often led on an overly ambitious trip by inexperienced leaders. The magnet for these groups was the myriad of beautiful lakes, often ringed with dangerous cliffs. One particular episode stayed with Max because it could easily have been avoided.

In the summer of 1973, a large church group checked out for Lone Lake where they spent the night with the intention of proceeding on to Rowe Meadows the next day. The disorganized crew got off to a very late start, leaving the children strung out on a long arduous scree slope in the heat of the day. They had no water and no backpacks. The sleeping gear consisted of a rolled-up blanket they carried over the shoulder—there may have been one or two sleeping bags among the lot of them. Some food, such as a can of beans, was rolled up in the blankets.

By the time the group had assembled in the meadows, the leaders realized that five of the children were missing. It was dark by the time they set out to look for them after sending for help. During the night, four of the kids showed up in camp, but one young fellow was still missing when a search party was organized the following morning. It was not long before they found him at the base of the Lineham Cliffs. It deeply affected Max, who felt the tragedy could easily have been avoided.

It was not the last time people would come to grief on the Lineham Cliffs. There existed a very precarious trail across the cliff band that was often taken by fishermen taking a shortcut to the hidden lake. The fishing was notoriously good there because it was hard to reach by the long route. It was so treacherous that the cable protecting the worst part of the face has since been taken out. The trail is now officially closed just before it leaves the spectacular waterfall that rushes out of the remote lake.

BY 1974, MANAGEMENT in western region knew they needed people with outdoor skills and hired over twenty seasonal wardens that summer who showed promise. The training previously given only to permanent wardens was now extended to new recruits in a special school, the Seasonal Warden Training School held at the Palisades Training Centre in Jasper National Park. The Palisades was a national training centre for Parks Canada and was actually a replacement for the old Cuthead College in Banff. It was also the year that "Affirmative Action" underscored the hiring standard and women *had* to be brought on board.

Two women were actually qualified for the Warden Service, but only one of them would go on to be involved with public safety. But before Kathy Calvert could start, she promised to go to Waterton to run the first Women's Conservation Corps for Max Winkler. The Conservation Corps was a government run youth camp set up to train students in several backcountry skills as well as provide a work program in the parks. It had been run successfully for boys for some years, but now the dreaded affirmative action required this privilege be extended to girls as well. During her interview, Kathy was able to convince the panel that she did have the background required for the job—which was not missed by the astute Max who was on the hiring board. If he had to have the program, he wanted someone who seemed to have an outdoors background to run it.

Kathy had, in fact, been convinced to send in an application by her friend Tim Auger. She had met him on a climbing trip to Lake O'Hara where he first began working in the park. In the early seventies there were very few women climbers and fewer yet who were brought up with outdoor skills. A healthy stint on the family farm taught her how to ride horses, but she made the list for women applicants when she added a degree in biology to the resume.

Other promising young climbers at this first school who became involved in the early public safety program were Jim Murphy and Traf Taylor who went to Banff. Kathy Calvert eventually went to Yoho, where her climbing abilities came in handy when Tim left. By 1974, Tim Auger was being increasingly pushed to join the ranks of the permanent staff and to "take the job seriously"— advice from Jim Sime who was looking for a commitment from him.

Tim did take the job seriously, but he was also having fun in Yoho with his good friend Rick Kunelius, who actually took over as the Lake O'Hara warden when Tim was pressed into more extended public safety duties throughout the park.

With life going well for him, he actually turned down several permanent job offers, which baffled many seasonal wardens eager to get full-time work. Andy Anderson, who was CPW in Yoho when Tim arrived—as well as friend and staunch supporter—had moved on to Banff to be replaced by Hal Shepherd. Shepherd was a product of the old school who had actually participated on rescues himself. He was also a colourful product of the Second World War and loved to come to work wearing a peaked cap rather than the traditional Stetson. He had a passion for spiffy uniforms, was a stern disciplinarian and liked things run in a snappy fashion. The military impression was enhanced by a beaked nose, a patch over one eye and a glint in the other one that could pierce steel when he was angry.

Tim recalls one frustrating episode on Cathedral Mountain when he was probably glad he was not looking at that one good eye. A father and his 14-year-old son had failed to register, so Tim went to investigate with Dale Portman, who had left Jasper to take the public safety position in Yoho. The two wardens found an empty tent below the face with a note pinned to the flap saying, "Gone to climb south face of Cathedral Mountain." The fellow had a history of being overdue and this was the third time Tim had had to go and look for him. With some weariness, they looked up at a narrow, ugly snow gully punctuated with telltale footprints. Tim thought it was "probably dangerous at any time of the day." With philosophical optimism, they climbed up on a huge boulder and began to "holler their lungs out" hoping, but hardly expecting, that they would get a response.

When none came, Tim got on the radio to Hal to explain the situation. The vast 760-metre rock face was impossible for two men to search without aid, and it would soon be a third night out for the pair. Quite reasonably, he requested a helicopter for the search. Tim relates there was a long silence on the radio then—with great authority—they received instructions from the Chief. In a booming voice he directed: "TIM! THIS IS WHAT I WANT YOU TO DO! PROCEED TO THE FOOT OF THE GULLY AND CLIMB IT UNTIL YOU ESTABLISH CONTACT WITH THE PARTY ... REPORT BACK TO ME!"

In baffled amazement at this military solution, neither Tim nor Dale knew quite how to respond. Tim could not imagine the reasoning that would caution the expenditure of money on a helicopter so obviously needed under the circumstances. Tim thought, "This is just Nutso!" Dale had a sense of Hal's disembodied good eye looking down on them, mindlessly surveying the scene from the sky. Suddenly, to their astonishment they heard a faint cry for help. Amazed at the turn of events, the young wardens had to comply with the mission to "proceed on foot" to the man and his son, now descending by a completely different route. But the outcome, humorous in hindsight, could have ended tragically. To Hal's credit, he never disputed a helicopter call from then on.

When Tim talked to Jim Sime about taking on a full-time job, he mentioned that he wanted to work in public safety full time, but Jim was not a proponent of specialized work, feeling that the strength in the Warden Service lay in well-rounded work. Nevertheless, that is what Tim wanted, and he did not want to take a position where that could not be accomplished. He was not interested in Jasper or in any of the small parks that had limited climbing action. Clair was already the climbing warden in Lake Louise. The only real option was to go to Banff, for it was becoming apparent—even for the most laid-back person—that any manager in the public safety program would need strong leadership abilities. The intensity of the work, combined with an individual approach, was bound to lead to tense situations or conflict that would have to be resolved on many levels. Strangely, it was this inner tension of balance, restraint and conflict that would provide the cohesion for the emerging professionalism soon to define the burgeoning public safety program.

The opportunity to move to Banff was provided by his friend Rick Kunelius. Rick joined the Warden Service in 1972 but quickly moved to Banff as a full-time warden in 1973. When Rick arrived in Banff, most of the public safety work was being handled by the wardens being trained by Walter Perren with the aid of one young warden named Bruce McKinnon. Bruce was a meticulous and accomplished climber who was thrilled with using the helicopter for rescues. The older wardens, however, were slowly withdrawing from rescue work, making room for younger men. Because Rick had some climbing experience with Tim in Yoho, he was put directly into the backcountry/frontcountry routine where he was teamed up with Earl Skjonsberg until Earl was chosen for the rescue dog program.

But even by that first summer, Rick noticed that accidents were occurring on steeper and more exposed places well beyond the climbing ability of most of the wardens in Banff. But then none of them were great rock climbers willing to tackle the outer limits of extreme climbing. In fact, they were getting scared. Peter Fuhrmann had been organizing all the rescues if they were at all technical. Peter's job though, was to ready the wardens to do the brunt of the rescue work rather than do it himself.

The gravity of being involved in mountain rescue became clear to Rick after responding to one unpleasant episode on Cascade Mountain. It was for a young cadet who had gotten off route while trying to descend from the top of the mountain, thinking it was a shortcut to the cadet camp (located toward Lake Minnewanka north of Banff townsite). The cadet camp often had mishaps until they upgraded the leadership requirements in the late eighties, and Rick initially thought it was just a routine call out. Unfortunately, the boy had slipped over a 90-metre cliff to a small ledge in the middle of the face. It was an exposed position to sling into, but that was not what bothered Rick. The boy's head had been split open from the impact and part of it had separated from the body. It was difficult for him to absorb at first, and he had to sit back for

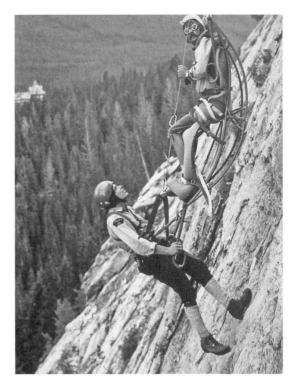

Rick Kunelius and Tim Auger with rescue stretcher.
BANFF WARDEN ARCHIVES

an internal dialogue before he could proceed with the recovery. He knew then, with absolute clarity, what he would be facing at any given time if he stayed in this function. He had to find some way of detaching himself from the brutal side of the work and that moment was upon him. He quickly reasoned it was not a body or a person any longer but a "package," not dissimilar from what he might pick up at Safeway. A package of meat that had to be wrapped and delivered to the customer. With a coolness that he remembers to this day, he used a yellow park garbage bag to scoop the separated skull and place it in the body bag with the rest of the remains. Within minutes, the operation was over and the team was back on the ground.

In 1973, Bill Vroom was still going on straightforward rescues, but the standard was increasing exponentially, and it would not be long before greater expertise would be needed. In

153

Rick's mind that was Tim. He was backed up in this idea by Andy Anderson, now CPW in Banff.

Tim was ready to move. By 1974 he was the first warden to achieve full guide status, setting the standard for most public safety positions in the future. Yoho had only minimal rescue work and as a seasonal, he could only make suggestions about how to run the program. It was small consolation that the senior wardens in the park took what he had to say seriously. Besides, he had just gotten married. Time to move on.

By now the ranks in Banff had been joined by another young warden who would become an integral part of the emerging Banff rescue team. Lance Cooper arrived in 1973 after joining the Warden Service in Kootenay National Park in 1972. He saw better opportunities with public safety in Banff and was happy to bring his creative mind to early equipment development. But he was particularly entranced with the flying end of the job. He developed a close association with Jim Davies who introduced him to all aspects of the helicopter. In fact he got into public safety work mainly because of the helicopter, though rescue work was important as well. This early experience would be a boon to the park for many years to come after he, himself, became a rescue pilot.

Keith Everts was the third man to form the small cadre of wardens at the core of the public safety team in Banff. He came to Banff from Rogers Pass after learning as much as he could about avalanches from Peter Schaerer. This solid grounding would more than qualify him to run the avalanche program at Sunshine and Norquay in the coming years. Though his forte remained in the avalanche field, he had tremendous organizational ability and was a dominant force in the structuring of the new team being assembled under Andy Anderson's direction.

Rick Kunelius recalls they spent another harrowing year through 1974 dealing with every emergency that cropped up before Tim Auger moved to Banff in 1975. By 1975 visitor recreational use had exploded, and sometimes there were three or four rescues a day, leaving the wardens reeling with work. Keith, who was influential with Andy, wanted to maintain the strength inherent in a non-specialized Warden Service (which he favoured), but could see the need for a dedicated public safety team. He backed Tim and soon the small group found themselves getting organized in the small rescue room in the basement of the warden office—and putting Lance's carpentry skills to good use. Tim was in heaven. It finally matched his idea of "what a serious mountain rescue place was really like."

A fifth person was also there to help smooth the way for the development of this team to full capacity. Peter Whyte, an unlikely looking warden from Yoho, moved to Banff in 1973. He did not fall into the lean and wiry category so typical of the mountaineer, being heavy set and not physically inclined to the work. But he had strong administrative skills and had an uncanny bent for facilitating awkward meetings or strained relationships.

When Tim came to Banff, it spelled the beginning of change in the hierarchy of response to rescues. Despite his efforts to fit in, the older wardens recognized the disparity between his capabilities and their own and knew he stood for a new order of business. He did not want to play the role of hero, but the altered nature of the public safety job made it difficult—if not impossible—to keep a certain level of elitism from creeping in. Peter Whyte recognized this and often stepped in to smooth misunderstandings. Everyone felt comfortable with him and brought him their grievances, which he would then translate to acceptable terms and pass to those to whom the grievances were directed. It was an invaluable gift that was sorely missed when he finally transferred to Kootenay.

Tim's efforts in developing a public safety team took him to a new level of professionalism. He accepted that the job had to be done on the terms dictated by circumstance and just went ahead and did it. His willingness to talk out matters and be available helped a lot. He established a professional relationship with Peter Fuhrmann that worked but was sometimes difficult. More important, they established a mutual respect that kept individual differences from hampering the development of the program. Again, tension promoted cohesion and they maintained a workable balance. Slowly changes occurred as they developed a local training program, revamped the rescue room and responded to endless rescues.

One of the things they all worked on was the organization and the hierarchy of involvement from the field level up to the rescue leader. Protocol was important to determine leadership and responsibility. Although Walter Perren had the mechanics of the rescue operation quite functional, Peter Whyte felt that clarification was needed. He was quite meticulous about using plans, a trait he had picked up from working with the Alberta Forest Service. He worked with Peter Fuhrmann on structuring a rescue plan from a command centre down to the field rescue teams and support crew. To begin with, it was trial and error, aided greatly by insisting on having a critique or debriefing after every event. Peter Whyte felt they "made immense strides in terms of professionalism and development of the program" in the first few years.

With Tim handling the training, rescues and development of the rescue room, Peter Fuhrmann was free to concentrate on perfecting the sling rescue gear and keeping abreast of developments in Europe through IKAR. It was an important connection that kept the young Canadian rescue unit current and up to standard. He and Willi often came back from Europe with the latest in rescue inventions, many which were invaluable in saving lives. An example was the versatile bean bag (Laerdal). He gleefully showed up in all the parks with this floppy sack full of round semi-hard objects about the size of beans. A volunteer was instructed to lie in the thing, and when he was sufficiently cushioned by beans, a suction pump was applied to the bag. When the air was sucked out, the adaptable beans compressed around the whole body, turning the sack into a body splint. The captive warden was immobile and could even be stood upright without being released. The sack fit nicely into the Jenny Bag, flew well and was invaluable in saving time with elaborate splints. It was also the answer to safely transporting victims with back and neck injuries. Jay Morton morbidly observed, "Yah, and if the patient dies, you still have a last impression you can send to the parents." Though black humour is often discouraged, particularly while on actual missions, it certainly lightened the atmosphere when Peter got long-winded on a favourite topic.

Peter also involved himself with upgrading the first-aid training in the early seventies and soon had field wardens obtaining EMT (Emergency Medical Technician) status. The extent to which medical care was expected in the field was and still is an issue of debate. The wardens would never become astute diagnosticians, particularly under the constraints found on a mountainside in bad weather and failing light. The idea of setting up IVs or administering drugs was bandied about, but in the end it was felt that in most cases just getting the patient off the mountain without adding to the injury was the best course of action. Jay Morton recalls one incident on Mt. Murchison where a climber sustained a serious head injury from rock fall. Some of the attending rescuers wanted to get quite elaborate about dealing with the injury, but it was obvious to Jay the man could not be helped up there. Finally he just said, "He's dying, for Christ sake! Let's just get him down before he freezes." This bleak statement closed the matter, and without another word, they slung the man off to the waiting ambulance. Jay was right though. He was dying.

Other things like oxygen and all supplies needed for the treatment of bleeding, circulation and stabilization were felt to be essential. Several wardens contributed to finding efficient ways of carrying these field items, and an atmosphere of teamwork prevailed in these efforts. The rescue plan was becoming established and it specified what roles different people were qualified for.

The original team had new additions in the mid-seventies. Dan Vedova arrived in Banff in 1976; Cliff White (who had actually started in Banff the summer before) and Gord Irwin both started working in Lake Louise the same year. These additions were welcome, because the work was intense and there was always some degree of burn out. Peter Whyte could not emphasize enough the need to work as a team. He states: "You had to work as a team or you wouldn't last. The guys had to depend on each other … it was so cliquish … but it had to be to survive." Indeed, some of the original team members soon went off to other jobs in the Warden Service, but the rescue plan, though refined through the years, remained the blueprint for all those who followed.

Tim was also determined about where his responsibilities lay when accidents occurred. Though there were distinct lines on the map defining boundaries, it meant little when agencies outside the park needed help. It was also not clear where Lake Louise and Banff responsibilities ended. As Tim admits, "There was Clair, who was a really strong personality out at Lake Louise, and no doubt there was a certain amount of territorialism," but they did all train together and mostly assisted each other if the work load got heavy or something major was underway. For Tim, "When there was something going on, you just pitched in, no question."

Clair Israelson had been managing standard rescues, like searches for lost skiers up Mosquito Creek, hikers up the Pipestone River and evacuations from Abbots Pass with little difficulty. The rescue at Abbots Pass was an exemplary example of the Banff and Lake Louise teams working together to save a young woman who had broken a leg while descending the steep ice slope below the pass. The accident was reported late in the evening, thus eliminating the use of the helicopter until the following morning. Because her companions had left her at the bottom of the "Death Trap" near a large open crevasse in an area heavily prone to avalanches, it was paramount to move

her to a safer location. A ground crew went in that night with a camp and hot food to stabilize her until she could be flown out the next day. Clair asked and got Banff's assistance on this from Tim, Jim Murphy and Lance Cooper. Ironically, the woman was only in the tent 10 minutes before the helicopter arrived in the wee hours of the morning to fly her out. Tim reflects that it took most of the night to locate the woman and set up camp under dangerous conditions. One interesting aspect of this rescue was the use of horses. Clair had spent enough time in the backcountry with horses and was happy to use them when warranted. He saved time and energy by arranging a horse party to take men and equipment as far as the Lake Agnes Tea House.

The rescue on the Super Couloir on the north face of Mt. Deltaform was decidedly different. This was a steep nasty place that became "very ugly" when the weather turned bad. Jerry Rogan and Jim Elzinga attempted the second ascent of this route, which was considered at the time to be "one of the most extreme climbs yet done in the Rockies." The weather was superb, however, and as they were very experienced mountaineers there was no initial concern. Clair was not overly worried when bad weather set in during the night of the 15th, but that changed when Rogan's wife called at 9:00 a.m., saying they had not returned. Fearing the worst, Clair called for the helicopter, but could not fly until noon when the weather cleared enough for him and Traf Taylor to check the lower half of the mountain. They located the expected tracks in the couloir leading to the steep part of the climb but found no one on any of the possible descent routes. They found the climbers' tent in the meadow, which strongly indicated that they were still somewhere on the face.

If Clair had nightmares of impossible rescue scenarios, this was one. He needed backup, and soon Tim Auger and Peter Fuhrmann were on their way from Banff with all the gear they could cram into Peter's station wagon. Tim ruefully recalled that Peter's driving was the scariest part of the rescue. "It was pouring rain … he drove like a maniac. It was a driving rainstorm on the Trans-Canada Highway, but his windshield wipers were so bad that they basically didn't clear the water off the windshield. All you could see were the shimmering headlights of the vehicles that were getting wider and wider apart as he would pass … he had this red cherry light on and he would pass despite visibility. I was terrified." That was nothing compared to getting up the Moraine Lake Road. "He still had his foot to the metal, and he went over a bump and landed so hard that the shocks ground out and both the front hubcaps let go at the same time and were rolling beside us before peeling off into the woods. I remember Peter just bearing down and driving on saying, 'Remember this place!' like we are going to come back and find the hubcaps on that featureless road."

As he wobbled out on the parking lot at Moraine Lake wondering how to avoid the return drive, Tim realized that the situation was indeed serious. More than that, he was dismayed to learn that the missing climbers were close friends. Despite the shroud of cloud that clung to the mountain obscuring the upper face, Tim and Peter flew another aerial reconnaissance but saw nothing. In frustration, they set down below the face and called up with a loud hailer. Faintly from high in the mist, two indistinct voices could be heard, confirming that they were somewhere on that vast freezing face and still alive. But little more could be done except prepare a survival pack to sling in if the weather cleared. Tim reluctantly drove home with Peter to get some sleep before tackling the problem early the next morning.

Clair spent a second anxious night debating the wisest course of action. He had asked Peter what he would do and was disconcerted with the answer: "It's your territory and your rescue. It's up to you." Though the weight of leadership settled on him like a shroud, by morning he was calm and prepared for the day. He was convinced that he was responsible for the rescue team and would not jeopardize anyone's safety. Tim had no notion of making dangerous decisions either, but when the weather had not cleared the next day, he suggested putting a ground team up as high as possible to see if they could establish contact. Clair, however, was not happy that they had no idea where the two men were. A lone climber could be hidden in any of the deep gullies or overhangs that riddled the face. So the waiting game, hardest of all to play, began as the anxious team settled in to wait for a break in the weather.

To keep the tension down, Clair kept everyone busy preparing gear for "all possible eventualities," which included setting up a base camp at the bottom of the climb. From this location, they heard voices again at noon. The weather then closed in with a vengeance, and nothing further could be done until the clouds scudded briefly away in the afternoon, allowing for a short flight, but again they could not find the men.

With pressure mounting to send a ground team up the regular route, it finally cleared enough in the evening to fly right to the top and over the back side of the mountain. Within minutes the wardens spotted the men struggling down the snow-plastered south slopes. This was fortunate, because the pair wouldn't likely have survived a third unplanned night. Both men were soaked to the skin, and the temperatures were below freezing. They had actually made the right decision to climb on and not wait for a rescue. Clair writes, "As conditions worsened, they realized that a rescue party could not reach them, so they decided to continue rather than sit and freeze to death." Constant rock fall and avalanches ruled out retreating the way they had come up, and climbing out to the summit was their only hope. They still might have died, however, had not Jim Davies been able to fly in and pick them up before they reached the deadly cliffs that ring the back of the mountain.

When Tim left Yoho, the wardens in that park were unsure who would fill his role as field rescue leader.

Dale was the only choice for this role as he had strong travel skills and was experienced in avalanche control after working in Rogers Pass. However, his mountaineering skills needed upgrading if he was to function well in this field. He accepted the challenge, knowing he had help nearby from the Lake Louise wardens should an incident occur that was beyond his skill.

Kathy had also moved to Yoho after leaving Waterton. Though Hal Shepherd agreed to take her, the men throughout the park system were a bit uneasy about this new experiment. What helped Kathy was her ability to climb and her solid comfort level with horses. She not only stayed, but returned the following year and for twenty-five years thereafter. One big reason was her growing relationship with Dale, whom she married nine years later.

Despite Dale's reservations about his new job in public safety, many significant rescue-recoveries were done in-house without the need to call in Lake Louise. Gordon Rutherford was experienced and active and other young wardens had come on strength who could be counted on for non-technical rescues. When an experienced climber from Golden went missing on Chancellor Peak at the west end of the park, locating him was the difficult part. The man, along with his son and his neighbour's son, was reported missing on the 13th of December of 1976 by his wife, who was angry that a rescue party had not been organized when she phoned. She felt the Warden Service should have realized that he was now well overdue as he was expected home the night before. A check of the registration book at the west gate, however, failed to turn up a registration slip.

While Dale was organizing the search, the duty warden checked the registration again, and this time found the missing sign-out slip in the middle of the book. For some obscure reason the man had decided to sign out in the middle of the book where it was easily overlooked. This provided the information about where to search—but there was an added cryptic note from the climber saying that if he did not return, the park was to contact Tim Auger. Dale did not contact Tim, because it was too early in the search to involve wardens from another park, and it was incumbent upon them to do what they could before taking this step.

With what light remained in the day, Dale Portman and Jim Purdy flew across the face until they found the climbers' tracks. They also saw evidence of avalanches released by goats moving across the face, indicating a high hazard. When the climbers' tracks disappeared in the remains of a small sluff, it was obvious where a series of slides had taken them. Portman and Purdy returned to base to rig up the sling gear. They located the victims strung together with the climbing rope in the avalanche deposit before the dog handler from Banff arrived on the scene. The rescuers never found out why the man had taken his son and his friend to climb under such unfavourable conditions. Possibly they had a desire to climb the mountain officially in the winter, thereby making it a first winter ascent, but it has remained a mystery, and to Portman it was all rather strange.

It was also during these years that the park became the magnet for ice climbers. The lower north facing slopes of Mt. Dennis created an ice fall paradise in the winter. With the sport in its infancy, accidents began to proliferate. Dale soon found himself on winter training schools learning how to ice climb in preparation for an eventual rescue for a stranded climber. However, most climbers fell to the bottom, making most recoveries fairly simple except for the constant hazard of avalanches. Most waterfalls formed in gullies, which are natural watercourses in the summer and avalanche routes in winter.

The other accidents in Yoho involved water. There were several drownings in the Kicking Horse River that tragically involved children, but it was the death of a young woman at Twin Falls that Kathy often remembers. The girl was on a two-day camping trip with her boyfriend when she fell over the 180-metre Twin Falls. The girl had innocently gone to a benign-looking pool at the top of the falls for a cup of water. When she reached down, her foot slipped on the rocks, and she disappeared below the surface. Her stunned boyfriend, who saw the accident, could barely take it in. She never reappeared, having been immediately flushed over the falls by the strong current beneath the surface. The next day saw all of the Yoho wardens and standby help from Lake Louise using grappling hooks in the torrent below, trying to snag the body should it be wedged in one of the many eddies. Kathy never forgot the poor boyfriend who stood transfixed, looking, hour after hour, at the indifferent water as it flowed over the cliff from the glaciers above. By the following day the family asked for the search to be called off, realizing the hope of recovering the body was highly unlikely.

ANOTHER WARDEN who started his career in Yoho was Darro Stinson, who took advantage of Tim's presence in the park to begin his climbing career. He loved climbing and went out with Tim on any occasion he could. He went on all the training schools he was given time for and even started to accumulate his own equipment. More important, Darro recognized that if he wanted to work in public safety, he would have to climb on his own time. Many wardens who had an interest in public safety climbed recreationally on their days off; In fact, it was becoming apparent that extracurricular climbing was required to achieve the standard needed for different rescues.

Things took off for Darro in 1975 when he was stationed at Sunwapta Falls Warden Station, Jasper. Stinson teamed up with other enthusiastic young wardens at the station such as Bruce McKinnon, who had moved up from Banff to be in charge of the Columbia Icefield area. Bruce was a careful but accomplished climber, who taught both Darro and Tom Davidson (newly arrived from Waterton) many of the basics of mountaineering. But it was Willi Pfisterer who became Darro's mentor. He recalls "Willi really took me under his wing and pushed me really hard at times when I was way over my head. Some days it amazed me." Willi would often call up and say, "We're going on a climb."

When Darro first arrived, he felt that there was actually more training going on in Banff. He later realized the casual but constant exposure to climbing at the Columbia Icefield in Jasper, either at work or on his days off, accomplished more than he knew, building a solid foundation of experience and skill. More important, he found that there was an acceptance of the work ethic surrounding public safety then. If he put in a hard 12- to 18-hour day climbing, no one minded if he showed up a few hours late for work the next day. None of the wardens ever thought of getting paid overtime, because work and recreational climbing began to seem like the same thing.

The wardens also learned a lot from the many accidents on the Columbia Icefield, some of them quite bizarre. The first sling recovery Tom Davidson ever did was for a tourist who had wandered up on the icefield by himself and had died of exposure. Tom had only slung once on a school, but now he was lowered down among gigantic crevasses to pick up the remains of the poor man from New York who had become disoriented in bad weather. On another occasion, they went in to pick up a man who had been killed after falling into a crevasse. The unconcerned party he was travelling with did not get too excited either about the dead man or the weather. Despite poor conditions, they carried on to climb the Snow Dome before returning to report the death at the end of the May long weekend.

In another similar instance, Murray Hindle recalls going up to see what could be done for a member of the British Army left in a crevasse by his teammates. The mountain rescue unit of the army had been up on the icefields to conduct a crevasse rescue training session when a snow bridge collapsed on a member of the team. Their experience must have been limited, however, as they did not seem to know how to help him.

159

Without further ado, they cut the rope, tied it to an ice axe and skied out for help. When Murray and crew got there, they went around to the other side of the crevasse where they could see he had tried to get himself out. If he had been brought up by the survivors, Tom and Murray would not have had to chip him out of the ice hours later.

Murray Hindle remembers another very cold situation that could have been serious for the rescue team. The weather was terrible when they flew in to the upper portion of the Athabasca Glacier. A man had fallen into a large crevasse, but by the time they reached him at midnight he was dead. In the haste to save his life, however, only the rescue gear had been flown in and Murray had not even had time to get his personal pack out. To keep warm and get some protection from any possible icefall, they dug a trench and hunkered down for the rest of the night, with Murray minus a sleeping bag. When light finally dawned around 5:00 a.m., they were more than eager for the support crew to fly them out. Rick West, the coordinator and supplier stationed at the highway, was a little more casual about the request for early morning pickup. Murray was in no mood for his reply of "Well, we're just having coffee and breakfast …" His short answer was an unequivocal "RIGHT NOW!"

DURING THE SEVENTIES Willi and Peter ran the regional schools, sometimes together, but often singly. Willi continued to take select groups of wardens up to Kluane National Park to ensure they were ready to work in that environment. Derek Tilson recalled one trip when they combined a training school with an actual rescue, giving them an opportunity to try out a newly purchased helicopter. They were on Mt. Steele, testing out their survival skills in the extremely bad weather that never let up, when Tom Davidson managed to cut his thumb quite badly on a can of bacon. At that altitude and in that weather the can was frozen and difficult to hold. It had slipped out of his grasp and sliced deeply into the base of his thumb. Willi wanted an excuse to test the new Allouette helicopter and give the pilot a chance to get experience with the new machine, so he flew Tom out with the next break in the weather, not a few of the wardens wishing they were going with him.

One of the elements that characterized the early training was the freshness and levity the younger wardens brought to the program. Though there was no question of where the expertise or authority lay on those early trips, it did not eliminate the inherent sense of fun often found in a youthful crowd. Both Peter and Willi, on one trip they ran jointly, were caught by surprise by how good humour prevailed. Jay Morton, Clair Israelson and Larry Harbridge, a warden from Waterton, felt it was time to show Peter—a connoisseur of good food and wine—how to manage a meal properly on a glacier. Peter brought the most impossible meals along when he could get someone to carry the food or if the trip was helicopter supported. On this occasion, the three, who were designated rope mates, embellished their own supplies with an array of exotic food. The only drawback was having to carry the additional goods in already heavy packs.

The three did not produce the booty until the second camp below the Balfour Col where they dined in style. They laid out the epicurean meal on an orange tablecloth over the snowy surface. The wine glasses were placed appropriately to receive the fine champagne, which they had carried with care to accompany the lobster, caviar and other delicacies. They toasted each mouthful with a flourish as fellow travellers ate barely chewable freeze-dried pork chops or canned beans. Everyone laughed except Willi, whom Jay Morton remembers being "rather pissed off at the whole affair." Willi was still working on his remarkable sense of humour on that trip. Dale Portman, who was tenting with Peter on the trip, remembers him being quite indignant as well. At minus 20 degree Celsius, Dale was more annoyed about trying to rehydrate the pork chops Peter had insisted they bring on the trip.

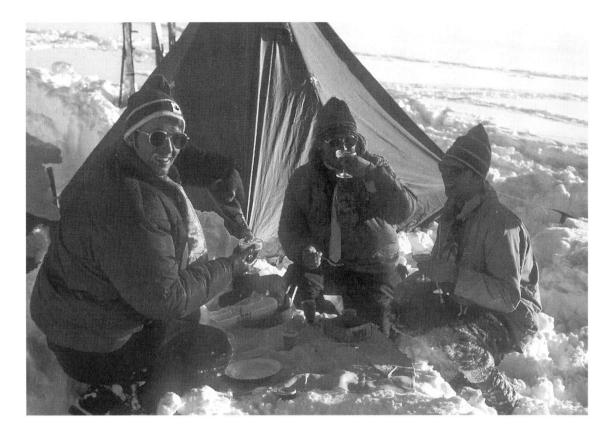

Wapta Icefields tea party. Right to left: Clair Israelson, Jay Morton and Larry Harbridge. DALE PORTMAN COLLECTION

Teammates kept that episode in mind when Jay went on another trip to the Peyto Glacier. Jay meticulously packed everything he was given the night before the trip, but trustingly left it in the rescue room overnight. At the trailhead he could not figure out why his mates were so eager to help him on with his pack, and he certainly felt the weight when they took off. He thought no more about it other than to assume he had spent more time in the bar the night before than he should have. The trip began with a descent to Peyto Lake across a slide path difficult to ski. Jay could not handle the weight and plunged down on one uncontrolled turn that took him to the bottom. He tried to pick up the pack to join the others but simply could not do it. When he took his water bottle out for a drink, he discovered two short railway ties crammed under the top flap. Well above, his teammates chortled with delight, astounded at how far he had carried it.

Another joint Banff/Jasper school that had light moments mixed with drama was a helicopter-assisted trip to the Freshfields. Duane Martin remembers this as an intense trip capped by an equally intense rescue scenario that turned real. After climbing in the area, Peter and Willi wanted to complete the course by setting up a crevasse rescue practice. Unfortunately, there were no crevasses anywhere close to camp. There was, however, a large extended cornice that loomed over the Howse Valley hundreds of metres below. It was a spectacular, scary place, and when Peter asked for a volunteer to be the rescue victim, only the Jasper boys did not step back. Suddenly Marv Millar,

161

John Strachan and Gord Anderson found themselves put "in an interesting situation," as Duane described their dilemma. The ever willing-to-be-helpful Marv was further volunteered as the victim, but he only smiled and waved wanly as they dressed him warmly and sent him over the edge.

The minute he leapt off, the whole cornice shuddered and settled with a "whump" down the entire length. At the same moment, the rope dramatically cut three metres back into the soft outer edge, dragging Marv's belayer Gord Anderson, almost to the edge. Fortunately, the rope cut in far enough to stop running and the rest of the crew were able to secure Anderson. Marv had prussic slings to stand in, but his legs still went numb after 15 minutes. Not having a radio to communicate with did little to relieve the stress, but after a while he saw the grinning face of John Strachan who was lowered over on a second rope. With everyone committed to the rescue, it still took most of the afternoon to bring him up.

Duane remembers having a fabulous meal that night, courtesy of Banff which always had money for good food if a helicopter was around. The overproof rum that followed, however, was a contribution from many sources and definitely took the edge off a very tense day. A wild snowball fight ensued, which ended in the collapse of many of the elaborately built snow caves.

The following day was spent rebuilding the caves and going on a final climb. The avalanche Keith Everts started that almost pulled another rope mate down with him was anticlimactic, as Peter held them both. There was a moment of silence, then Dale, standing next to Peter, gave a cheer and raised an imaginary score, Olympic style, yelling, "5.8!" Cheers followed with other scores ranging from 5.6 to 5.9.

Peter was becoming increasingly concerned about the growing popularity of ice climbing and decided that winter schools would have to focus on the unique rescue challenge it poses. With characteristic bravado he settled on Takakkaw Falls—one of the most demanding ice climbs around—for his first rescue practice. They created a simulation of a stranded climber halfway down the frozen fall by lowering Derek Tilson down the ice on the cable. He didn't go alone, however. Lance Cooper went down with him as his rope mate. All was fine until they tried to bring them back up. Derek recalls a jerk in the cable but he did not move. In fact, they did not move for over an hour. This began to get uncomfortable with the rushing of the water just beneath the ice curtain. They were also getting cold and had to continually dodge falling ice as the crew above worked on the cable problem. Derek thought they had trouble freeing the swivel connector, but that was minor compared to the fact that the cable was a bird's nest above the connector, because more cable had accidentally played out. The cold and lack of tension on the cable had caused it to unravel, creating a mess that could not be wound back up until it was freed.

Difficulties like this were discouraging to the rescuers, now beginning to view using the cable on a major rescue with some trepidation. The two men were faced with the possibility they would have to down climb the tricky waterfall, a concern, since they were not experienced ice climbers. Ultimately the cable was freed, and the pair were brought up but no one was happy. Subsequent rescue practices on other waterfalls were more successful, but the cable did present special problems that had to be considered.

By the late seventies taking the Association of Canadian Mountain Guides course was a serious consideration for those who wanted to excel in public safety. When Clair Israelson completed the full guide's course in 1981, he realized how important the training was in setting the standards for mountain rescue. Both Peter and Willi knew the importance of this training and felt that the park should back other young wardens who showed talent and commitment. Darro Stinson and Tom Davidson were chosen to attend the first courses from Jasper, and Gord Irwin and Gerry Israelson, Clair's younger brother, went from Banff.

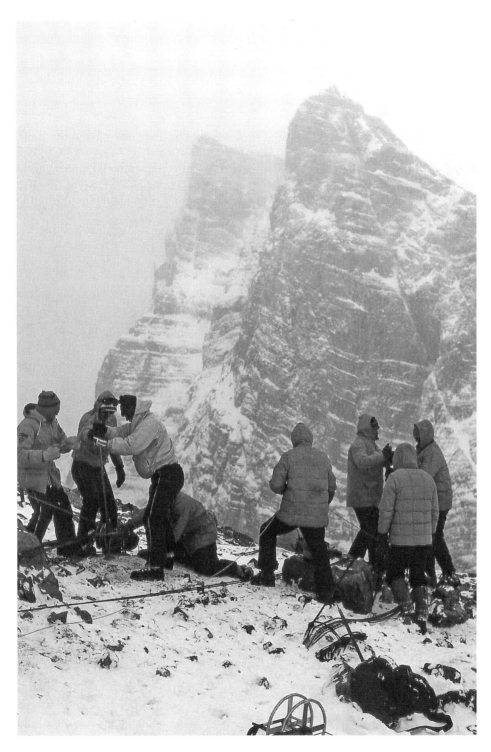

Kananaskis Country rangers and Kootenay wardens joint training at Helmut Falls. KANANASKIS
COUNTRY PUBLIC SAFETY ARCHIVES

Gerry certainly became aware of the park warden job through Clair, but it was his upbringing in the mountains that attracted him to the job. Gerry had the ambition and the talent to become a very good climber and teacher in the field. He actually started with provincial parks in B.C. but was hired on with federal parks in 1976. He reflects that it was ironic that with his climbing background, he was sent to Elk Island National Park (along with fellow climber Al MacDonald) before he was able to transfer to Yoho National Park. Once in Yoho, Gerry took off. There he worked for Dale Portman in the public safety function until he transferred to Lake Louise to work with Clair at the ski hill.

When Gerry moved to Lake Louise, he met and soon married his wife Leslie, who was particularly skilled with a sewing machine. During these early developmental years of exploring new equipment and tailoring gear to specific needs for heli-sling rescue, her talents were invaluable. Gerry was delighted when she was able to design such items as sling packs for first-aid gear and other bags that could be carried by the rescuers for various missions. It was a great time for those in the field to come up with new ideas for specialized equipment—most of which is still in use today.

Gord Irwin came to the Warden Service through the park's Interpretive Service. His uncle was a world-renowned climber who had worked in mountain rescue in New Zealand, which influenced Gord's decision to start climbing. He grew up in Edmonton, but he wanted to be in the mountains and eventually arrived in Jasper National Park in 1969 as part of a campground cleaning crew. He was hired in Yoho National Park as an naturalist before eventually retuning to Jasper to work in that function at the Columbia Icefield. This exposed him to the Icefield and more climbing opportunities on that icy expanse. Already well into the adventurous world of climbing, Gord took advantage of the opportunity to learn and took courses in crevasse and rope rescue. He was even able to get involved in early sling rescue practices when Willi noticed his interest. He soon

realized his vocation lay with the Warden Service, but more specifically in public safety. He applied to become a warden, was accepted and began climbing in earnest. With natural ability that lent itself to the public safety profile, he also realized that becoming a guide was important and was soon in the program.

By 1976 there was a young contingent of wardens in all the parks who were capable of doing the routine work of rescue with expert help close at hand if needed. And rescues abounded, keeping everyone on their toes.

DURING THIS PERIOD Peter took opportunities to keep wardens exposed to the realities of the work. One of his concerns was that the public safety field looked glamorous but could at times be quite unpleasant. He thought one of the best ways to see if they were cut out for the job was to send them on a rescue that would test their fortitude. This happened to warden Dan Vedova during his second year in the field.

It was a particularly tragic mishap on Mt. Assiniboine, involving a young climber with little experience and worse gear. He was approaching the top of the climb when he decided to unrope from his partners. The circumstances were not clear to Dan, but it seemed that he had gone over to the north face, possibly to look for the route, when he slipped (threadbare boots may have had something to do with this). Not being roped, he fell over 300 metres down the north face. When Peter got the call, he decided to send in Dan and Rick Kunelius for what was most likely a body recovery.

When Dan and Rick slung into the ridge as close to the body as they could get, reality was staring them in the face. The climber had been torn apart by the fall and was scattered over the immediate cliffs above. Rick was happy to let Dan pick up the more distant pieces; his mind was already drifting toward work as a wildlife biologist within the Warden Service. Dan was still committed to rescue work and diligently packaged the remains in the body bag. But it was an effort for him as the sight of the mutilated body strongly affected him. It was his job to sling out with the victim, but he nearly suffered the same fate as the climber in the process. As the ring came toward him from the helicopter, he reached forward to click on when a sudden downdraft pulled it just out of reach. But he was already committed. As he fell forward off the mountain, with the weight of the dead man pulling at him, all he could think was, "This fellow is going to kill me too!" But somehow during the downward fall his carabiner had closed over the steel aperture just before it pulled away. With a feeling of euphoria and relief he realized he was going to live. When he completed the mission, he flew back to where Rick was on the mountain, just for the sheer joy of survival. Despite the experience, Dan stayed in the field over the years as a solid member of the public safety team in Banff.

Dealing with the mangled bodies of unknown climbers was often bad, but later that year some wardens had to deal with the death of close friends. The brunt of the trauma was experienced by Tim Auger, who went in to Mt. Assiniboine again to recover the body of good friend and climbing mate, Bugs (Alistair) McKeith. Tim had climbed with Bugs on many occasions, but most notably on the first attempt to climb Takakkaw Falls in winter. They were not successful due to fiercely bad weather on the climb, and had a miserable trip out characterized in the *Calgary Herald* as a "seven-day ordeal of freezing temperatures, unexpected mountain snow and rainstorms and brushes with killer slides." Such trips create stronger bonds between friends than most people develop in a lifetime.

Bugs' tragic fall down the north face of Mt. Assiniboine was reported by his rope mates, who discovered him missing after they unroped for the last 30 metres to the top. He had gone on ahead of the other two, but had fallen through what was first thought to be a cornice before reaching the summit. Tim described the feature as "a horrible

sucker hole ... there should be a sign there because it's so dangerous." Bugs was walking on bare rock but fell when he stepped onto the snow patch obscuring the cleft below. Tim noticed, "It was exactly like falling in a crevasse ... he would have fallen about three thousand feet."

The flight around the base of the mountain brought rescuers to the base of the north face where they spotted some equipment on the surface of a small glacier. They landed on low angle ground and geared up prepared for crevasses, but they did not need to go far. Earl Skjonsberg had come in with his search dog Faro, and he saved them the trouble of a prolonged search. According to Earl, it was one of the easiest recoveries in his career. The dog jumped out of the helicopter and went immediately to where the body was and started digging. Tim was grateful for both the quick recovery and the presence of good friends Rick Kunelius and Lance Cooper, who were there to collect the crumpled body from beneath the layer of snow which covered him. He was one of the first climbers to die in the close-knit climbing community between Calgary and Banff that included people in the Warden Service.

OTHER THINGS WERE CLICKING into place by the second half of the seventies. The ski hills were becoming the place to be if anyone had serious aspirations of guiding or working in public safety, because this was where people gained the needed skills. Mike McKnight was now area manager in Lake Louise, a person Clair could rely on after he broke his leg skiing.

One scary event with bombs occurred when Clair was laid up with his broken leg. The guys working at the hill had been learning to operate the avalauncher, but it was complicated and often seemed more so in the wee hours of the morning. When Clair heard nothing and asked what had happened to a bomb that never exploded, he was not happy when no one else had heard anything either. After several seconds that seemed like minutes, a small sound like a distant thud was heard from behind the hill. That was followed by a short radio communication from the ski patrol hut asking if they were missing a bomb. It had gone off on the lower slopes of the Eagle Run, close a group of Japanese skiers. The laconic comment from the patroller was, "Funny way to welcome our out-of-town visitors." No one was hurt but that was just good luck. Or bad luck. The chastised group of avalanche personnel scurried back to recheck their settings, thinking reading glasses were the order of the day.

Sometimes it can be hard to get paths to slide after a storm. Jim Murphy and Scott Ward had been trying to get one of the avalanche chutes to slide, using every means at their disposal to settle the snow. They had thrown bombs throughout the entire snowpack over several days with no results. They even ski cut it manually to see if that would release the built-up snow. Nothing worked. The ski patrol continued to pressure them to open up the area or to at least let them ski it to make it safe for the public. Knowing that everything possible had been done, it seemed the best course of action; at least the patrol was semi-responsible for the consequence. With a yell of excitement, the patrol launched into the gully, providing the impact needed to release a significant avalanche. Everyone went for a great ride that took all but Jim and Scott, who were watching from a rock outcrop. Though no one was hurt, it was a reminder of the underlying dangers of avalanche control.

This happened during the period the ski hill at Lake Louise was expanding, opening new runs with unknown avalanche problems. It was happening at Marmot Basin as well, and at Sunshine and Norquay in Banff, and it left the wardens on a steep learning curve. The pressure was always enormous from managers who wanted to satisfy the skiing public's ever-increasing demand to access closed areas. This finally ended in death when a person was killed in an avalanche at Lake Louise after a closed run was opened up. Again, every control method had been employed to stabilize the run, and it was thought to be solid when it was opened to the public. The inquest left no blame with the Warden Service, but it added a level of consequence to the job that dampened some of the levity experienced in the past. As many controllers were aware, it was not closing an area that created the problem, but the decision when to open it again. The job had a serious side, and the consequences of a mistake were equally serious.

Other aspects of avalanche control also had their moments. Helicopter bombing was a good alternative in Alberta because good flying conditions were more prevalent than in British Columbia. Also, colder winter temperatures in Alberta often tightened up the snow pack immediately after a storm, reducing the hazard, which reduced the need to try and release avalanches during a storm. Peter liked the fact that a helicopter was quick and could get close to the trigger zones to drop the bomb. There was always a concern that the person handling the bombs be experienced. Working in a small, confined space could be tense when trying to put everything together quickly and in the correct sequence and get it out an open door into a howling wind. On one memorable occasion, Peter was putting the bombs together, then handing them to Monty Rose to toss out. Somehow one of the bombs landed on the helicopter skid and obstinately refused to be shaken off. Cursing the perversity of fate, Rose had to quickly get out and kick the volatile package off before it exploded.

Though wardens made no attempt to do avalanche control in the backcountry, it was still a concern when snow stability deteriorated. Big natural avalanches were always an occurrence in the backcountry, affecting skiers now travelling in droves to obscure destinations. They were going in search of good snow, exploring valleys leading to high glaciers or meadows all along the Icefield Parkway and the Trans-Canada Highway. Though the year 1977 did not see a lot of snowfall, extended cold weather in the early part of the year caused a significant layer of depth hoar to form, creating a bad avalanche hazard in the later part of the winter.

It seemed that once March arrived, there were close calls everywhere, but a couple were noteworthy for what was learned, if not by the rescuers, then certainly by the travellers. On March 19th two young men set out to climb Bow Peak after camping the night above treeline on Crowfoot Pass. The avalanche hazard was considered high, and when they checked with the warden office in Lake Louise, they were told to avoid any wind-loaded west-facing gullies. With this in mind, they did stay on the ridge for the ascent but forgot the warnings when they opted to glissade down the west facing gully. The inevitable happened. The second man triggered a slab avalanche that engulfed his friend some metres below, sweeping him out of sight. After a few minutes of shock, the survivor kicked steps down the face. Remarkably, he found his friend still alive. He was able to dig out his upper body before the snow consolidated around his legs. After digging for half an hour, he gave up.

At this point, exhaustion and panic began to affect the decisions the survivor made. He did not think he could get his buddy back to the tent if he were freed, and so he opted to go for help, thinking he could get to the highway in half an hour—a distance of over five kilometres in poor winter snow conditions. He added to his difficulties when he left behind his hat, his gloves, down jacket and most important, his snowshoes. Without any footgear he was soon wallowing up to his waist in snow, making progress almost impossible. He struggled on valiantly, now with self-preservation rather than rescue in mind. By dark he finally reached the Bow River but nowhere near the trail they had come in on. In desperation he tried to cross on the ice, but repeatedly fell in. Miraculously, he made it to a snowmobile track. If his judgement wasn't seriously impeded before, it was not improved by the condition he was in now. With unbelievable determination, he followed the fruitless track for over three kilometres before it

doubled back on itself. Exhaustion finally took over, and with frozen hands, he laid down a few spruce bows and went to sleep. He must have had an amazing constitution, because he woke up in the morning still alive and found their original snowshoe tracks leading to the highway. In 15 minutes he was picked up and taken to Lake Louise to report his tale of woe.

There was, of course, no way his friend could survive being left in the avalanche for that period without protection. The wardens found him pinned in about 50 centimetres of snow and covered with the down jacket that his partner had thought would insulate him from the cold. It was after recoveries like this that parks realized some education on travel, winter or summer, was badly needed. But proactive programming was still not part of the arsenal of accident prevention.

The second avalanche tragedy that winter followed quickly on the heels of the Bow Peak misfortune. By the 27th of March, the avalanche hazard was posted at extreme because of continuous spring snowfall, and travel in avalanche areas was strongly advised against. Unfortunately a group of 20 guests from Sunshine Village (joined later by three other skiers) had asked a guide to take them to Citadel Pass from where they would fly to Assiniboine Lodge. Helicopter skiing is not allowed in national parks, so the group had to ski to the park boundary for the helicopter pickup. The group did not check with the Warden Service about the avalanche hazard, presumably because they were with a guide, and they left that detail up to him. Unfortunately, the practice of checking with wardens was not fully ingrained with guides, and in this instance it was not done.

The distance as the crow flies to the pass is not far, so they were comfortable getting away by 10:00 a.m. The party set out on the regular route across the meadows, but after an hour, the weather deteriorated badly, making it difficult to make their way above treeline. The guide now looked for an alternative. He felt they could still make the rendezvous by dropping below treeline into Howard Douglas Creek. Here things took an ominous turn. There were some small, steep slopes in the trees that the group had to cross, and at one point a small avalanche released, taking one member of the party on a short ride. He was unhurt, but now the guide was alert to the avalanche situation. They stopped for a brief lunch then continued on more cautiously. When at last they came to a much larger opening, the guide told the main body to stay in the trees while he skied out to test the slope. Unfortunately, he was still hampered by poor visibility and could not assess the extent of the open area above him. He only got 15 metres when the slope fractured and began to slide. With a warning shout of "Avalanche!" he turned downhill and out-skied the running snow. He and two others made it to the safety of a rock outcrop, but the avalanche he triggered released a much larger one from the slopes above that swept through the trees, hitting seven members of the party and burying five of them. Only quick action on the guide's part saved all but one. With controlled speed he immediately found one man whose ski tip was showing. Yelling instructions to the survivors, he had them probe quickly in the most likely areas for any other survivors. In almost the same breath, he dispatched two of the skiers to Sunshine for help. Three more women were found around the bases of trees, but a fifth woman was not located for another 45 minutes. No amount of artificial respiration could save the victim, who had simply been buried too long under two metres of snow.

The guide did not slow down in caring for the injured survivors and the rest of the party, now tired and suffering from shock. He soon had a base area stomped out with a fire for everyone to keep warm, rest and take stock of the situation. His timely dispatch of the two skiers meant that a rescue party was able to mobilize and set out for the accident site by 5:00 p.m. They arrived in excellent time around 8:45 p.m. with enough gear and food to keep the injured victims comfortable for the night until they could be evacuated by helicopter in the morning. The main party and the guide skied back to the meadows where they were picked up by a Sno-cat and taken to Sunshine Lodge.

The inquest that followed the accident ruled the woman's death was accidental, but the inquiry recommended that a minimum of two guides should be present for groups of that number, that an electrical homing device be carried by all members of the party (the Pieps and Skadi had been on the market for a number of years and were extensively used by most heli-ski companies) and, finally, that all guides be required to check the avalanche hazard information.

THE FOLLOWING SUMMER saw the last of the mountain rescues done with the aid of horses. Dan Vedova was now working in the backcountry but had come out for a shift in September just in time to be called in to a body recovery on Mt. Temple. Some people who had been hiking down from Sentinel Pass saw what looked like a body off the main route on the mountain and reported it to Moraine Lake Lodge. Prior to this a local doctor had reported his nephew missing on the tourist route, and it seemed likely that this might be the missing man. The winds were too high to fly, so Clair and Dan set out on foot and soon found the climber on a steep and broken slope. Since the weather still did not permit flying, Clair decided that the old-fashioned method perfected by the wardens in the sixties would do just fine. Consequently a large ground crew brought the man down. Using a improvised rope lowering system, he was taken the rest of the way by pack horse.

By the end of the seventies, the warden rescue teams in each park were coping with all the major accidents that came their way and had embarked on a training program that was slowly raising the warden climbing standard to that of an average good climber. The public safety function now had people in each park who were dedicated to the work full time. The bar had been raised in Banff and Jasper to a minimum of two professional guides in the program. They were in the process of attaining this goal with the intent of having six for all the mountain parks in the future.

With the public safety program developing in fine style, Willi felt it was time to accomplish his cherished goal of putting a warden team on top of Mt. Logan, and he opted to climb the more demanding east ridge. Since it was important to have Kluane wardens along on this training climb, they set out in May of 1980 with 13 climbers. They lost two men in the first week when one man injured himself and was flown out along with a Native trainee who chose not to continue the climb. Other problems plagued the team when they discovered that the conditions between Camp I and II were more ice than snow, and that not everyone was equipped to climb. Despite this, they still managed to both supply Camp II and establish Camp III from which a summit attempt could be made. The summit team selected to go consisted of Tim Auger, Tom Davidson, Peter Perren and Murray Hindle.

They had help from Willi Pfisterer and Ron Chambers in setting up Camp III, but Murray recalls that the four were occupied mostly with hauling loads for the summit push. Though it snowed heavily on the lower slopes of the mountain, conditions remained good on the upper half, giving the team the break they needed to go for the summit. Murray remembers struggling with a violent headache and cold feet the day they went for the top, but he was cheered by getting there and sharing a chilly can of peaches in celebration. He does not add that the descent was livened up by a close slip by his teammates behind.

Just before Tom set out on the trip, Bev Hunter, the warden secretary and close friend in Jasper, had a dream that something bad was going to happen on the climb and warned him to be "very careful." Tom recalls ruefully that when Peter Perren was knocked off his feet by a sudden gust of wind on an icy section of wind-blown ridge, he thought this was what Bev had foreseen. Certainly

it was desperate enough as they slid over 70 metres before stopping short of a major cliff. Thanking their good luck, they tucked in behind Tim and Murray, who were well down the ridge heading for Camp III. It certainly did not dampen the cheers over the radio when they relayed the good news. Unfortunately, bad weather now settled in at the upper camp, delaying the summit team from descending immediately to Camp I.

The reunited team now only had to reach base camp. That morning Murray decided to rope up with Tom, who was ready to leave. He had previously been partnered with Tim for most of the climb. Tim and Peter, however, were right behind them when they set out for camp.

Though the exposure off the ridge was spectacular, the climbing was not difficult, and all parties climbed short-roped along the descent ridge. No thought was given to this until they reached as short steep down step to the ridge that was fairly icy. Both Tom and Murray recall with clarity the condition of the ridge at this point. For Tom, the ridge was spectacular, dropping off over 1,200 metres on the left and more than 600 metres on the right, covered with thigh-deep snow in many places but blown clear and hard where the step was. Murray was about three-quarters of the way across the exposed section when he suddenly heard Tim holler. As he turned at the shout, he saw Peter jam down his ice axe, but he had very little time to react. Peter later wrote: "I quickly positioned myself to arrest his [Tim's] fall. The rope snapped taut and for a brief moment I thought I had stopped him. But then, just as suddenly as Tim had stopped, the kinetic energy of arresting his fall catapulted me into space and I instantly travelled the length of the rope past Tim." Tom had seen the rope go tight as Tim sped toward the gully on the south side of the face and tried briefly to run back to Peter, only to see Peter fly into space as though flung out by a giant arm.

At this point Willi and Ron Chambers were a bit farther down the ridge and neither saw nor

169

heard Tim fall. Murray remembers being stunned by Willi's reply when he shouted: "Willi, Willi! Tim's fallen!" Willi irritably yelled back: "Well, tell him to get up!" After a moment this sank in and Murray had to clarify the awful reality. "No! I mean … he's *still falling!*" As the drama replayed itself in his mind he realized that the small ice step off the bulge had broken when Tim stepped down, causing the initial fall. Suddenly Willi was exclaiming: "Oh for Christ sake!" as Murray watched both men free fall, hitting rocks and starting small avalanches in their wake. Then they were lost to sight. All of them had seen enough rescues to know the consequence of what they were seeing.

Peter Perren will not forget "bouncing head-first down the hill" hoping the rope would hang up on a rock outcrop before they were swept over the cliffs below. But the fall started a wet avalanche that engulfed them. Peter's recollection never wavers: "I remember feeling more and more snow coming in around me as the avalanche grew larger." They did not bounce over the hard rock surface but rushed downward on a cushion of snow that eddied over the sharp edges, sending them into free fall over vertical faces, cliff after cliff until they came to rest at the bottom 600 metres below the ridge. At one point "between the second and third free fall" Peter felt his leg snap, tearing the patellar tendon and most of the ligaments at his knee.

Immediately after Willi saw the climbers fall, he sent most of the team back up to Camp I to set up the VHF and radio for help. He then proceeded down the mountain with Tom Davidson and Ron Chambers but knew that it would take hours to get to where the climbers must have fallen. No one could believe what had happened, particularly after the success of the trip. Tom recalls Willi being really concerned by the turn of events as they slogged down the ridge, knowing that survival was next to impossible. After three to four hours they heard the helicopter arrive as they made their way to where they hoped to find the

fallen climbers. To their complete astonishment they suddenly heard Tim shout, and a few minutes later they saw a small figure waving at them. It was Tim and he was alive. A second figure moved and with astonishment and relief they realized that both men had survived their incredible fall. Willi still did not know what condition they were in—he had been to many an accident where the people were alive but had died on-site or on transport.

By a miracle the avalanche had cushioned their fall, and the only major injury was Peter's mangled knee. When the avalanche left them on the slope, Tim was completely buried but Peter was left on the surface and despite his bad leg, was able to dig Tim out. Little was said. The immense relief was evident, though the survivors were still in mild shock. With no time wasted, Tim and Peter were loaded directly into a helicopter and flown to Whitehorse, Yukon. The rest of the team was also picked up later that day by a second helicopter bringing in another climbing party. Murray recalls that this was actually a questionable operation as the weather started to fail just as the helicopter arrived. The weather socked in for three weeks following their escape, and the party that had come in with that flight were pinned down for the duration. They never did leave base camp.

It took Peter several months to walk again, and his knee never did fully recover.

TIM SURVIVED HIS ORDEAL on Mt. Logan and was back that summer to resume his duties in the field. His work in the public safety program continued as before, but one thing that hovered in the air was the possibility of having to deal with a truly challenging north-face rescue. Apart from Deltaform, there had been no serious accidents on any of the formidable faces requiring any serious rescue effort. The wardens did not think that would last, and so they were not surprised when two young instructors from the Cadet Camp in Banff went missing on the north face of Mt. Bryce in the Columbia Icefield.

The two men were considered "moderately experienced mountaineers," who had more experience being rescued than succeeding on big face climbs. They had started off to do the climb at the end of a cadet climbing camp in the area. The pair were reported overdue on the 4th of August to the Banff warden office, who passed it along to Clair in Lake Louise. A subsequent helicopter search revealed they had headed for the face across the Castleguard Glacier to the base of one of the biggest faces in the Rockies. It is an extremely ambitious climb that requires moving fast over steep terrain in the few hours of the day when the face is not bombarded with rock fall. Unfortunately the pair were not able to climb the steep fifty-degree ice on the upper face before afternoon warming turned the route into a bowling alley of ice and rock fall. One of the men was hit by a large rock which left a compound fracture of the left arm and a badly bruised hip. Unable to go up or down, they dragged themselves to a relatively protected rock outcrop where they set up a bivouac and prepared to wait for a rescue. After two days without food and not knowing a rescue was coming, the unhurt climber continued on to the summit ridge to see if he could climb out from there for help. With any luck at all, this would still have been a two-day marathon as there was no easy way off the mountain and the walk to the highway was still a good day away.

When Clair and Tim flew in to check on the missing party on the 5th, they feared they would find them well up the face. Clair's worst nightmare came true when they spotted (on the last pass before the clouds rolled in) the injured man in the middle of the face, waving at them as they flew by. Not quite sure if he was glad the man was alive or not, Clair started mentally putting together a plausible rescue scenario. The weather now began to turn bad, but it was not the clouds that were the problem so much as the intensely high winds. The clouds were too low around the upper part of the mountain to find the other climber so they returned to the Columbia Icefield to set up a strategy. The big north-face rescue was upon them, and Clair decided he would need all the help he could get. He contacted dispatch with word to round up the best that were available. The result was one of the first multi-park rescue amalgamations undertaken by the wardens.

While people like Darro Stinson, Tom Davidson, Willi Pfisterer (from Jasper), Gerry Israelson (Yoho), Hans Fuhrer (Kootenay) and Lance Cooper (Banff) were being recruited, Clair and Cliff flew back to the mountain to get a better look. When they got there, the clouds had lifted and they were able to spot the uninjured man on the summit. With great relief, the overjoyed climber was picked up by the rescuers, who were able to sling in for him. From the survivor they learned the extent of the injury suffered by the man on the face. It was not encouraging. They had hoped he would be able to climb out under his own steam, avoiding the possibility of having to do a cable rescue.

By now other conditions were conspiring against them. Jim had to return to Banff, as his helicopter was due for service. He was relieved by Gary Forman from Jasper, who showed up with enough men and supplies for a siege. Meanwhile, Clair and Cliff worked their way down to a small glacier partway down the face to set up base operations. Though hampered by intermittent radio contact, they established a landing area marked with stones in time to greet Tim Auger and Darro Stinson. Displaying some fine flying through bad winds and swirling snow, Gary got both men in with more gear and a camp. He then went back for the climber and after several attempts was able to fly him off to the meadows below.

The four rescuers now took another look at the situation and decided the best move was to set up a static line across the face to the stranded man beneath the poorly protected rock outcrop. They were still hoping that the injured man could be slung out, but initially it seemed likely he would have to be carried out. How, exactly, was not clear. It was a long way, and they would be constantly exposed to the rock and ice fall that had caused the accident in the first place.

Late into the day, Clair and Cliff began to work across the steep 50-degree slope that Cliff remembered being mostly hard snow. Clair does not recall such great conditions, saying in his report that "The ice on the face was very poor quality making climbing slow and causing problems establishing adequate anchors." The continuing problem of ice fall plagued them all the way across the exposed, unrelieved slope. As they went they placed ice screws for Tim and Darro Stinson, who began to place a fixed rope for the return trip. After the second team had crossed about a third of the fall, a substantial piece of ice-encased rock knocked Tim off his feet and left him suspended from a nearby ice screw. When the debris hit him, Tim initially thought it might have broken his back—or at least his leg. He was all right, but the unnerving episode encouraged the men to make haste. Throughout, squalls of snow and hail lashed at the team, sometimes limiting visibility to 45 metres.

Finally after 4½ leads of tense climbing, Cliff, now in front, reached the injured man, who indeed was incapable of climbing on his own. Desperately hoping Gary could get in with the sling, Clair and Cliff got the victim into the Jenny Bag then called for the helicopter. Fortunately, they had an opening of good weather and Gary gave it a try. To their relief, the line came in, and the man was plucked from the side of the mountain, dramatically swinging into the vast space above the glacier far below. The two rescuers then cleaned up the gear and flew down to the meadows, now hot in the afternoon sunshine. With dispatch, everyone was flown back to the Icefield Centre to step down the rescue operation. "Quick and dirty," as Cliff said when it was all over. It was fortunate for everyone that Gary was able to individually sling the rescuers and victim off the face before the weather closed in again. The rescue report laconically states: "The last flight came in [with Auger and Stinson] at 20:00 hrs. At 21:00 hrs, the Columbia Icefields were obscured in a storm."

The possibility of serious north-face rescues surfaced again the following year on one of the most difficult faces in the Canadian Rockies—the north face of Mt. Alberta. Seen from any angle, the isolated monolith is intimidating, with no easy route to the top. It stands alone, penetrating the sky at 3,619 metres, just south of the Columbia Icefield, usually coated in snow and ice year-round. The view of the north face must have been particularly terrifying to behold. It would have been intimidating to any climber on seeing it for the first time. It certainly was for Tobin Sorenson who set out to do the first solo ascent on October 3rd, 1980. It was a strange time to attempt the climb, because it was late in the season, with short cold days edging on the start of winter storms.

Sorenson was a young, intensely religious man from California who had tested his abilities on several difficult world-class north faces in Europe and North America. The most outstanding of these was the third solo winter ascent of the north face of the Matterhorn and the first solo ascent by an American of the north face of the Eiger Direct in Switzerland. At 25, he could also add to this list eight first major ascents, a solo winter ascent of Mt. Robson and the north face of Mt. Kitchener. He had the credentials and experience to attempt the climb, but may have been awed by the extreme isolation of the mountain. Mt. Alberta is not easy to get to. The approach is made difficult by the distance, the steep terrain over Woolley Col and the glaciers surrounding the mountain. The time of year added to the loneliness of the vast, empty valleys that surrounded the mountain.

The Jasper Warden Service was aware of Sorenson's attempt and fervently hoped he would be successful. When he failed to return on the day he was registered back, they accepted that a search was called for. On the morning of the 8th, Al MacDonald, who was still a fairly green warden at Sunwapta, set out with pilot Gary Forman and dog master Alfie Burstrom on an initial reconnaissance flight, hoping to find the man on his way out.

They did not find Sorenson, but they did find his tent between Mt. Alberta and Mt. Woolley. Gary set down while Al checked for evidence of fresh occupation. In that interim they flew up to the shoulder of Alberta, looking for an escape, and the weather turned bad. The clouds clamped down in earnestness, leaving them stranded on the shoulder at 3,000 metres overlooking the valley below the north face. The disgruntled Burstrom passionately hated being stranded above treeline, and the enforced three-hour confinement in the chilly helicopter buffeted by 120 km/hr winds and driving snow almost caused him to bolt for the timber where he could at least light a fire.

Al recalls: "When the weather finally broke, after about 5 hours, I think, the helicopter wouldn't start because the battery was so cold. I remember Alfie got out … and he actually pushed the blades. And that was just enough to get the momentum so that the battery could turn over and start the engine." With the ceiling lifting, Gary was off, spinning over the huge drop above the valley, quietly muttering: "Now hang on because I don't know if this thing is going to fly or not …" Calling on his considerable skill as a pilot, Gary did fly the helicopter off, and soon they were back to the warm security of the Sunwapta Warden Station.

The next day brought renewed good weather and more people to join in the search. Duane Martin went in on the first flight around a mountain he had long been intrigued with. The flight took them across the massive north face which "left the indelible impression of black concavity." He found it inconceivable that anyone would want to climb such a godforsaken place of dark rotten rock and steep, blue ice. But when they found his body at the base of the mountain, they found out that Tobin Sorenson had gone there to be closer to God. Though the crumpled body told a short story of failed pitons, his letter to his girlfriend, found under deep layers of clothing, told more. The letter, now attached to the rescue report, is a remarkable insight into a journey taken by a man into the forbidding territory of the solo climber.

Tobin *had* been impressed with the mountain and the loneliness of the place. It inspired him to pray throughout the trek as he observed the beauty of the country, adding, "It's also very lonely— there isn't even a trail up here. Tomorrow I will be going across a glacier and that's scary alone." His first impression of the mountain certainly coincided with Duane's thoughts. He reports: "When I first came over Woolley Pass and saw Mt. Alberta I about died. I just shouted out loud 'Oh no!' It looked much too difficult and very BIG."

Tobin refers to the cold as well, even before reaching the base of the climb: "My fingers are freezing and the candles are getting low." The other thing that concerned him was the difficulty of the retreat if his climb was successful. By the time he reached the base of the climb, he was having considerable doubt about having the strength for the task. One of his main concerns was getting back. He notes: "If I can get up the thing I've also got to get down it. And the descent looks horrendous." Despite this, at no time did he entertain the idea of turning back. Things improved once he was rested after a satisfying supper. By the end of the first day he had completed the lower ice portion of the climb and was prepared for the difficult exit through the steep overhanging rock face above. A cheery note indicates that all was well at that point as he adds: "Once again I am in my little cocoon, warm and cosy …" Throughout his writing, he is strengthened by his faith in God: "Our lord Christ is truly renewing in my mind and heart. I've got to know God."

This did not last. The writing fades in size as his predicament deepens upon reaching the rock where the route becomes uncertain. "It took me an hour to figure out which way to go up the rock. There were two possibilities. I finally decided for the route on the left. Now I think I have made a mistake because the climbing has been outrageously hard. But I'm committed now, and there is not much I can do but keep going." The last entry indicates that the weather was beginning to change for the worse which caused him more anxiety. But his determination was unwavering despite his growing weariness and fear: "I am very committed on a route that has probably never been done. I was cold and tired and frightened. In fact I almost started to cry. Everything is wet. My legs are cramping out, but at least I'm warm now, tucked away in my sleeping bag and bivouac sack. Oh, I hope it doesn't snow. I've got to go now. You should see this place, everything is hanging all over the place."

The next day his fears were justified. The knotted rope and bent piton indicated that he had finally reached a pitch too difficult to climb. When he fell, the belay piton failed, and he plunged to his death hundreds of metres below. His final words reveal a powerful will to live and serve God, but most of all, to return to his deeply loved family and fiancé. The body was reverently placed in the Jenny Bag and flown back to his family in California. Whether Tobin was within his limits to tackle the north face of Mt. Alberta in October can only be assessed by climbers of his stature who would choose to go there themselves. As it is, his accomplishments guaranteed him a revered place in climbing history and helped establish a scholarship for excellence in a college that many aspire to.

7

Reality of Rescue

WHILE THE SEVENTIES WERE A TIME of learning and experimentation, the eighties saw a period of affluence that enabled the public safety function to thrive and expand. By 1979, the wardens were still the only professional mountain rescue organization in Canada. They were learning what people were capable of under difficult conditions, as well as the limitations and abilities of those involved in the program. They also learned that even the most experienced people are subject to accidents.

The 1980s would bring a continuation of the same work ethic, but the function became more streamlined with an added seriousness. The young, brash wardens hired in the early seventies were no longer brash nor young. Most were approaching their mid-thirties and were married; some had families. The challenge of pulling off big rescues such as Mt. Bryce had a sobering effect.

One of the elements that made a significant difference was the refinement of teamwork, which can only be developed with time. It was the binding glue that made training and rescues work, and it was always a source of concern if good people left the program. During the late seventies and early eighties this was not a problem. Several people came on strength who

were eager and talented and prepared to put in the time needed to meet the standards of the public safety program. The most significant of these were Gerry Israelson, Gord Irwin, Mark Ledwidge and Pat Sheehan. All four men became involved in the ACMG guide's program early in their careers through the support of Parks Canada. During this period Dianne Volkers began active work in public safety. Dianne was the second woman to be assigned to the public safety program after Kathy Calvert in Yoho. In the fifty-year history of the program, only two other women would play noteworthy roles in this function.

One of the growing factors limiting wardens from becoming involved in the public safety program was a greater leaning toward specialization. The helicopter made rescue work much more efficient, resulting in fewer people being called out for rescues. The wardens assigned to public safety were expected to climb at a higher standard and were given opportunities to develop their skills. The development of specialized gear demanded that rescue personnel be trained constantly in this field.

Despite a trend toward specialization, many wardens still got out on training schools during the early part of the decade. Peter and Willi's trips continued to be noteworthy and challenging and quite memorable for some. Rick Ralf recalls travelling with Peter Fuhrmann as one of the highlights of his career saying: "I enjoyed Peter's company and some of the challenging trips that he's done over the years. It was a lot of fun." Peter had a tendency to travel late in the day, but one particular school Rick attended was deliberately planned as a night excursion. He claims it was a typical Fuhrmann school. When he arrived in Banff they were sent up the trail to the Beehive in Lake Louise where they sat until it got dark. Rick began to suspect something was wrong, but once the sun went down Peter gave them the scenario. It turned out to be a night rescue practice. He recalls: "So we had to go out in the middle of the night, and do a rescue practice to see how it went at night. When you think back, that was good training because a lot of times you got a phone call in bed, and it's two in the morning or whatever— but you have to get up and get organized." In the end, he adds, "Those Fuhrmann scenarios were never easy."

Peter was not the only one who saw the value of nighttime training. Kathy and Gerry showed up from Yoho for a school in Jasper with Willi Pfisterer, who had plotted out an even more ambitious night exercise. Willi decided it was time to see how difficult it would be to travel through the night for a crevasse rescue on the third icefall of the Athabasca Glacier. It was obvious that the helicopter could not be used because it was dark, and there was the added assumption that it would not be called the next day because of bad weather.

The "victim" was sent up with a climbing party and told to find a convenient crevasse as far up as they could without undue exposure to the ice fall from The Snow Dome. Around eleven o'clock, the "accident" was reported and the first rescue party was dispatched with light gear to move fast and plot the way through the maze of huge crevasses that laced the first and second icefall. It was fairly clear to the heavily burdened second party, now laden with the bulk of the rescue equipment, that no one had really seen much of this route in midsummer. Or at least, not at night. With perplexed amazement, the slower rope teams wound their way around the huge crevasses barely lit by headlamps.

Kathy was happy she had been training when she was given one half of the rescue toboggan to carry. The aluminum ladders were the key to crossing the larger crevasses, but it was slow work. One finally gave out, however, while Kathy was belaying Ian Syme across a particularly large expanse of blackness. It broke right in the middle, sending him down clinging to the far half of the ladder. Fortunately, it never quite parted at the break, and he was able to climb out the other side. The rest of the party now had to climb down the broken bridge and up the other half. Everyone made it, and by morning most of the rescue team arrived to save their "victim." By the time he was loaded into the toboggan and brought out, it was almost mid-morning. The debriefing gave everyone an opportunity to review the success of the exercise, and it was agreed that if a helicopter could be used at all, it was the best recourse. The ground party should only be sent up if prolonged bad weather set in—the exposure of a large party to extremely hazardous terrain was not the best first option.

Some schools did not escape without casualty, however. Dianne Volkers remembers Peter had a penchant for training in the Lake Louise area. Since her first assignment was in Lake Louise, she attended quite a few of his schools. Dianne was one of the few wardens who had a strong background in climbing before she started with Parks Canada. She grew up in Vancouver, where she learned to climb, and soon found she had an interest in rescue work. Like Tim and Clair, she worked with a mountain rescue group in North Vancouver and had acquired some knowledge in that field prior to being a warden. She was a talented skier as well, which made her a strong addition to the Lake Louise staff.

Dianne's most vivid memory of a training school was the traverse of Mt. Victoria. It stood out in her mind because it seemed plagued with small accidents every day. It was a large school with 12 participants, including a couple who were RCMP officers with little mountaineering experience. The number was quickly reduced after the first climb on Mt. Lefroy, when one of the climbers was hit by a rock and had to be flown off. Before traversing Mt. Victoria, two more dropped out when one of the members got sick and was taken down by one of the wardens. Dianne actually enjoyed the climb, because she was partnered with the one remaining RCMP officer who happened to be a reasonably good climber. However, the day did not seem to end. Mt. Victoria is a long, broken ridge; progress was painfully slow. Dianne recalls that some rope teams were not having such good rapport. She could hear the various teams yelling at each other throughout the day as communication became difficult. After 12 hours they finally reached the col between the main summit and Mt. Collier following a difficult descent over rotten rock. It was 8:30 p.m. and getting dark when there was a dispute over the next course of action. Peter wanted to continue down in the dark, but Gord Irwin disagreed. But as Dianne put it, Peter "loves it when things get a bit difficult and people have to sort things out a bit." In this case she concurred with Gord adding: "I love Peter, but he does push a little bit." However, if a team leader could present a good argument, that was all that Peter required. They spent the night out and were out early the following morning.

Ice climbing was growing in popularity, and soon there were schools cropping up to train the novice. With big routes still not climbed, it was

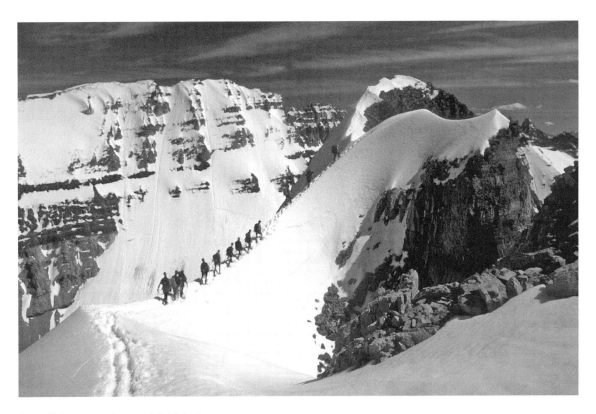

Peter Fuhrmann school on Mt. Victoria. GREG HORNE COLLECTION

an open challenge to the better climbers to gain some first ascents. The concerned wardens closely monitored these climbs, knowing that the chances of being called to a rescue were pretty good. The greatest danger to the climber in these natural water funnels was from avalanches.

One of the big objectives in the early eighties was a route called Polar Circus. It was also where Tim Auger lost another close friend. On the day of the accident, John Lauchlan was attempting the first solo climb of this route. Unfortunately, he chose to go during a period of high avalanche hazard. Friends wondered why he set out under such unfavourable conditions on February 5, 1982, but the pressure from competing climbers to capture this plum may have been a motivation. When his car was still at the road at four o'clock in the afternoon, two other friends, Jim Elzinga and Albi Sole, who were climbing in the area, became concerned, particularly after they spotted fresh avalanche debris covering his tracks on one small slope. They drove immediately to Saskatchewan Crossing Warden Station where they reported the possibility of an accident, then returned to check it out further. The rescue report states: "At approximately 1,825-metre elevation they found the missing man at the base of the first ice pitch." Meanwhile Tim set out from Banff to meet dog handler Dale Portman at Lake Louise, thinking an avalanche search was a likely possibility. When they met the two climbers at the Saskatchewan Crossing, Tim's worst fears were realized.

The following day the weather was brilliant and clear as Tim and Dale flew up to recover the body and attempt to discover what had caused the accident. From the helicopter the men found John's tracks leading onto a small steep slope, halfway up on the climb. He had released a slab avalanche as soon as he tried to cross, which swept him down over 100 metres of moderately angled steps, then over a 25-metre waterfall. This had not killed him however. Drag marks to the top of the next pitch suggested he had sustained serious injuries but that he was conscious and was attempting to reach safety. He managed to set up a rappel anchor, but his body was found at the bottom of the large waterfall he was trying to descend. It was not clear if he fell while setting up the rappel or if the anchor had failed while rappelling. John was found with the rope wrapped around his body, but incompletely, as though he were trying to do a body rappel. One arm was badly broken, making any attempt to rappel difficult, but there was little else he could have tried.

Thankfully, dealing with the loss of friends is not always the outcome of rescue work, and successes often stand out in people's memories more than failures. Tim was able to look back on many successes made easy with the helicopter, but there were occasions when it could not be used. One such occasion cropped up when Tim had to do some difficult climbing to rescue the victim.

A tourist had heard a man hollering for help near the bottom of Tunnel Mountain and had reported it to the warden office late in the day. Tim and his team drove out to the trail leading to where the man was stranded, but by then it was dark. The man was about 23 metres up, which was more than enough to kill him if he fell, but not a long way to climb. Thinking all he had to do was get to him and lower him off, Tim began to climb up a corner with only a headlamp for light. Right away the corner turned into a series of cracks that got thinner and thinner but continued to lead right to the man. It was now very difficult, requiring the use of pitons and aid slings. Tim peered up to the terrified man who was crouched on a steep slab inside a small corner and wondered how in hell he had got there. Tim recalls: "He was facing out with one hand in this crack, kind of holding himself saying 'Hurry up, I'm not sure how long I can stay here!'" But now the crack Tim was working up began to peter out. He was standing in the aid slings on dubious pin placements, wondering if he could hold the fellow if he slipped off. This was very doubtful, and he had no choice but to radio out for someone to send for a bolt kit from the rescue room. Time dragged by for both of them, but finally the kit arrived twenty minutes later. He soon whacked in a couple of bolts to the cries of, "Hurry up, hurry up!" from above. With a decent anchor in place, he reached the grateful man and tied him into the rope. With another bolt placed just above, it was "a snap to lower him down." It continued to puzzle him how the fellow had got there in the first place. Once they were down, the shaky victim explained he had traversed in from above on a ledge that was not obvious in the dark, then found he could not return. He had not climbed the crack at all.

During this time, Clair was having mixed success on Mt. Temple. The east ridge and the Greenwood-Locke route were proving quite popular but were definitely challenging when it came to rescues. One climber impressed Clair with her fortitude and climbing ability when her partner suffered a fall in the Black Towers on the east ridge. The Black Towers are easily the crux of this climb if people try to climb through them instead of skirting around their base. They are rotten and steep, requiring tedious belaying and delicate climbing. Clair was flying by on a reconnaissance flight when he spotted a single climber frantically waving and apparently in trouble. They could not get in immediately because of bad winds, but they were able to get close enough to drop a bag with a radio to establish communication. This turned out to be a challenge as well, but soon they enlisted the aid of Greg Yavorski, a Cadet Camp instructor who spoke Japanese and was able to translate for them. It was quickly established that her partner had fallen while trying to lead through the towers and had been seriously hurt. Hoping to get help, the young woman climbed on through "difficult and extremely exposed rock unroped to reach the summit icefield." The winds abated enough for John Flaa and John Steele to get in and assist in slinging her down to the staging area.

Getting her partner out was another matter. When the woman had left him with her spare clothing, he was alive. This would be a much more

technical rescue so Clair enlisted the aid of Gord Irwin and Tim Auger. Because the man was possibly still alive, Clair took the unusual course of enlisting Dr. J. Boyd working at the Banff hospital, who also happened to be a good climber. He brought in Jim Davies from Banff to fly the tricky mission, and soon they were on the precarious towers above the victim. They had spotted him hanging from a rope during a bumpy fly by but could not tell if he was alive or dead. Once the station was established, Dr. Boyd was lowered down to the man, but there was nothing he could do. The dead climber was slung out to the staging area. Although they were not in time to save the man, the rescue stood out for the success of operating in such difficult terrain and for the pluck of the young girl who had survived. Clair was always impressed with the malevolent nature of the aptly named black towers as, no doubt, was everyone else.

THROUGHOUT THE LATE SEVENTIES and early eighties, cable rescue was considered an essential tool in the mountain rescue arsenal and practice with this equipment was ongoing, though it was never really used in any big rescues. But using one single cable left some people uneasy about reliability, and they sought a better safety margin. The answer was to work with a dual cable system. Jim Murphy recalls heading out for the Devil's Thumb above Lake Agnes on the first dual cable-rescue practice with Tim. They were lowered over the face with winches working side by side attached to each other with an umbilical cord (a rope connector about 1.5 metres long) to see if this was practical. Although it increased the safety should one cable fail, it was difficult to co-ordinate. It was helpful in lowering a stretcher, because both men could work together to manoeuvre the victim over difficult terrain, but communication remained a problem, particularly in getting the teams to work in unison. The helmets with an imbedded microphone did not work that well and often garbled such essential commands as "slower" and "lower."

The other problem was the umbilical cord, which repeatedly got hung up on rock outcrops. They had to continually go over and free the cord while trying to get the team above to stop lowering so they could effect the manoeuvre.

Another major problem with the cable was its tendency to unravel with long lowers. This particular scenario happened on a rescue practice on the north face of Mt. Athabasca using the dual cable method. A dual lowering system was set up on the summit with the purpose of sending down the men with a stretcher right to the bottom of the face. Brad White and Gerry Israelson confidently set off waving a cheery goodbye, hoping to sail smoothly to the bottom. But the north face of Mt. Athabasca is not all that smooth nor is it that steep. Several rotten cliff bands, where the cable would run over the soft, crumbly rock, had to be negotiated. It was one of the first times such a long lower had been tried and it proved the limitations of cable. As Gerry later explained: "The cable is essentially a twisted strand. Like screws, when the cable starts to run in grooves [ice or stone] or runs over any surface that grabs the cable, the twist in the cable causes it to turn. The swivel at the end would counter this effect. However, the swivel can only remove the tension [twist] up the line as far as it is free hanging. So the bottom end of the cable is usually OK. It is the middle and top where the tension builds up. The cardinal rule is to always keep the cable fully loaded so that the upper part of the line can't kink. The rescuer is dependent on the team up above to manage the line. And the team depends on the rescuer to keep the line loaded until they reach the accident site. For shorter practices, this worked. However, on a long lower, there are many more potential problems.

"On long lowers where the cable problem is exacerbated, there are multiple contact points that may be great distances apart. The grooves in the stone turn the cable as it descends and the reverse should happen as the cable is brought up. I'm talking about the middle part of the line … not the end. The bird cage [unravelling of strands] occurs when a section of the cable not affected by the swivel comes back up. The tension is not reversed as quickly as it is normally, so the cable starts to open up more and more. We did not see this until we started practicing on big mountain faces and the problems were discovered quickly."

This, of course, happened. Again, communication and distance were a problem. In this case, though, Gerry's cable was affected first. Suddenly Brad was moving down while Gerry stayed put. The umbilical cord between them was becoming taut leaving them in a precarious situation. They tried to let those above know the predicament before it was critical, but the radio connection was poor and the message was not received. The weight of the cable was now sufficient to create its own load, and the people above continued to let out more and more cable thinking the boys were having an uninterrupted trip down the face. Finally as the cable piled up, the message was received and the men were brought up. It was an interesting critique at the end of the day when these limitations were considered. Despite these setbacks, the dual cable was considered an improvement and a safer way to go.

A couple of changes on the horizon were the availability of longer cables, now used in Europe, and a new rope product called "blue line." This heavy-duty rope now being considered for rescue work had far less stretch compared the regular climbing ropes. The advantage of cable was its compactness for carrying to the top of a climb and the fact that it was slender, thus less susceptible to rock fall. It also ran with considerably less friction over rock, making it easier to raise and lower. The blue line, by comparison, was very bulky and could easily be nicked or chopped by rocks. It was heavy and created a lot of friction when in contact with the rock. Even with less stretch, the men had to bring up quite a length before the actual load came on the line and the rescuer began to move. On the other hand, tests showed it would sustain considerably more shock before snapping. A new combination was being worked out where the cable would be the principal lowering and raising tool, while the blue line would be used for backup as a belay anchor. The combination would provide the attributes of both while minimizing some of the drawbacks.

THE PUBLIC SAFETY PROGRAM was moving forward and keeping abreast of the expansion in climbing and other risk-oriented sports, but that was not always a guarantee for unquestioned support from park management. By 1983 the federal government had created several new northern parks that also had a public safety mandate. This coincided with drastically escalating helicopter costs (from approximately $150/hr to $400/hr in a matter of a couple of years). So the Assistant Deputy Minister for Parks Canada was asked to review the matter. He created a Program Management Committee (the much dreaded committee) to investigate the allocation of money, announcing: "Concern has been expressed that the program may be overextended in the provision of search-and-rescue services to the public, particularly in relation to high-risk activities such as mountain climbing." The committee wanted to know what other countries were doing, what alternative agencies (such as the RCMP) could handle rescues, how Parks could recover money from high-risk adventurers who needed rescue, and what the long-term policy should be.

In accordance with this disquieting inquisition, a fairly long report was submitted to the committee, and the superintendents of each national park across Canada were asked to submit a set of recommendations. The report indicated that several significant advances had been made in the mountain parks with regard to avalanche forecasting and control; that an effective double cable system had been developed to facilitate rescue on difficult rock faces; and that the helicopter was effective in rescue and backcountry search operations. It also recognized that a public safety program was much more difficult to maintain in newer parks in remote locations, especially in northern Canada. More significant, it was pointed out that "Parks Canada Policy provides no clear direction on what levels of mountain search-and-rescue service should be provided to the public."

Prior to this paper coming out, the parks in the western region had decided to get together annually to review different rescues in each park, the state of the equipment and various policy changes, as well as programs for the next year. It was called the Public Safety Advisory Committee and representatives from Parks within the western region attended every year to keep in touch. It certainly was the arena to look at policy affecting the program. The committee had already concluded in 1981 that "several directives related to public safety in national parks … were badly out of date, weak in content and in need of complete revision." One policy sweepingly indicated that Parks had an objective of providing aid to all visitors feared to be in distress or potential danger and that this aid should be extended to those outside the park if requested.

Though there were questions about legal responsibility and cost recovery, most of the field personnel just wanted to know if the program was going to continue and if so, under what direction. After evaluating if any other agency in the region could do an adequate job (and concluding they either could not or would not), and admitting that some form of public safety program had to be maintained, the analysis promoted the second of three recommendations: that the status quo continue with limited resources to be provided in parks located at the extremities of normal visitor travel. The public safety program was allowed to continue and even expand to meet the demands of increased recreational activity, but some were alarmed it had ever been questioned in the first place.

DESPITE THE REVIEW, leaders in the public safety field once again looked at the problem of the north faces. Most of the truly scary ones were in Jasper, prompting a meeting to be held at Tangle Creek near the Columbia Icefield. By this time Darro Stinson had taken over the public safety position from Tony Klettl in the park. Gerry Israelson had moved up from Lake Louise to work with him, making a very strong team for that park. Rick Ralf was also active in the program and recalls flying around Mt. Kitchener, the North and South Twin, the face on Mt. Columbia as well as Mt. Alberta and Mt. Bryce—virtually anywhere people could get into big trouble. They looked at all the routes, judging the potential for rescues: where cable would reach, where the helicopters could fly to, where teams could be located and evacuated from. It was a sobering look at reality. In the end they realized some rescues just might not be possible, particularly if bad weather was a factor. And on big north faces, bad weather was usually a factor. Gerry observed: "We came to the realization that as an organization, there may be circumstances when we really can't do anything … you know, if the risks were just unacceptable." The responsibility of the public safety team was to handle 95% of the routine events in the park rather than an improbable rescue that might happen infrequently. The week-long meeting was over, and everyone went home hoping that a worst-case scenario never developed. And in the end it never did. The anticipated interest in the north faces from extreme climbers never materialized to the point where anyone got into trouble.

A lot of rescues had little to do with north faces—or even climbing for that matter. Water rescues and searches for missing persons were always part of the job. Searches were often interesting as they tended to involve some sleuthing. One of the key elements in a search is the mental outlook of the missing person, and the relationship he or she had with friends or family. Sometimes people were simply trying to get away from a family crisis and were unaware that anyone was looking for them. These people often just went home. This was never the case for lost children, however. One search for a missing child also revealed that poor initial results came from underestimating the range that a lost child could travel.

Such was the case of a "small thin" boy from Germany who spoke no English missing from Rampart Creek campground on the Icefield Parkway. Clair Israelson was alerted by the campground attendant that the child had gone missing around 6:00 p.m. wearing only green shorts and sandals with no other clothing or gear. A search was implemented immediately after an initial hasty search by the local warden revealed nothing. Luckily it was the 28th of June, with fine warm weather and clear skies. Gord Peyto was called in with his dog, soon followed by Alfie Burstrom and the RCMP dog handler Gary McCormick. It was not long before a second search party arrived, and with the help of volunteers from the nearby youth hostel, they were able to assemble two teams. The main search areas identified right away were the cliffs below the hostel to the east and the muskeg north of the campground. Rescuers were also concerned about the banks of the river. Although the search continued through the night, no evidence of the missing boy turned up, nor was a track picked up by any of the dog handlers.

By the following day, the grid pattern extended more to the south and east of the campground, but now it was felt that a thorough search of the river was required. Kayaks, the jet boat and foot patrols were sent out to scour every centimetre of the bank. A fourth dog handler, Scott Ward, was brought in to give the other dog teams a break. A very discouraged Clair brought in more wardens from Banff, Jasper and Yoho to relieve the ground crew. By noon, even the British Army was employed but still to no avail. Finally, the search was extended north to Norman Creek, a small tributary well away from the campground. None of these possibilities brought any results. The traumatized parents thought that the child may have been abducted. Most of the searchers worried he had drowned. Suddenly a call came in from a motorist who had found a young child sitting under the bridge at Saskatchewan River Crossing. It was 4:15 p.m. when the search was brought to an end, and the relieved parents were reunited with their son.

Everyone was amazed that the boy was found 30 kilometres from where he had first gone missing. With the parents translating, they were able to determine what had happened. The young child had gone to the washroom shortly after they had pulled into their campsite, but when he emerged, he was not sure what direction to head. Then he saw a camper pull out onto the highway travelling south. He thought his parents had left him behind, and he ran after the departing vehicle. But rather than stick to the road, he took a shortcut through the bush thinking it would lead to the highway. Once in the bush, he became completely lost and soon came to the river. He was smart enough to avoid the water, however, and continued downstream throughout the night till he came to the bridge sometime the following day. A passing motorist had been alerted to the search, and when he spotted the boy under the bridge, he immediately picked him up and reported to the Warden Service.

A number of lessons were learned from this search, not the least of which was to not underestimate how far children can travel. Also, the boy had been taught on the trip over from Germany not to talk to strangers. That, plus a normal fear of being lost, may have encouraged him to hide when searchers called out his name. Reviewing psychological parameters became an essential component of future searches.

Kathy Calvert kept the lessons learned from this search in mind the following summer when she was notified of a man missing on Mt. Hunter at the east end of Yoho National Park. Kathy was now in an acting position, running the public safety program in that park after both Gerry Israelson and Dale Portman had left for more fertile fields in Lake Louise.

The man did not return late in the day after hiking on the trail to the Mt. Hunter Lookout, and by the following morning his concerned parents reported him missing. The main problem was that the missing man, though well into his forties and equipped with warm clothing in a day pack, was mentally challenged, and no one was certain how he would react. The search extended well outside the area the man had gone missing from, largely because PEP was called in and many people volunteered. Unfortunately he was not found soon enough. He had wandered down off the trail in the dark through steep bush and had lost his eyeglasses. He was blind without them. He then probably attempted to cross the Kicking Horse River on hearing highway traffic on the other side. His body was found washed up in an eddy on the trail side of the river the following morning.

Water-rescue capability was also expanding, particularly by those wardens who had an interest in scuba diving. Murray Hindle, who had been diving for many years, thought this expertise could be used in water-rescue situations. Other wardens who took up the sport, such as warden Bob Hansen and warden John Woodrow, agreed. The possibilities were explored with more enthusiasm after Pat Sheehan joined the Warden Service and moved to Jasper. Pat was an energetic young climber, skier and scuba diver with an Irish background. He was infectiously popular with everyone and was soon in the public safety training program where he worked closely with Gerry Israelson and Darro Stinson. His interest in scuba diving coupled with his role in public safety gave him the ear of his mentors, and he was able to convince them that water-rescue training should add to their expertise.

A new jet boat was added to the water-rescue arsenal. The scuba training was limited to those who had their dive tickets, but the boat training was open to all who wished to pursue this sport. The jet boat was the one expensive item that needed a lot of training to handle well in whitewater. To get this expertise, the boys took it out when they could but also scheduled regional schools to train others. It was actually one such school that almost "sank" the program.

The new Jasper boat was brought out for a joint Banff/Jasper water-rescue school put on at Becker's Bungalows just south of Jasper townsite. The river curves close to the highway at this location, which has some of the biggest rapids in the river. It was an ideal spot to launch the boats and do repeated body pickups and to practise driving the boats in high waves. The Jasper boat had shipped some water during repeated trips down the river and had begun to ride lower and lower. The driver felt the boat was sluggish but decided to try for one last pickup before returning to shore. It was once too often, however, and a wave swamped the boat. Though everyone made it to shore, it was a while before the jet boat was replaced.

Though the jet boat remained a necessary part of the rescue artillery, the scuba diving soon faded out. There were not enough rescues to justify the in-house expertise, and if a dive team was required, one could be brought in from the Calgary or Edmonton Fire Rescue Teams.

The divers did get called out a few times before the program collapsed. Pat Sheehan was sent down to Panther Falls to retrieve the body of a man who had fallen over. Pat had to go down on a cable to access the pool beneath the falls. It took several attempts to reach the body, which was being cycled through the back eddy. With

great difficulty he finally secured the man and the wardens were able to bring them both up.

The divers also created opportunities to train and extend their experience. Bob Hansen suggested they search the bottom of Athabasca Falls in winter for the body of a man who had gone missing the previous summer. He was aided by fellow warden divers Murray Hindle, Pat Sheehan and Ivan Philips. Recovery efforts that summer had brought no clues to the man's whereabouts, but winter provided a rare opportunity to see if he was trapped at the base of the fall. It was an experience Bob never forgot. Previous training had taught him to be prepared for a face looming suddenly out of murky water, but he was unprepared for how the cold affected the equipment. It was so cold that he had trouble keeping the regulator valve open. The amount of oxygen in the frothing water kept it colder than the surface air temperature, and his gloves kept freezing to the valve. The eerie blackness, the powerful current and the thunder of the fall under the ice added to the surreal conditions, which he described as "spookier than hell," and after the others had spelled him off, they called it quits. They had been able to explore most of the pool and were glad to report to the family that the man was not there. It eliminated one more possibility of his whereabouts, and they felt the effort was justified, even if it was almost foolhardy.

BY THE MID-EIGHTIES, it was apparent that rescues in the national parks would not be handled by any agency other than the Warden Service. The volume of incidents was also rising with the increase in tourism. This meant helicopter use was increasing as well, not only for rescues but for routine jobs, making the park contract much more lucrative to several newly formed helicopter companies. The very thought of having to fly with an unknown pilot unnerved most of the wardens, who justifiably felt they left their lives in the hands of the man flying the machine. Conversely, the pilot trusted the rescuer to do his job properly

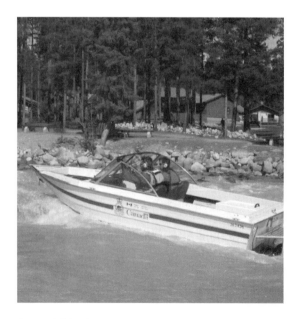

Jasper jet boat. JASPER WARDEN ARCHIVES

and not kill them all. The bond between pilot and rescuer was implicit and vital to the success of every operation.

Jim Davies had devoted his life to developing heli-slinging as a practical life-saving rescue procedure and during the seventies was the only pilot who had the expertise to fly some of the missions asked of him. Jim Murphy's experience on Wenkchemna Peak brought home to him just how important the bond between pilot and rescuer really was, when they were required to pluck a dentist off a rather delicate ice serac. It was a late call for help that came to the warden office as he and Cliff White were leaving for the day. Two climbers had set out to climb Wenkchemna Peak near Lake Louise but were badly off route and had wound up in a terrifying tangle of hanging seracs. They finally got hung up on one spindly serac from which they were trying to surmount a second. The second serac was seriously overhung, preventing them from reaching the top. Realizing they were not going to make it, the dentist opted to jump back down to the serac from which he had just escaped. In the process, he hooked his crampon strap on the other leg and literally fell onto the top of the serac. Only now he had a broken ankle and was stuck on top of the icy spire that was vertical on all sides and little over a metre and a half at the top. His partner was able to find a way down and scuttled back for help.

Jim and Cliff flew in with Davies under rain-soaked skies to see what could be done, just as it was getting dark. They found the man huddled on the pinpoint of ice (Jim felt that just finding him was amazing) and knew all they could do was sling in and try to set a belay while hanging from the rope. Cliff went in and set up the anchor, making it safe for Jim to come in with the stretcher. Cliff had actually established the anchors on the side of the second serac so that the belay was from above, leaving more room to work, but Jim still smilingly recalls: "It was very crowded on the top of this serac." It was now getting quite dark, and with the threatening weather Davies was not

sure if he could get back in. It would have been precarious for the three to spend the night on the tiny pinnacle. Knowing this, Davies decided to try. With huge relief, the two wardens and the victim heard the familiar whop of the rotor blades as the precious sling hung from the barely visible belly of the helicopter. Now came the crux of the rescue. They had to attach the stretcher and rescuer to the sling while freeing everything from the protection of the anchor. It was this dicey transfer that required quick work and delicate flying. If one anchor was left in place, the machine would crash when he tried to fly off. Everything went smoothly, however, and Davies was able to get back for Cliff, now feeling very alone on the lofty perch.

When other helicopter companies came looking for the same work they were told, justifiably, that they did not have the pilot that could do the job. At the time, Jim Davies was hired on what was called a single-source contract, and the work was not put up for bid. They were able to do this because the contract specified the company must supply a certified rescue pilot, and Jim was the only one available. But it was a government contract—usually required by law to be open for tender—and this argument only stalled the bureaucrats for a few years. As the competition grew hungrier, the demands to open the contract for bid intensified until the wardens were slowly forced to produce standards by which others could be tested.

Cliff White recalls an event that helped prolong the continuance of the one-source contract. The occasion was a night rescue on Cascade Waterfall in winter. It was a rescue Davies remembers well, because it was a challenge not usually encountered during normal rescues. Two young men had completed the climb and were descending when they were hit by an avalanche. One man was seriously injured with a broken leg, but his partner was unharmed and able to go for help. By then it was pitch dark. Normally, such a rescue would be left until morning, but the man may not have survived the night. White discussed the situation with Davies, and they decided to try a sling that night. Jim remembers: "I had a landing light [that shone] straight down and one that [shone] ahead, and once I got over the waterfall, I was able to put the lights on and go straight in. I followed the trail this kid made on his way out and we found the victim that way. I was slinging the wardens at the same time, floodlighting the whole area with the helicopter … and it worked very well. There wasn't even a moon that night, it was absolutely black."

It was a first night rescue using the helicopter in the mountains, and it was a success. But Cliff White noted that it also came to the attention of the Director General, Jim Raby, in an unexpected way. Raby was driving to Banff that night and happened to see "the light show" on the side of Cascade Mountain. He came over to see what was going on, and as Cliff says, he "got an earful about why they needed a rescue pilot who can do this work at the top end of his game." All discussions of putting the work out for contract were put aside until more consideration could be given to pilot expertise.

But by this time, flying using vertical reference was becoming more commonplace, as pilots learned this skill while logging or moving equipment at gas well sites. Called long lining, it entailed flying loads at the end of the line attached to the cargo hook. It was not so much a technical leap as a mental leap for new pilots to go from flying static objects to live cargo, and they were eager to try the work.

One of the other government requirements was that the lowest bidder had to be accepted as long as he met the terms of the contract. With Jim's contract now on the horizon, companies with deeper pockets than his were prepared to undercut him once they had the right pilot. All they needed was a certification process. The day came, Tim Auger recalls, when "Fuhrmann came along and said, 'Well we're going to have to go out and test these pilots.'" They had no recourse but to consult Jim Davies, since he was the only one who knew what was required. There were other standards that

could be thrown in, however, such as thorough knowledge of the park geography. This actually worked one year when Peter asked the candidate to verbally describe the location of several well-hidden backcountry lakes. This kept the wolves off for a while, but it was a rather poor fence. Finally one company complained to Ottawa, and the wardens were told to solve the problem.

Near panic and rebellion set in as wardens realized they might have to commit their lives to an unknown pilot. It is interesting that Jasper was not going through any of this dilemma. Gaby Fortin, now the CPW in Banff, was not wrong in saying that Jim Davies was the only certified pilot in Banff, but this did not include Gary Forman, flying for Yellowhead Helicopters in Jasper. Gary had actually gone through a simple test with Peter Fuhrmann shortly after he moved to Valemount, B.C., and he began to fly rescue missions for Jasper National Park in 1980. Jim Davies was quite happy with this arrangement, because it was too far for him to fly for rescues and the work load in Banff would have prohibited this anyway. Yellowhead Helicopters also had a second qualified pilot when Todd McCready joined the company. Jasper was too far off the beaten track for competing companies, who did not find it lucrative enough to compete for.

Ultimately, Banff had to provide a test that was equable to any company wishing to submit a pilot for certification. They could even point to Gary and say this had been done in the past. Though the park was able to insist the pilots have high flying standards, the requirement of having to take the lowest bidder was still unsettling. The wardens needed help, and they got it from a person working for Supply and Services who was responsible for helicopter services for Canadian government jobs. He was in full sympathy with the dilemma and was one of the few who seemed to understand that they were asking for commitment and an ability to bond in a team environment where lives were at risk. He was able to advise them that they could be choosy as long as they were very specific in the contract's "terms of reference." Knowing that the future of a safe program now hung on the outcome of establishing a valid test, the wardens carefully outlined the flying parameters. For this, they relied on Jim's expertise to a limited extent. If he were seen to be too deeply involved in the process, they could be justifiably accused of a conflict of interest.

However, Jim set the de facto standard that had to be met. He was the first Canadian pilot to receive the Robert E. Trimble Award for outstanding mountain flying in Dallas, Texas, in 1975. As Tim recounts, "We dreamt up this test that had these various components that you would have to be a Jim Davies or Gary Forman to get through." But throughout they had to be "squeaky clean." They could not be seen to be protecting Jim if they wanted the program to survive.

With the doors now seriously open to the rivals, the companies marched in with their pilots—and their lawyers. The debate, by now, had even reached the House of Commons. With a seriousness that was never a part of the heydays of the seventies, Tim and Clair and Peter laid out the test requirements, knowing that if they failed a pilot they'd better have a good reason. Still, with a risky combination of guts and trepidation, they did fail pilots. But who could complain? Their lives and the lives of casualties depended on their decisions, giving them a strong "bucket of blood" argument for those who objected. The companies, of course, did object strenuously to the point that Transport Canada finally sent in inspectors to see just what the problem was. One fellow was "sent out with orders to make sure the thing was cleaned up," leaving the boys with little choice but to show him what they needed. He was flown on a rescue scenario on the north face of Mt. Victoria over the "Death Trap" in semi-whiteout conditions. The flight was enough to convince the man that they really did need the best they could get.

Todd McCready, now flying for Gary in Jasper, was always impressed with what it meant to be part of the rescue team. He had the advantage of being raised in the town and being the son of

Tom McCready, a local outfitter and skier. Through working with his dad, he had an intimate knowledge of the park before he ever started to fly, and he was well known to most of the wardens. By the time he went to work for Gary, he was good friends with several of the wardens on the rescue team, and he formed a close bond with them over the years. He had a healthy respect for the work, especially when flying "live cargo." But his first challenge was to "get on the same wavelength as the rescue team itself … it was a totally different language to me." It was a matter of being familiar with the jargon so that he could figure out what was happening. That led to smooth flying for everyone, and slowly a subtler form of communication developed as the men began to form a unified team.

He reflects: "I think the biggest psychological thing in the sling rescue was the fact that you were hauling live cargo. And again, I guess it's funny how your mind works. You could do a recovery of somebody who is deceased, and you could fly them and it was a totally different mind set because that person is dead. And then you go back for the rescue team, and they are wandering around, and you pick them up and fly and again … it's live cargo … it's not really like a light switch that you turn off and on, but there is definitely a difference."

When Tim and Clair were looking for that sensitivity in a pilot, they had good reason to look hard. All they had to do was recall a frightening incident that happened in the Bugaboos to Peter Enderwick, a warden working with Hans Fuhrer in Kootenay National Park. They had been called in to look for a person who had drowned in a stream crossing on the way to the upper camp and were ending the mission when the mishap occurred. Hans recalls the pilot was very good and well trusted, but on this occasion radio interference almost resulted in a fatality to a rescue. He picked Peter up and was returning to the lodge when he was contacted by the RCMP about details of the drowning. The radio

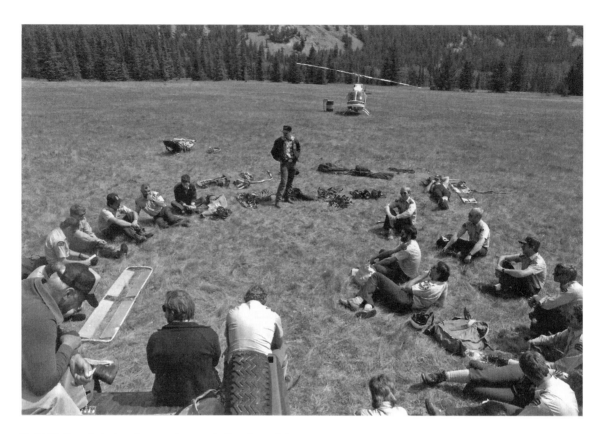

Todd McCready instructing wardens on helicopter safety. TODD MCCREADY COLLECTION

communication to Peter was now cut off, and he could not get through as they rapidly approached a building. In fact, the communication with the RCMP was so distracting that the pilot forgot he was slinging a live person. At the last minute he remembered that Peter was still attached to the line and pulled up just before he was slammed into a wall. Peter was madly trying to detach from the line and was actually able to do so as soon as his feet touched the ground but it was a very close call. From that time on, all communication except with the person being slung was eliminated until the rescue was over.

Both Tim and Clair knew they needed stable careful pilots with enough confidence to go "into situations that could be very, very difficult." Not all pilots had the ability or desire to fly into dangerous terrain in bad weather with a live

cargo permanently attached to the machine—and for brief seconds, be permanently attached to a mountain. "Our test had to go beyond that because it recognized that there are some situations that some people can [handle] and some can't [handle] as well. We want only those people who can." The emphasis from the beginning was that the pilot would be part of a team working together under difficult conditions where an individual's actions meant the safety of the team and victim. Many pilots flew well, but not all were able to work well as team members under those conditions.

Finally a company called Quasar came forward with Jim Stone, one pilot who was outstanding. After going through the regular test, they had him fly through an actual scenario on Cascade Mountain that Tim described as having "a bit of a sting in it." It looked easy from the ground, but they had asked him to go into a location that was prohibitively dangerous due to gusting, quirky winds. Stone waved it off, saying it was too dangerous to get into. Jim Davies, now working for Okanagan Helicopters, was asked to fly the mission as well. When he called it off, they knew they had a pilot who passed at every level. With Okanagan Helicopters unwilling to underbid their rival, the contract finally went to another company.

Despite the high standards, Jim Stone passed the rigorous test and the wardens had to honour their commitment to the process they had established. Tim knew then that his days of flying with Jim were over, saying: "The world became a new world at that point." In fact they entered into a nightmare world where pilots came and went with alarming frequency because of the volatile world of helicopter companies. In the mid- to late eighties everyone seemed to have a company that lasted for only a few years before being bought out by another.

The contracts Banff signed automatically affected both Kootenay and Yoho national parks, because they came under Fuhrmann's jurisdiction. This was often frustrating for the wardens in Yoho, who preferred to fly with Don McTighe (who did not work for the company with the contract) because he flew out of Golden, B.C. for Okanagan Helicopters and was significantly closer and more experienced. Meanwhile new pilots would regularly show up for rescues. Whether it was the bureaucracy of fair play or greed that led to the new condition, the fallout left a field of lost friendships and bitter feelings. However, one good result was the establishment of a testing program that would ultimately save lives. In the end, Tim was able to say: "I don't think we'd be here today if it wasn't for the pilot test."

Aside from the problems with helicopters, the number of accidents continued to mount, with 1986 being almost a record year for big events throughout the parks. That summer saw

a challenging rescue successfully concluded on a remote mountain in Jasper. Mt. Bridgland is a spectacular-looking peak north of the Yellowhead Highway in Jasper that became the objective of a group of climbers from the Edmonton section of the Alpine Club. They set out to climb the peak on a hot summer day around the end of July and were almost successful until the leader took a nasty fall just short of the summit. By the time two members were able to hoof it out for help, the weather had turned foul. Overnight, the rain set in, turning to snow in the early morning hours. By the time Gerry Israelson flew in with a team of three other wardens (John Niddrie, Darro Stinson and Greg Horne), they could only fly partway up the lower half of the mountain. Not knowing when to expect a break, they decided it was best to climb the rest of the way with enough gear to provide food and shelter for all until a retreat plan was in place. The climbing was terrible on steep rock bands covered with a centimetre of verglas overlaid by fresh snow. They succeeded in getting to the injured climber, who had broken his leg in the fall. In short order, they had a tent erected and the man stabilized. Fortunately the weather changed enough for Todd McCready to test the limits of the helicopter and sling them off. It was a memorable experience for both the Alpine Club members and the rescue team, who felt quite good about their achievement.

Though the number of routine rescues continued unabated, several stood out for being unusual in scope or merely tragic. The worst snowmobile accident to date occurred at the end of March, 1986, in the Clemina Creek valley south of Valemount where four people were killed. This accident was also alarming because of the number of people involved displaying utter ignorance of the dangers of avalanches. The group of eleven from Drayton Valley, Alberta, did not even get to the fun part of driving up the avalanche slopes. Merely driving up the valley across the runout path under the extreme hazard was sufficient to release the huge avalanche that buried six of them. Although two were recovered alive, the other four were deeply buried under four metres of snow. Two of the victims were found by a probe line when Willi Pfisterer arrived from Jasper with a team of wardens to conduct the search. The other two, who were buried very deep, were not found until the following day. It was a difficult search for the dogs because of extreme gas contamination from the tumbled snowmobiles that neutralized their scenting capabilities. One thing Willi was happy about was developing a more effective way of digging deeply buried victims out rapidly. He set up the digging in a tiered fashion starting over a wide area at the surface that was reduced by layers as the digging progressed downward, much like strip mining.

The final analysis of the accident indicated that a new class of clientele was on the horizon. The wardens were actually quite surprised to learn that the "group had no suspicion whatsoever that they were placing themselves at risk. It appeared that they were totally unaware that avalanches could possibly occur, and in any case, were unable to recognize avalanche terrain." From that time on, Willi made it a point to visit each group of visiting snowmobilers when they arrived in Valemount to instruct them in the ways of avalanches, avalanche prevention and rescue techniques.

The second accident that spring was not unlike many crevasse accidents that happened frequently enough on the Columbia Icefield, but it was singularly tragic in that it easily could have been prevented. Inexperience and youth certainly played a role in the outcome as did the reaction of the victim. Two young men from Edmonton set out to climb a relatively moderate ice route on Mt. Andromeda but got into trouble before even reaching the mountain. They knew about roping up but did not consider the glacier to be as hazardous as it was. Due to poor route selection they wound up in heavily crevassed terrain. After the first boy almost slipped through a snow bridge, they decided to rope up. In the process,

the second boy fell through the snow bridge he was standing on and went down 15 metres. The shocked 18-year-old left on the surface responded quickly by rappelling down to his buddy, but with no training in crevasse rescue, there was little he could do. Despite his 15-metre fall, the victim was unhurt except for an injured shoulder. It was four-thirty in the afternoon when the accident happened, but instead of going for help, he chose to stay with the victim. He did what he could to keep the boy warm, but nothing would stave off hypothermia for a person wedged in ice. Though the boy was terrified of dying, and did not want to be left alone, he was still alive in the morning when his partner went for help. Unfortunately, it was too late, and he died before wardens could reach him. Though it was commendable for the partner to spend the night with his dying pal, a quick rescue would have been better as it would likely have saved a life.

In stark contrast to this were the actions of a small girl later that year in Banff National Park. On August 15, a family from California ignored the warning of local pilots about poor flying conditions and headed for Kalispell, Montana, from Banff. They departed from the Banff air strip and immediately got lost, heading up toward the Sunshine Village Ski Resort instead of staying in the main corridor. The severe downdrafts in the side valley doomed the small aircraft, and shortly after being seen flying low over the Bourgeau Lake parking lot, the plane crashed approximately 150 metres below the main trail crossing Healy Creek. The parents were killed on impact, but the two daughters survived. The oldest daughter had a skull fracture, a broken jaw and a broken arm. The younger girl, who was only six years old, had an injured shoulder and the heart of a lion. She realized immediately that her parents were dead and her sister was hurt. Acting with perception beyond her years, she pulled her sister from the wreckage and then set out for help.

Not knowing there was a trail, the child headed downstream two kilometres through the dense bush until she entered a canyon, where it became too difficult to proceed. At this point she yelled for help. This is a popular hiking trail in the summer, and her cries were heard by three women hiking above. They could not locate where she was, however, and went immediately to the gondola to report the cries. Scott Ward was the first warden to get to the scene; he flew in with Sean Meggs. They spotted the little girl from the air, then slung in from a nearby staging area. Scott had originally thought the person was an adult and was shocked to find a little six-year-old. The little girl showed huge presence of mind when Scott asked her where her parents were. She was able to say, "They're dead. Our plane crashed but my sister is okay." She then told him where to find the plane. When they reached the plane, the sister was found in a sleeping bag near the bodies of her parents and, though suffering from injuries, was still alive. Tim Auger later summed up the situation saying: "If those hikers hadn't heard her, this rescue would have had very different consequences. We didn't know that plane crashed—no one did. We wouldn't even have started looking until today. Our feeling is that the 11-year-old wouldn't have survived the night." It is not likely the small heroine of the affair would have either. When Scott found her she was already shivering with the onset of hypothermia. It rained heavily that night with cool temperatures, which would surely have sealed their fate without the child's courageous action. She was given the Presidential Bravery award by Ronald Reagan upon returning to the United States.

August rumbled on with its series of fateful events. On August 28th a young assistant mountain guide set out to climb Mt. Baker on the Wapta Icefield with a party of four who were participating in an Introduction to Mountaineering school sponsored by Yamnuska Mountain Adventures near Canmore. They ascended the mountain by the northeast ridge and reached the summit around noon. Unfortunately, they had encountered difficult icy conditions on the ridge, and

the guide did not feel comfortable retreating with four inexperienced people down the problematic ground. He thought it would be better to continue on to the east face, which, though steep, would allow a straightforward vertical descent that could be protected by the rope from above.

It is a long face, however, and it was time consuming to have the clients climb down individually while he belayed. It was now two-thirty in the afternoon and the snow on the face was softening up alarmingly. Hoping to get off the treacherous ground more quickly, the guide proceeded to lower the group together down the 50 degree slope. With no other gear at hand, the guide tried to secure the belay by stamping out a platform and planting the ice axe vertically into the snow near the rear of the stance. With an Italian hitch and an additional wrap into a carabiner for friction, he stood on the head of the axe, placed the rope over his shoulder and proceeded to lower the party. The pull of four people on the axe, however, was too great to sustain, and the anchor pulled out before the party moved very far. The collapse of the belay sent everyone tumbling down the steep face, pulling much of the soft, heavy snow with them. Attempts at self-arrest were futile, and the fall was only finally stopped by the bergschrund near the bottom of the face.

When the guide was able to assess the situation, what greeted him was something no guide ever wishes to encounter. He could see only two of his people, and they were partially buried in snow. As he tried to extricate himself from the now hardening snow, he realized two clients were completely buried. It took 10 minutes before he was free and it took 10 more minutes to dig out the first man he reached. The guide then followed the rope down to the missing clients. With the help of the two boys using ice axes, hands and climbing helmets they finally reached one of the missing climbers. During this time they spotted a party from the Canadian Army and signalled to them for help. It was a corporal from that unit who finally got word to the Warden Service to send assistance. The survivors continued digging and soon found the body of the fourth victim, but all of this had taken over an hour and a half. Neither of the two buried persons were found alive.

The first wardens to respond to the call were Clair Israelson and Mark Ledwidge, who got to the scene shortly after the fourth person had been excavated. One body was still partially buried, and it remained for the wardens to free him from the now well-hardened snow. The devastated survivors were flown out, as were the bodies, but Clair and Mark remained to assess the cause of the accident. Because it was a professional school that involved a guide, it was paramount to establish exactly what had happened. In the event of a death on a professional outing, an inquiry was inevitable and the information had to be correct. Accordingly they inspected the point of anchor failure, measured slope angles, took a profile of the snowpack and recorded everything on film. The main outcome of the inquiry was a recommendation that guides operating in national parks must carry park radios. This was actually a fairly major step forward at the time, a significant perk for the guiding community. It provided a real safety margin for activity within the park and even areas beyond the park if they could trigger local repeaters.

ONE OF THE MOST DRAMATIC and important rescues in the history of mountain rescue in Canada occurred only three days later on Mt. Robson. It was an epic that Willi Pfisterer must have anticipated all his working years in the public safety program, because he was certainly prepared for it. Not only had he climbed the mountain over 15 times himself (guiding), but he had also made it a point to get public safety warden teams to the top as well. He had made several attempts to get a team to the summit, but bad weather had always kept them off. The first relative success on the mountain had been a year earlier when Willi cajoled eight wardens across the Black Ledges under less than favourable conditions. The team had managed to get fairly high on the mountain but was forced to sit out several storms that saturated the already deep snow plastered on the mountain above the ledges. The ledges were covered in a combination of snow, running water and ice mixed with bare rock. Kathy Calvert certainly had trepidation about the whole adventure after reading "ledges of death … ledges coated in ice … formidable ledges" in the log book at the hut the previous day.

At two-thirty in the afternoon, the whole team sat down for a conference on whether to proceed or to turn back before things got worse. As constant snow slides peeled down the mountain, each warden calmly said it might be better to return before anything big decides to fall off. That decided, they returned under a constant barrage of ice coming from the huge icefall that looms over the ledges. Here Willi dramatically told them to unrope and climb free through the short gully. Once he was over, he timed each warden saying: "Go … you have seven seconds to get through!" Kathy was not sure how many of the others glanced down at Kinney Lake 1,500 metres below, but she did and was impressed. Although they did not make the summit, Willi had achieved part of his goal. He at least had got the team over the ledges, so they would know the route, which he felt was critical.

He returned the following year, again with a similar combination of public safety wardens to try again for the summit. This time they were successful, though Dianne Volkers recalls feeling very relieved when they got down. One of the highlights of that trip was rappelling directly off the mammoth icefall above the gully that Kathy remembers skittering across unroped. It must qualify as one of the most spectacular rappels in the world, with the airy view of Kinney Lake so far below and the Rocky Mountains spread across the horizon. Willi now had a group of wardens who had made it to the top as well as across the slippery ledges. This knowledge was the armour they had to be an effective rescue team on the mountain.

When Willi was notified at 10:45 a.m. on August 31 by the Valemount RCMP that a group of four climbers was overdue on the north face of Mt. Robson, he hoped to get in for a simple snatch and grab rescue and be down before any serious weather eliminated this option. Willi promptly sent Brian Wallace, Pat Sheehan and Murray Hindle off to investigate, but by then the weather closed in, and they could not get close to the beleaguered climbers. They were, however, able to reach a couple of climbers who had heard voices yelling for help from the vicinity of the north face.

It seemed that a group of four men had climbed to within a few hundred feet of the summit ridge which would take them to safety, then they had sat there through three days of good weather. None of them reported any injury but neither had they moved from their perch, and they were now calling for help. It turned out to be a classic case of overestimating their own ability and underestimating the mountain, leading to a series of mistakes. They set out on Tuesday, the 26th of August, for Berg Lake where they spent the first night. With good weather prevailing, they made it to the base of the face the following day and were up early on the 28th to begin the climb. The trip organizer set off strongly in the lead for two rope lengths. The second pair of climbers then took over to about three quarters of the way up the face where they stopped to assess their position. For the last few rope lengths, the leader had been complaining of feeling unwell and was slowing down. Despite this the four men convinced themselves that they were better off to keep going. The summit did not seem that far away—despite the worsening ice conditions—and they felt they had a chance to get off the route the next day. Not wanting to jeopardize the team's chances of making the summit, the sick man agreed to keep going.

The leader of the second rope plowed on, now burdened with the brunt of the work—only now the ice began to deteriorate, making it difficult to place solid anchors. By now the sick man was

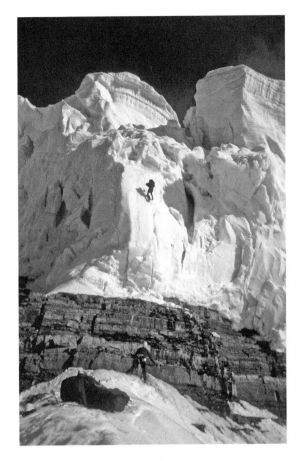

Rappelling off seracs on Mt. Robson. GREG HORNE COLLECTION

much worse, but fortunately under failing light, they found a small crevasse to set up a crowded bivouac. The spirits were high for the three who thought they would escape the following day, but the fourth man continued to get sicker as the night wore on.

The following day the weather worsened, discouraging any real attempt to exit to the ridge. The previous day's leader made an effort to get to the ridge but could not place an anchor he felt secure with. The rain and the poor condition of the fourth man led to his decision to sit out the day, hoping for an improvement in both the weather and his rope mate. Despite the weather turning fine that day, none of them felt strong. The sick man simply got worse with time and could barely sit up or eat. The seriousness of their situation was rapidly becoming apparent, leading to discussions of retreating. Though they tried once more to get to the ridge, nothing had changed and again the lead man retreated to the bivouac site.

Help was on the way, but Willi delayed sending in a ground team until it became obvious that there would be no break in the weather. The forecast was anything but encouraging, with foul weather predicted until the end of the week. There was a brief moment of hope when the cloud cap cleared off almost enough to land a team, but it was not enough. Meanwhile, there was a fury of activity below, bringing in more men, supplies and equipment to a rescue base established at the Mt. Robson park headquarters for running the rescue operations and strategy planning. A team disembarked at the ranger station on Berg Lake to monitor the weather on the north side of the mountain, but Willi now felt their best hope would be to get a team in on the south side of the mountain. He was right. Clair Israelson, Mark Ledwidge and Gord Irwin, who had arrived by helicopter from Lake Louise, reluctantly agreed. They realized the best option was to fly a rescue team in as high on the mountain as possible, equipped with a camp and supplies to effect a rescue from there.

With amazing good fortune, the weather cleared again, giving them a chance to reach the Robson Hut and sling a camp in from there. Israelson, Irwin and Ledwidge found themselves above the ledges at four in the afternoon and proceeded to climb the mountain. They left the main camp gear pinned to the slope for a follow-up team to use when they could be brought in.

Because none of the men had climbed the mountain, they relied on Willi's incredible memory to stay on route. They had to negotiate what Gerry Israelson (who later joined the team) described as "the maze of wild ice formations aptly called gargoyles."

Willi recounts: "So I tell them from down below where to go." After they got up the first hump Willi's instructions were: "Go over onto the glacier and then there is the big ice ramp on the right side … then the seracs. Well, you have to turn right now under that serac. But watch it! There is a big crevasse to the right." It was dark by the time these instructions filtered over the radio. Clair confirmed his location, adding: "Now what?" Willi unhesitatingly replied: "Turn left, go up that icefield and there is a big crevasse … Then there is—straight up and down—an ice face." Clair again said: "Yah. What do we do now?" The reply was "Is the ice face in front of you? Then you have to go down a little bit. And then you cross a crevasse and you go straight up. It's very steep and then you get up on the ridge." The trio continued until they were able to say: "Ok, we're on the ridge now."

The relentless instructions continued: "You go a little bit to the left and you end up on the ridge at the big chute." Clair again called down saying, "There is a snow obstacle here." Willi replied without a break: "Go to the left, you can get around it and there is one more steep bit then it eases off. When you get on the ledge above, go on that a little bit because that could be an avalanche slope." On they went, trusting the heavily accented voice they knew so well. "Then you go on … you're going to feel the wind coming the other way, but you'll be going up the summit ridge … it goes downhill and as soon as it gets uphill, there is a big crevasse and most likely you will get across." Willi paused a moment when Clair came back on the radio saying: "Now what, it's down everywhere." With his irrepressible good humour, Willi could not resist saying: "Shit! You screwed up … you're on the summit." Everyone at base camp broke out in peals of laughter. The boys had made it through with the combination of teamwork and skill, and they felt good.

Willi's next piece of advice was more than welcome. He counselled: "Is that crevasse down below? … that is most likely the best place to spend the night." Which is what they did.

The next morning, the bad weather continued unabated but did not prevent them from making their way down the Emperor Ridge to where they could make voice contact with the beleaguered climbers below. Irwin recalls: "The upper part of the Emperor Ridge isn't the worst part … below us would have been worse, but it still wasn't good. There was no decent place to build anchors or anything like that. It was crappy snow, and we had to take some time to develop decent enough anchors to lower the rope down to the guys. We used all our resources." It was an epic getting all four men to the ridge with much yelling back and forth in the reduced visibility. The biggest problem was the poor condition of the stranded climbers. They were so weak they could barely come up on a fixed line. The leader of the second rope was the strongest and was able to climb over to the rescue team and secure a line for the others. Moving with a full pack in their enfeebled condition, however, was impossible for two of them. At one point, Irwin told them to ditch the packs and climb free. He thought they would just attach them to the end of the rope so they could be hauled up later, but in their weakened condition, all they thought of was to jettison them entirely. Despite this, Gord was alarmed when one of the men pitched over backward in a complete faint, landing head downward. The rescuers were now yelling fiercely at the men to move up to the ridge. They had to make that distance with the aid of the rope or they would be finished. Gord recalls, "After a few more episodes like this we got everyone back onto the ridge." From there, they proceeded slowly to the summit.

Once in the summit bivouac, the famished climbers, who had eaten very little in the past few days, devoured everything they were given—the most important of which was fluid. While they scarfed the hot drinks and food, the rescuers evaluated their options. The weather, which had never been good, began to deteriorate to near whiteout conditions. Clair wanted to get the whole party back down and over the ledges that day if possible, knowing the forecast showed no improvement in the coming week. To their dismay, once they left the small cave they found all their tracks had been obliterated by the blowing snow. To add to this, the batteries on the radios were fading, limiting conversation to emergency communication only. They had only reached the large bergschrund four hundred metres lower than the summit when everything started to run out: visibility, stamina and daylight. With little choice, they made the decision to hole up in the bergschrund for a second night.

They found it to be a most pleasant place—beautiful, in fact, with its stalactites hanging from the ceiling and crystals of ice glittering bluely in the soft filtered light. To save batteries they turned the radios off and heard nothing from below. But just after getting settled, Gord thought he heard a helicopter. He was by the entrance brewing yet more tea when he looked out, and to his astonishment saw Todd McCready waving for him to get on the radio. The summit cap of dense cloud had freakishly parted, allowing the pilot a short window to fly in, and he now thought he had a slim chance to get them off. With haste they radioed back saying that the four weakened climbers should go first. While Todd returned to the hut to set up the sling line, the boys packed the gear belonging to the climbers and with no time to spare had them ready to sling out.

The summit cap may have cleared enough to give Todd a visual reference for the stranded team but the flying conditions were still extreme. Todd recalls: "There were horrendous winds, very heavy cloud cover mixed with freezing rain and snow … and then there was the altitude. You're kind of pushing the limits of the aircraft."

With the winds swirling around them, the exhausted climbers only knew that one minute they were sitting in a snowy hole at 3,500 metres and the next they were in a warm hut being greeted by other rescuers. Gary Forman was there with a second helicopter to ferry them down to base camp.

Meanwhile, Todd went back to try and get the rescue team. Todd felt that the first two flights were rough, but with two men on the line, he had had the weight he needed to stabilize the line. Now he had to fly Mark Ledwidge out on his own, in order to leave two men behind in case the helicopter could not return and they had to climb their way down. Todd explained: "Of course, just being the one guy on the hook, it was a little bit lighter and the weather and turbulence was such that there was feedback through the hydraulics. There was one point where we just hit a big vacuum and away we went. You're just on for the ride." Todd did not think Mark was aware of their situation: "Yah, he was enjoying the ride, he didn't know what was going on." Todd knew he was going to come out of the drop but added: "When you do, you're going to get *hammered*. And we did. I was on my way down and Mark was on his way up. You look at the rope and there is just a big loop in it." For an instant Mark was looking into the helicopter, then he was flying slightly above, knowing this was not where he should be. Mark had flown many times under the helicopter but this was one ride he had no illusions about. Enjoyment was not a word that came to mind when he thought of that flight. Terror was a little more accurate. Todd later described it as "pretty wild, yah, pretty western." That was the end, however. The clouds rolled back, encasing the two remaining rescuers in their ice palace for another night on the mountain. Fortunately for them, Todd had managed to bring in the ubiquitous bucket of Kentucky Fried Chicken during the flights, the solace of all Parks rescues.

While tragedy was skilfully being circumvented on the top of the mountain, Willi was wasting no time putting together a support team to bring the men on top down if conditions did not improve. One of the reasons they were having so much trouble retreating was that they had not brought wands with them to flag the route. Mark later reflected: "It would have been a significantly different outcome if we had wanded the route." Possibly, but they still had the major obstacle of getting across the black ledges under appall-

ing conditions. Gerry Israelson was contacted in Banff to hurry back to Jasper to help on the support team. He was well qualified for this role, having just successfully completed his full guide exam that day. But nothing on the exam came close to the ultimate test of climbing through the ledges with Greg Horne to fix the route for the descending party.

Willi sent in Al MacDonald and John Niddrie with Gerry and Greg, hoping that four men would be enough to establish a good retreat route. The crew brought up enough static line to fix the route right across the ledges. When they got to the ledges they received a call from Clair asking them to come right across to the camp and gear flown in earlier, on the far snow arête. They had not planned on doing more than fixing as much line as they could before returning to the hut, where all their gear was left for the night. But Willi also realized that the men above needed help in finding their way down the upper half of the mountain and concurred.

Greg thinks there must have been a long pause on the radio while they ruminated over this latest development. He looked at the snow-plastered ledges and realized they were in a horrible condition. And the short little gully under the icefall presented the same commitment it always had. It was too dangerous to fix ropes through there or even have the comfort of a belay because of debris plummeting from the ever-active icefall above. Greg later named the feeling of having to cross the ledges under these conditions "real sphincter factor," but there seemed to be little choice. He certainly had good reason for the sphincter-tightening reaction. As he was crossing the gully unroped, he got too high on the route and had to down climb. Greg recounts: "I remember where the pick of my axe was stuck in the cracks in the rocks and you look between your legs and there's Kinney Lake, like 1,500 metres below … and actually, somewhere there, one of the picks pulled out, and I kind of experienced the old barn door trick where I had one crampon [on the ledge] and my other arm and leg swung out in the air over Kinney Lake." This hair-raising episode was probably missed by Gerry, now laying out the fixed line to be placed over the rest of the slippery ledges.

When they reached the cache, all they found was a couple of duffel bags that miraculously were still there in the now howling winds. It was blowing so fiercely that one lens of Gerry's glasses was blasted right out, leaving him slightly blind for the rest of the climb. At that moment they heard the helicopter coming in for the rescued men above, but when they looked up they saw to their astonishment two figures on the Wish Bone Arête route up the southeast side of the mountain. This made no sense if it had anything to do with the rescue mission they were on. The swirling clouds obscured the scene minutes later, leaving them wondering if they were seeing things. A brief conversation with Clair above did little to enlighten them other than to confirm it was not their party. It slowly dawned on them that there was a third party that no one knew about wandering around the summit of the mountain.

They had little time to contemplate this latest development. The storm was much worse for them without the protection of a cozy snow cave. With great difficulty they managed to dig out the tent, but to their dismay, the "full camp" did not include sleeping bags. There was a Therm-a-rest, a stove and some cabbage rolls and crackers for food, but little else. The wind was way too powerful for them to remain where they were, so they moved the camp higher to a slightly less battered location and settled in with only the tent fly for a cover. In the middle of the night, the tent actually threatened to blow right off the mountain. In desperation, Gerry went out to get some sort of anchor in by using their helmets as a deadman in the snow, leaving Greg inside to hold things down. Greg, who was a skinny individual, ruefully commented he wasn't sure how the "light man" was going to do this, but the makeshift anchors held, and they made it through a very cold night.

By morning, nothing had improved. Willi conferred with both teams and felt the best strategy now was for the upper team to continue down and meet the support team fixing the route below. Since the battery supply for the radios had been replenished when the food was flown up, communication was less of an issue. The lack of wands was the problem. But if the camp had not come with sleeping bags, one thoughtful individual had thrown in a bag of cutlery. There was also a pile of yellow garbage bags (what these were intended for was never discussed). The ingenious pair gleefully cut the bright yellow plastic into long strips and tied them to the cutlery to act as markers for the descent. With some difficulty they finally met the upper team and followed the cheerful yellow strips back to the flapping tent camp for another night on the mountain. Gerry recalls that he and Greg were actually in worse shape than the other two because of the miserable night they'd spent virtually in the open. But now the two chilly men were buffered by the sleeping bags that Gord and Clair had, making it not quite so cold.

The following day tested the fortitude and climbing skills of all the rescuers, but particularly Gord Irwin. In the rush to fly the weakened climbers off the day before, his crampons had somehow been flown out. He now had to negotiate the iced-up ledges without them. Most of the going was actually not too bad because of the fixed ropes and fresh snow, but the short gully under the icefall had no protection. Gord, recalls with understatement, "It's not hard climbing but it was tricky … it was full concentrated climbing at that point."

Once across the ledges, they encountered more fixed line left by Al MacDonald and John Niddrie, and soon they were back at the Robson Hut. They received a warm welcome from the men waiting their return, and in short order the pilots had everyone back at base camp. Willi was extremely proud of what they had accomplished and knew his work as the alpine specialist was justified.

The question of who the men were that Gerry and Greg had seen stumbling toward the summit was also solved. They turned out to be Daniel Bonzi, the guide from Banff, and his client Paul Mesrobian, also from Banff. During their descent, the boys had actually established voice contact with them but were unable to direct them down. The rescue report filled for the officially overdue men states: "At approximately 16:00 hrs Bonzi and Mesrobian found the camp and stayed there the night. Radio contact was made. Thursday the pair descended the mountain via the established route and reached the base of the mountain at the same time the helicopter began to search the lower half of the planned descent route."

FOR WILLI THINGS HAD NOT SLOWED DOWN for a minute. On Monday morning, long before the rescued climbers were evacuated, Willi had received a report of an injured woman at the Whitehorn Ranger Cabin. She had been climbing with friends but had fallen and broken her leg. Her companions were able to get her to the hut, which was fortunate, as weather was so bad in the morning that Todd could not even fly up the valley. While this new development was being considered, Gary Forman announced he had to fly off to a plane crash. The RCMP staff was also taxed. When that plane crash call came in, most of the members were tending to a highway fatality down by the bridge near the turnoff to Robson Provincial Park. Gary flew off with what RCMP members could be liberated.

That afternoon, while taking a much-needed break from the media circus outside the tent, Willi found himself scrambling to launch another, more serious rescue for the crew of an overturned raft in the Robson River. He must have thought God had mistaken him for Job with the endless series of catastrophes placed at his doorstep that weekend. In this instance, a group of five men with a river guide had decided to raft the Fraser River between the Robson Park Headquarters and the Moose River 16 kilometres upstream. The whitewater goes quickly from class II rapids to class III just near the park. When the raft entered the turbulent water, it swamped under one very large wave and overturned. The guide and one other man managed to get to shore, while the raft and the four remaining occupants plunged downstream where they were caught by a large sweeper.

Fortunately, the accident happened close to the highway and only five kilometres upstream from the Robson Park Headquarters. The guide reported the accident immediately, but must have been astonished to find a full rescue team with helicopters ready to jump to the scene. Willi, now on an adrenalin high, leapt into action, getting

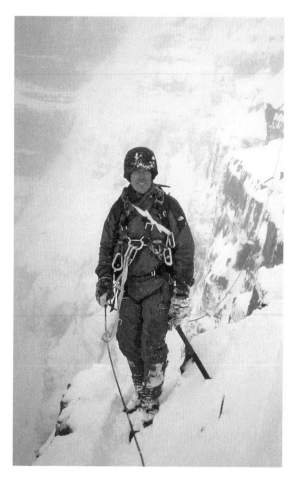

Gord Irwin on Black Ledges on the Mt. Robson rescue.
GREG HORNE COLLECTION

the men and helicopter organized with both sling and rope rescue gear. Within minutes, a shore crew using ropes managed to pull in two of the hypothermic rafters clinging to the sweeper. The remaining two men still on the overturned raft were picked up by a rescuer who slung in with Todd and brought them out individually. The RCMP were impressed with the performance, indicating that it was likely lives were saved by the quick response.

While this occurred, the rescue team was still on the mountain with the four climbers. It was not much later, however, that Todd and Gary were able to bring down the rescued men plus Mark Ledwidge. The successful rescue of the four men created media headlines and for most of the reporters, this was the end of the story. Suddenly the once teeming parking lot was empty. The journalists departed along with the still-overwhelmed climbers, now in the company of the RCMP. Both Willi and Todd were surprised over the lack of interest in the welfare of the rescuers struggling to reach safety themselves. Even the rescued boys never said thank you, although one statement to the RCMP indicated gratitude for the live-saving effort. Gerry philosophically reasoned that they were undoubtedly appreciative but "were probably a bit embarrassed."

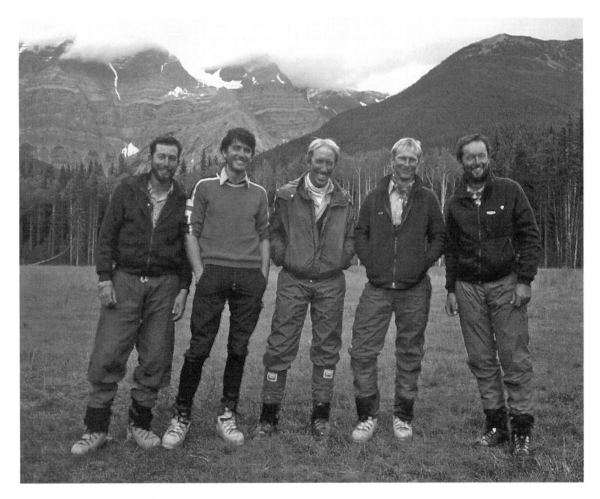

(L to R) Greg Horne, Mark Ledwidge, Gord Irwin, Gerry Israelson, Clair Israelson. GREG HORNE COLLECTION

What was much worse, though, was the lack of appreciation from their own park. When the team finally assembled down at the parking lot, the monumental work of returning equipment to the rescue room and sorting out gear began. There also needed to be a debriefing, but before that was undertaken, the now well-bonded group felt a burger and a few brews were in order. Since this was an interim break in the down staging of the rescue, it seemed appropriate that the meal be tabbed to the park. To their disappointment, this was refused. It was almost a slap in the face, and it reinforced the perception that management was often out of touch with what was required risk-wise on a serious rescue. Word got out quickly about the parsimonious attitude of "Her Majesty's Service" and the assistant superintendent himself came down to foot the bill and offer congratulations. Never was a gesture more appreciated.

One man who was very much appreciated on the rescue was Todd McCready. As Gerry Israelson noted, it was "above and beyond the call of duty when Todd went in there and flew those guys out." Gary Forman was also very proud of Todd but had a mixed reaction to the extreme conditions he flew under, saying to Gerry, "I didn't know whether to congratulate him on a job well done or boot him in the ass." It was pretty clear to the rescue team, though, that Todd deserved their congratulations. Willi and the rest of the team nominated him for the Robert E. Trimble Award, given for courageous mountain flying by helicopter pilots throughout North America. Like Jim Davies prior to him, Todd was selected over all the other nominees and went to Dallas, Texas, in 1987 to receive the award.

In many respects, the Mt. Robson Rescue was a pinnacle in the story of mountain rescue in Canada. Gord Irwin considers it a "landmark" in that it was a joint rescue on a big, serious mountain that "brought home years of work" needed to develop a professional rescue team. Although it was not the first joint rescue on a big mountain, the conditions tested the depth, commitment and skill of the Warden Service and pilots to the limit. Unfortunately, pinnacles are often followed by losses.

The loss, in the early part of the year, was the death of Fred Pfisterer, Willi's young son, who was in training to become a full guide. Fred had completed his assistant winter guide course and was working for Mike Wiegele at Blue River, B.C. when the accident happened. On March 23, 1987, Fred, with a group of nine skiers were dropped off by helicopter, well above treeline, off to one side but not far from the summit of the slope. Fred wanted to take a quick profile of the slope and in particular look at and test a surface hoar layer that had formed over two weeks earlier. The slope had not been skied since the beginning of the early March avalanche cycle, and even though recent stability indicated in other profiles prompted an evaluation of "low hazard," another check was needed before the area was pronounced safe for skiing.

Six of the nine skiers were strung out across the slope behind the guide as he prepared to dig a test pit. If Fred had been able to finish the profile, it is quite likely they would not have skied the slope at all. He would have found an unstable surface hoar layer that when combined with wind loading made for a potentially large avalanche. They were off the steepest section of the slope and all might have been fine if a second helicopter had not landed with another party. The helicopter landed hard and appeared to initiate a fracture in the stressed slope, causing the release of a huge avalanche. Fred was only able to call, "Get out of the way" on his radio to the lagging skiers before being pulled down the slope with the first group. One of the three lagging skiers was also dragged a short distance before he was buried up to his waist. Fred and the six others were carried down 250 metres where they came to rest on a broad depressed bench that converged with the slope.

All seven were deeply buried. The guide from a second group quickly organized the remaining skiers into action. After skiing down to the bench, they picked up the beacon signals and began to dig. Unfortunately the deposit was very dense and hard to shovel. The victims were all buried from two to four metres down, and none survived.

Unbelievably, Willi was one of the first to hear of the accident in Jasper and rushed out immediately. This was an oversight as the people at Blue River had been asked not to call Willi if they had an avalanche accident just to avoid this very scenario. Having Willi come out at all was unfortunate; there was nothing he could do as the evacuation was complete when he got there. Alfie Burstrom who had volunteered to go along with Willi was denied permission by park management concerned about his absence during a cycle of high avalanche hazard.

One of the hardest things Willi ever did as a rescue leader was drive his own son's body back to Jasper alone. It was also the last rescue he attended. Although he had indicated before Fred's death that he intended to retire, the accident clinched his decision. Later that spring public safety saw its second loss when Willi hung up the red socks that symbolized his status as one of Canada's first alpine specialists.

Though the Jasper team knew the day was coming, it took some adjustment. He had been a mentor and father figure to everyone in the field and it was difficult to let go. Willi stayed on in Jasper for a while, eventually retiring on a small acreage near Tete Jaune Cache not far from Valemount, B.C. He was always available to give advice if he was at home, but for several years, that was not often. He took up gold prospecting in the Yukon in the summer, relieved by trips to Thailand in the winter. He did not lose all interest in climbing though. He was active in developing early guiding schools for the fine climbing found on the karst limestone hills in that blue, sunlit haven.

GERRY ISRAELSON HAD MOVED to Jasper in the public safety field position under Darro Stinson, who had replaced Tony Klettl. With Pat Sheehan and Bill Hunt in the public safety training position, the unit in Jasper was very strong, especially at the Marmot Basin Ski Area in the winter. Rick Ralf was also part of the team at the hill and happily recalls skiing with the numerous rotating seasonal warden staff from the valley. It was a productive, active period when the Warden Service was a leader in avalanche control work. Darro Stinson put it succinctly saying: "In my mind, that was a pivotal point in our ability to be leaders in the field in terms of forecasting in the snow business." This was a direct result of the close exposure to snow every day and the solid training from the avalanche courses put on by the Canadian Avalanche Association that Willi helped found. Darro felt that being called in by the coroner to investigate significant avalanche accidents such as the one at Blue River was a testament to the professionalism of the Warden Service.

This was also true in the Lake Louise and Banff areas where avalanche control at the ski hills was a big part of the public safety job. Gerry worked at the Lake Louise ski hill before moving to Jasper and recalls that period as "a pretty exciting time for everybody … you were learning lots and there was a physical and mental challenge. We were opening brand new areas that we had no experience in before … we didn't even know what the terrain looked like in the summertime."

The ski hills all felt that expansion was necessary if they were to remain competitive. As the heavy snow years of the seventies and eighties began to decline, the resorts had to make snow, forcing the cost of lift tickets up. They needed the avalanche-prone runs open to justify the large dollars it now cost to ski. When exciting runs such as "Delirium Dive" were closed, both skiers and management at the ski hills protested.

All this activity served to remind Parks Canada that the ski hills were, in fact, private businesses operating in national parks. Although private enterprise was not restricted in the park, many park managers began to wonder why Parks Canada was actually supporting an expensive control program for them. As the expenses mounted and the involvement of the Warden Service grew, so did the questions. With the ski hills united in wanting to conduct their own avalanche control programs, defending the work of the Warden Service became increasingly difficult until finally a full review of the program was undertaken. Bruce Leeson, the environmental consultant for Parks Canada, was involved with several of the discussions, mostly concerning the expansion issues. In the end, he recalls: "Parks Canada took the position that we were going to get out of the business of avalanche control … because it was a matter of finances … and it was a costly program." They decided to taper off the involvement over a two- to three-year period, allowing the ski hills time to properly train their staff.

None of this went over very well with the Warden Service. In fact it was quite a shock. The ski hills had provided a learning, training and employment ground for the Warden Service since they had begun working there in earnest in 1964. Gerry Israelson saw them as a place where young wardens were able to pick up essential skills such as learning to ski, gaining a feel for avalanche terrain, and above all, managing risk. They had to accept the responsibility of safety for others and learn to work as a team—a vital part of all public safety work. The wardens were on their skis daily, constantly thinking about what was happening in the snowpack and transferring that information

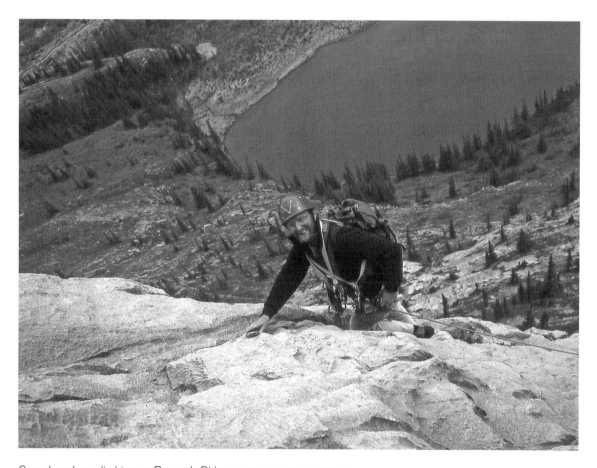

Gerry Israelson climbing on Benson's Ridge. HANS FUHRER COLLECTION

202

to the backcountry. They collected the data that was the backbone of avalanche forecasting for the public information bulletin. For Gerry it was "a tremendous period of growth in the public safety program," and he was not alone in this perception.

Gerry had moved to Jasper early enough to be part of the avalanche control program before it was cancelled. He was a younger, lighter version of Clair, with an offbeat sense of humour that always eased the tension in doubtful situations. He was a very skilled climber and skier with an unusual talent to find the right route on a difficult mountain. His greatest gift might have been his ability to inspire confidence with the people who worked for him, and in this respect, he was much like Tim Auger.

During the transfer period, the wardens stationed at the hill worked closely with the patrollers. Eventually, time gave perspective to the changing roles, and most wardens now understand that handing the program over to the ski hills was part of an unavoidable evolutionary process. The new staff took the responsibility to heart and developed a very workable program. It was a totally different style of avalanche control but in the end it proved very effective.

The loss of the winter avalanche program left a huge hole in the public safety program. Wardens now had to find a way to maintain their skills in some other fashion. Mark Ledwidge always maintained that skiing was the one skill most difficult to acquire, because it took years to learn properly. They also lost access to propagation zones that gave them a clear understanding of what was happening in the snowpack. As Stinson put it, "You had your head in the snow daily, and you knew what was going on. When we left the ski hills, the edge was gone and many people feel it was never regained." Certainly, the opportunity to train younger staff in this aspect of public safety was lost, as were the employment opportunities. The transfer process was fairly long, however, particularly in Jasper. Wardens were informed of the change in policy in 1987 but continued to

work at the hill and monitor the transfer as late as 1992 when they finally left for good.

Changes at the ski hills, however, did not alter the direction of the regular public safety rescue work. People continued to get lost, break ankles or have heart attacks. And there were always serious rescue challenges. Ice climbing was becoming more popular than ever, and the routes being undertaken often had significant hazards. Since waterfalls are the outflow of water collection basins, they frequently channel avalanches in winter. The Cascade Waterfall, which forms below a particularly large collection basin, is often swept by avalanches. Tim recalls one particular incident in 1988 during which the victims were fortunately spotted by wardens as they were being swept off by a fairly large avalanche.

The accident occurred at 1:00 p.m. as two young climbers from Britain were deciding the conditions were becoming dangerous and it might be a good idea to retreat. They arrived at that conclusion too late to avoid a large avalanche that originated hundreds of metres higher up the mountain. It knocked the leader off, sweeping him by the second man who was able to momentarily stop him on the belay rope. The force of the avalanche actually broke that rope, and the leader did not stop until arrested by a second rope tied to the anchor station. Fortunately for him, the second rope held, allowing the main avalanche to continue down where it collected in debris 7 to 10 metres deep. Even more fortunately, Bill Browne and Al Westhaver were out checking the waterfall for climbers. When they saw the accident they immediately reported it to the warden office and in minutes a rescue was organized. The pair were reached at 1:24 p.m. and evacuation was underway by 2:00 p.m. The leader who was caught in the avalanche was in the hospital within the hour, where doctors treated him for severe internal injuries. The prompt evacuation more than likely saved the man's life. The pair had come to Canada expecting cold temperatures, but did not give the avalanche hazard much thought. As it turned out, they were climbing during a period when the avalanche hazard was posted at high to extreme. During the weeks prior to this incident, unstable conditions and warm temperatures had increased the hazard, contributing to two deaths four days earlier at Lake Louise.

WATER RESCUES AND SEARCHES increased during the late eighties. Most water rescues are actually searches confined to riverbanks, and fall more readily into that category. By the end of the nineties a review of critical incidents left the wardens with a better appreciation of what affects river searches. A very extended search for a young man from Japan produced no results for over a year, until spring floods flushed the body from the accident site at Athabasca Falls. A summary of accidents involved with rivers revealed that 99% occurred at tourist attractions such as Maligne Canyon, Athabasca Falls or Sunwapta Falls. People who go over waterfalls, either in the main river or in canyons, often are held down by strong undertows. It is not until the spring floods come that the bodies are flushed out, often the following year.

In June of 1990, an accident proved the exception to this rule. The water in the Athabasca River was high, and a young offender who was participating in an obligatory canoeing exercise actually survived his tumble over the fall. The group was paddling from Moberly Bend to their camp at the Whirlpool. They knew that the falls were somewhere in the middle of the stretch and planned to portage around them. However, few of the paddlers had advanced canoeing skills, and when they hit the first set of rapids above the falls, most of them took on water. Three of the canoes headed for shore to empty out the water, but the boys in the fourth canoe swamped before they could make the bank. One of the boys was able to swim out, but the other was too numbed by the cold water to make it to shore.

Though the entire incident was seen by a family from California, they did not report the accident when it happened. The following day they checked in at the Sunwapta Warden Office to see if anyone had been hurt. The father stated that they "thought the canoe had been in trouble for quite a distance." They could see the boy being carried down by the current, then making a sudden attempt to save himself at the brink of the falls, but his efforts were "feeble and ineffective … like one already numbed by the cold." And that is the last they saw.

Showing panic or sudden presence of mind, the survivor ran to the bottom of the falls where, to his amazement, he saw the boy float by. He immediately pulled him to shore and checked him over. The boy was unconscious and did not appear to be breathing, but did finally respond to artificial respiration administered by a paramedic who happened to be nearby. He was hypothermic but he began to regain consciousness when he warmed up. The Warden Service was notified but most of the "saving" had been done. It was the first time, and so far the last time, anyone had gone over Athabasca Falls and lived. The canoe, retrieved the next day, was split in half and pounded to pulp. The wardens also recovered two life jackets and a baseball cap but refused permission to one of the group leaders to enter the canyon to recover a white bucket. One miracle was more than the group deserved.

BY THE END OF THE DECADE, the wardens would put their search procedures to the test in the biggest avalanche recovery effort up to that time. The Healy Creek avalanche created conditions that rescuers had never encountered, and it became a benchmark on the learning curve. The accident occurred on Sunday February 11, 1990, on the trail to Healy Pass, a very popular ski outing that begins at the Sunshine ski area parking lot. Five older experienced skiers set out for the day, intending to get as far up the trail as they felt comfortable with, given the poor weather and deep snow. They were following a broken trail forged by two independent parties a couple of hours ahead of them, which made it easier to keep going.

Despite the broken trail, they were slow because of difficulty with the wax due to warm temperatures and wet snow. One party member, who was tired from a previous day's outing, was having difficulty keeping up with the others. She was not worried when she lost sight of them partway up the trail; she continued at her own pace, but was startled by a deep rumbling farther up the valley around 12:15 p.m. Possibly because of continued tiredness, she turned back at this point and headed for the parking lot. On the way, she ran into another party of two and asked them to keep an eye out for her friends.

The two skiers continued on, despite having also heard the rumblings, and within a short time they could account for them. The fresh ski tracks they were following led straight into a huge avalanche deposit that had obliterated the trail. The avalanche had no doubt just come down—the overwhelming spruce smell of freshly smashed trees and shattered limb debris told them that. Even so, it was already hard as concrete. They did notice older ski tracks emerging from the other side and covered with new-fallen snow, distinct from the tracks they had been following. The pair continued up the trail until they encountered the first group returning. They had not seen the missing group of four, and now everyone was alarmed. They discussed the matter briefly then turned back to investigate the avalanche. When they reached the monstrous slide, they did a hasty search but saw no sign of the missing skiers. They felt something was drastically wrong, however, and decided the best thing to do was to alert the authorities. They skied out to the parking lot with all possible haste to inform the employees at the ticket wicket. This was passed immediately to the Warden Service, who had been receiving reports of avalanches all day.

Tim Auger took this latest news very seriously and initiated a full scale search at 4:30 p.m. Mark Ledwidge, working at the ski hill, left for the parking lot immediately to talk to the reporting individuals. There he met Tim and Scott Ward with his dog Smoky. Clair Israelson was notified in Lake Louise and calls went out to put rescue personnel in other parks on standby. Other wardens continued to arrive, while Tim and Scott took advantage of what visibility was still available to fly the valley looking for signs of the missing party. All they saw was what looked like a class III avalanche across the trail and two heavily laden skiers who did not fit the description of whom they were looking for.

The size of the slide was discouraging, but they still had to proceed as though people were still alive. Mark Ledwidge and Peter Enderwick headed in with skidoos, which proved to be a daunting task, but they needed a broken trail to bring in rescue workers when the helicopter could no longer fly. Before the light failed completely, searchers flew to the deposit and began probing where natural traps might pin a body. They searched the surface for any articles that may have been overlooked, but nothing. Well after dark, the ground search was called off, and everyone headed back to the warden office to debrief and to develop a contingency plan for the next day. Many things had been taken care of in the meanwhile. Personnel had been assigned to various tasks such as supplies and equipment, liaising and dispatch, organization of volunteers and camp coordination.

The Banff dog team (Ward & Smokey) searched the deposit that first afternoon and well into the night; they were soon joined by the Glacier/ Revelstoke team (Peyto & Baron). They covered as much of the open deposit as they could in the time they had before nightfall, but they also found nothing. This was unusual since it supposedly involved four people.

The next day, Gord Peyto and Scott Ward were joined by Dale Portman and Cody and an RCMP team from Cranbrook, B.C., Gord Burns and his young dog Griz. During the early part of the second day, the temperature dropped dramatically to minus 30 degrees Celsius. When the searchers went back the following morning, they finally got a good look at the enormity of the slide. Two days before the accident, it had snowed nearly 70 centimetres at temperatures near or just below freezing. The avalanche deposit was 185 metres wide where it crossed the ski trail, making the new avalanche path 67 metres wider than before the giant slide came down. It consequently took out many of the large Engelmann spruce that had defined the old path. The slide extended down into Healy Creek itself and cleared a swath 70 metres up the other side of the valley.

The open area of the deposit was split into search units where probe teams worked alongside the dogs. Scent starts to freeze at around minus 20 degree Celsius so there was very little or none coming to the surface. The dog teams were rotated throughout the day, worked for two-hour stretches then warmed up and rested in the large wood-heated tent that was set up on the edge of the deposit. The dogs came up with nothing, and frustration was beginning to set in.

The weather change also brought clear skies, and Tim was able to fly once again to see if by some remote chance the skiers might have gotten lost and wandered off the trail. He was also able to see what had caused the avalanche and to check the first path to see if further stabilization was necessary for the safety of the rescue workers. By the end of the day there was not even a hint of the skiers in the debris. At the evening's debriefing, everyone was registering frustration, particularly the dog handlers. No one had ever been on a slide worked so consistently by so many people with absolutely no result. Tim was heard to say, "It is almost inconceivable for four people to disappear without a trace, but on seeing the avalanche, we quickly recognized that possibility." They upgraded the search and brought in wardens from other parks as well as rangers from nearby Kananaskis Country. The moment a person was brought to the site, he or she was assigned a group and a location to search.

Early the next morning, Tim had the first slide path bombed to eliminate any hanging threat of secondary avalanches. It was a good call. The avalanche that was released swept down over the trail and wiped out the helicopter landing pad. This was quickly re-established, as was a large camp close to the search area, but well enough away to avoid scent contamination. There was a propane-heated warming tent for workers as well as a second heated wall tent for hot food and drinks. In those temperatures, this was a constant cycle, and only two people developed any frostbite. In the morning of the third day at temperatures of minus 33 degree Celsius the four dog teams and probe lines started searching again.

With no evidence of surface articles to indicate where people might be buried, the rescuers began to wonder whether they were searching the right avalanche. After thoroughly searching the open areas assigned to him, RCMP officer Gord Burns and Griz reluctantly moved on to search the treed area west of the slide path. It was covered with broken tree branches releasing strong evergreen vapour balm that was noticeable to the handlers. These broken branches were well mixed into the snow, making it difficult for his dog to work.

But dogs often amaze their handlers, and at about nine-thirty, Griz indicated the tip of a ski just under the snow and then indicated something buried farther down. The probers quickly confirmed the presence of a body two metres down, but it took considerable time to shovel down to the victim. At last the dogs were finding something despite the appalling conditions. Gord continued searching in the trees and succeeded in turning up several articles of clothing and a pack. With the discovery of the first body and the articles, the search master realized the trees had to be the prime search area. Everyone also began to realize that probing the area seemed to help the dogs by allowing the scent to reach the surface more easily. With Gord covering the trees, the other three dog teams remained working the main deposit, because it could not yet be eliminated.

At about three o'clock one of the probe lines in the trees located the second victim at about the same depth. It was again difficult to dig down to the victim, and they had to use steel shovels. By the end of the day the entire area had been coarsely probed and some parts had been finely probed. The next day all the dogs concentrated their efforts there.

The media finally had something to report. Perry Jacobson and Keith Everts, both assistant chief park wardens, were the liaison officers for the media and family—a job not envied by anyone, but for which they were highly praised. They showed discretion, tact and compassion, particularly for family members. Two families went home having some closure, but two more bodies remained to be found, and the snow gave them up reluctantly. At the end of the third day, they still remained entombed in frozen silence.

On the fourth day, the dogs began turning up more articles of clothing. When the sun's rays finally warmed the air up a bit, Griz enthusiastically indicated in another area of the timbered deposit, and the two remaining victims were found together under a log. The probe lines had covered this area the previous day without luck. They had probably hit the log instead of the bodies and discarded the find.

By now the course of events started to become clear. The friends had crossed both slide paths and were probably intending to return to the parking lot after having their lunch right around noon. They had moved well into the stand of old massive trees where they must have felt safe. Some of the trees were so big it would take two people to encircle them, indicating no evidence of slide activity for decades. Evidence of food in their mouths indicated they had been eating when the slide hit. The slide was released when one of the large cornices on the ridge well above the valley broke off and hit the wind-loaded slope below. The resultant slide was so massive that the wind blast alone would have hurled them down into the surrounding forest. The trees that were thought to provide safety had been stripped of branches as high up as eight metres by the wind blast.

The impact was sudden and complete. The skiers may have heard the immediate sound of the exploding avalanche as it plunged downward with a fearsome velocity and may even have looked toward the slide path expecting to see it go by. Nothing prepared them for the huge slide that mowed down the protective ancient forest where they ate their last meal.

In the end, the rescue workers concluded that the skiers had done everything they could except stay home. The critique did point out that they were not wearing avalanche beacons, but that would not have saved them. It would, however, have expedited the search, making it less risky to the many searchers exposed to a possible avalanche from the first slide path. Reports also carried a strong recommendation that people continue to use their beacons. The critique pointed out areas of improvement for the future, as all critiques should—no search is perfect—but it was undeniable that the Warden Service had reached a new height in the ability to handle large complex rescue scenarios involving multi-agency cooperation. Communication was handled well, but Tim thought one of the best keys was delegating tasks early and well. Egos were left at office doors and tent flaps, giving Kevin Blades, in an article for *Viewpoint Magazine*, a reason to compliment all involved for their professionalism.

THE SUMMER THAT FOLLOWED the Healy Creek Avalanche was dotted with rescues that benefited from the growing professionalism of the Warden Service and the skill of the pilots. But weather and circumstance on big mountains can always make for interesting rescues when helicopters cannot be used. Mt. Robson never lets much accident-free time go by, and in August of that year, a series of near tragedies was avoided, not by the Warden Service but the fortunate presence of two young Yamnuska Mountain Adventures guides.

It began with a pair of very inexperienced young climbers from Ontario who unwisely failed to take adequate precautions during their descent. Perhaps they were so elated with their success that they paid no attention to the greater difficulty of getting off the mountain, and in their haste to get down, did not belay over the treacherous ground they had climbed over. They did stay roped up, but they moved too quickly on the steep face below the summit. The higher man fell, pulling the second down a 75-metre fall only arrested by a large crevasse that broke the ankle of the second man. Fortunately for the inexperienced pair, the mountain was teeming with climbers. One party was already below them when their cries for help attracted the attention of a third party heading up the ridge. The upward bound Colorado climbers yelled to the descending party to go for help. After checking the injured pair and giving them advice on how to dig a bivouac, stay warm and wait for help, the two proceeded on to the summit.

The pair from Colorado were definitely optimistic if they thought that the boys below could get through the night without help. As they were going down, they passed close by and hollered out to see how things were going. By that time, the survivor, who had only cuts and scrapes, was descending to retrieve gear for the night. The man with the broken ankle was now in pain and quite cold. The Colorado climbers managed to lower him down to his partner when they realized just how inexperienced and ill-equipped the pair were. They, themselves, had no extra food or bivi gear to get through the approaching night with a storm clearly brewing. As they sat there they noticed two climbers heading for the Kain Face. They were Barry Blanchard and Troy Kirwan, guides from Yamnuska Mountain Adventures, coming to help. They had received word of the accident, and realizing things could get ugly with the deteriorating weather, they had immediately headed up with emergency supplies. They were able to leave a stove, food, fuel, a tent and some sleeping bags, saying they would return the following day to help the boys down.

The two Colorado climbers decided to stay in the bivouac with the young boys and retreat the following day when the guides returned. Poor weather, however, kept the guides from reaching them again till late the following afternoon, when with care, they were able to lower all four men to the camp below.

In the meantime, word of the accident had been received and Darro Stinson quickly was able to do a flight that day. Though they could not get a team on the north side of the mountain, they did sling a radio in to Blanchard. Rescue wardens from Lake Louise also showed up that night prepared for the worst. One team was flown to the Robson Hut where messages were relayed, and by the following day the wardens knew the men could be picked up at the lower camp. The weather improved enough for Gary Forman to reach the camp with Frank Staples, but was immediately stranded when the swirling clouds returned. Just after realizing he could not fly out, he heard cries of help from above. A third party who had summited the day before were desperately trying to get down. Fortunately, they were able to get themselves off the Kain Face and make it to the now-crowded sanctuary of the guides' camp. Barry radioed down that he had three more distressed climbers making a total of 14 people stranded for another night.

Gary Forman does not mind flying around the mountains, but he was never thrilled at having to spend the night on one. Unlike the incident on Mt. Alberta, he was not going home and had to make do with what comfort the camp offered. To everyone's relief, the weather finally cleared enough the following morning to evacuate the whole crew in stages, leaving the mountain to its solitary isolation in fog and ice. Gaby Fortin, now superintendent of Jasper National Park, sent letters of thanks to the helpful guides for their efforts that may have saved lives. It certainly saved the wardens from another epic adventure.

Gerry Israelson remembers one incident on Mt. Robson that stood out because of the bizarre way the victims were located. A pair of climbers attempting the north face were reported overdue after a two-day storm had hit the mountain. With a sense of urgency, Gerry and Pat Sheehan flew in with Gary Forman to see if they could locate the missing men. The weather had cleared after the storm into bright sky-blue flying conditions, giving them great visibility. The storm, however, had left most of the mountain under 25 centimetres of new snow, covering any tracks left by climbers on the mountain. If the rescuers hadn't realized it before, it became abundantly clear how big a mountain Mt. Robson is, as they flew for hours looking for any sign of life. All they knew was that the climbers had set out to do the north face; if they had successfully reached the summit, they had a choice of several descent routes. They could also have fallen off in any number of places. But the new snow not only covered tracks, it also covered any fresh avalanche debris. After hours of flying, Gerry decided they had to wait for the new snow to melt off before clues might surface.

As they headed back to a lower elevation, they spotted tracks for the first time that day on the Robson Glacier. The tracks were unusual, however, emerging from a moraine above the heavy timber and heading straight up "like an arrow shot." It did not seem possible that they belonged to a climber as no one in their right mind would take that route up the mountain. But it occurred to Gerry that they could belong to a scavenger such as a bear or wolverine. Sure enough, closer inspection revealed the imprint of a wolverine. The tracks went unerringly upward till they disappeared in the maze of crevasses formed just where the glacier toppled over a steep edge from a relatively flat upper bench. They found the startled creature crossing a large snow bridge as it turned toward them snarling in the blowing snow. Gary took the machine directly upward from there, and on the bench not far from the animal they finally found the missing men. Or one anyway. The lone survivor was waving feebly at them as they acknowledged his presence and flew to a nearby flat area to assemble the sling gear.

When they reached the man, Gerry was struck by his condition. He had never recovered a survivor who was so completely exhausted, mentally and physically. He was utterly spent. He was also considerably broken up by the fall he had taken with his partner when they released a small slab avalanche during their descent. His partner had been killed in the avalanche, but he had somehow lived through two nights of exposure despite his broken ribs, smashed pelvis and a possible spinal fracture. Gerry could only imagine the mental torture the poor man must have endured as he hopelessly watched the helicopter fly by repeatedly throughout the day. It was almost enough for him to give up his tenuous hold on life when the machine appeared to be leaving that evening. There was no possible way he could have survived a third night out. Gerry had not the heart to tell him that they had only found him because an errant wolverine had caught the scent of his dead pal and was on his way up for an easy meal.

THE LAST BIG RESCUE EFFORT at the end of the eighties actually occurred the following summer in 1991, but it marked the end of the reign of the alpine specialists and as such came at the end of a significant period in mountain rescue for Parks Canada. The experience gained on the Healy Creek Avalanche was drawn upon for the biggest cave rescue in Canadian history. It began when four men, all rangers in Mt. Robson Provincial Park, set out to acquaint two novices with Arctomys Cave, the deepest in North America. It was quite a challenge, but Rick Blak and Ron Lacelle were both experienced cavers who had been in the cave before. Chris Zimmerman had no caving experience but was a good climber, able to adapt to the environment. The fourth man, Hugo Mulyk, had some caving background and was an experienced mountaineer as well, leaving Rick little doubt that they would all do well. They undertook the exploration on October 17th when they expected the cave to be relatively dry compared to the wetter summer months. They took advantage of nearby Yellowhead Helicopters to ferry them in the 20 kilometres to the mouth of the cave above the Moose River. They did not plan to spend more than a day in the cave.

Blak and Zimmerman went down first as a team, followed by the other two a couple of hours later. They met at the large "Straw Gallery" approximately two kilometres into the cave system at a depth of 418 metres—well into the cave but not quite at the bottom. Rick and Chris had run out of rope for the spectacular descents typical of deep caves and were returning to the surface. The ascent was often slow, particularly at the bottleneck which was just above them at a ladder pitch blessed with a very cold waterfall (aptly named The Refresher). Rick went first using the fixed hand line to avoid the water, but when he pulled on the rope, the rock anchoring it broke free. It was a large 400 kilogram boulder that had seemed stable, but now it came crashing down on Rick, crushing his pelvis and knocking him unconscious.

When Hugo and Ron arrived 15 minutes later, Rick was conscious but in great pain, exacerbated by the flow of cold water. It took the three of them over 40 minutes to move him up to another site called The Elbow, where it became too difficult to go any farther. It was obvious that the time it took to move him that short distance meant they would never get him out by themselves. He was in far too much pain, and the difficult passages ahead entailed long raises interspersed with tight tunnels. It was also obvious that time was running out. They had very little equipment with them: a basic first-aid kit—which was of no use for that injury—and one fading lamp. What they needed was warm clothing, food, and camp gear as soon as possible to stave off the encroaching hypothermia, the anathema of all cavers. They decided that Ron and Hugo could move the quickest, while Chris, an experienced first-aider, would stay with Rick. But things looked bleak. It was a long way out and much of it entailed jumaring with only one temperamental lamp up

free hanging pitches between tortuous, water-soaked tunnels.

Chris was not used to caves, and suddenly he had to stay behind in the freezing blackness with a dying friend. With tremendous mental fortitude, he said goodbye to his teammates and the last source of light he would see for some time.

It was a difficult trip, and they were not out until the following morning, only to find the camp smothered in 25 centimetres of new snow. In despair they discovered the radio they brought in to contact Yellowhead Helicopters for the flight out failed to trip the park repeater, leaving them with no outside contact. It meant they had to go out on foot to instigate a rescue. When they realized their predicament, Hugo suggested he go for help while Ron returned to the men below with food and sleeping bags, but they found Ron did not have enough batteries to return. It was apparent that they both had to hoof it out over 20 kilometres of snow-covered trail to get help. After a short break to eat and warm up, they headed out, but it would be a heart-breaking nine hours before they got to a telephone.

Their terrible message elicited a response in the caving world like nothing seen before. Park Zone Manager Wayne Van Velzen immediately contacted Phil Whitfield in Kamloops to see what cave-rescue resources were available. Whitfield was the Provincial coordinator for B.C. Cave Rescue who sent out the call to all resources in Alberta and B.C. It was already late in the day, but people worked through the night, and by morning a team of cave rescuers were in Valemount, B.C. This was not an easy task, as the airfield had to be cleared of the new snow to receive the government jet carrying the 12 rescuers who were picked up from Vancouver Island and flown to the small town. In addition, PEP, in conjunction with Parks Canada and the RCMP, sent another 11 fairly experienced cavers. John Donovan, an Alberta caver, organized that group and had nine more men sent in. By daylight, a hodgepodge of teams were ready, but they needed organization and a coherent plan. Clair Israelson came in from Parks Canada as did Tim Auger, but in this instance, with an open ear to Tim's experience on the Healy Creek rescue, Clair took over base command and quickly had things running smoothly.

Clair knew he was no caver, but he knew the logistics of a major rescue, and as Tim had learned, the best operation runs with well-delegated teams. He had the cavers assess the situation and provide the expertise to oversee the underground work. They now had the daunting task of lowering a 90 kilogram stretcher down 418 metres of slimy, water-soaked, twisted tunnels and vertical drops. Once they were down, the whole process would have to be reversed, with the added burden of a man's weight. In addition, radio communication was not possible through solid rock with the normal VHF radios. They would have to string com-munication wire for radio transmission almost the whole length of the cave. The rescue summary bleakly states: "It was clear that if the stretcher were to be moved continuously, a tremendous amount of underground manpower would be required." The bad weather that is the constant companion of a major rescue operation continued to hamper all efforts made to bring people in and establish the base rescue camp.

Nevertheless, by the end of the first day a rescue team was headed into the cave hoping to reach the injured man before hypothermia or the injury finished him off. They had not gone far before they met Chris Zimmerman. With buoyed hopes they learned from him that Rick had still been alive when he had seen him last. But this was an artificial hope. Chris had actually returned to the surface without aid of light to preserve his

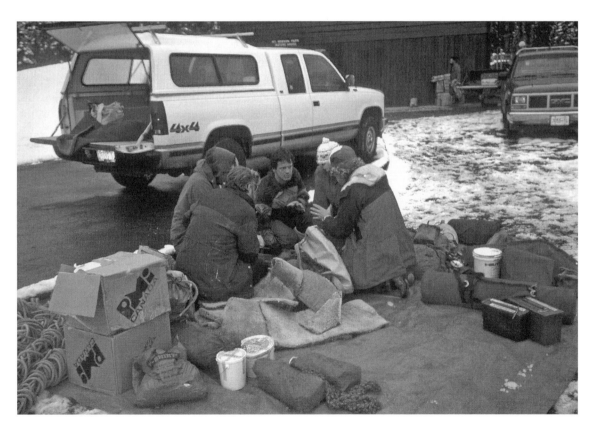

Organizing for Arctomys cave rescue. GREG HORNE COLLECTION

own life after hours of staying by his friend's side. The rescue team actually saved Chris who was disoriented and hypothermic when they found him. Zimmerman did not want to dash everyone's hopes, but he knew, as did Rick, that his hope of survival was highly unlikely even if help arrived. Rick was weakened and very hypothermic, but the injured caver knew he had to send his friend to the surface, or they both would die. This unselfish action was not a surprise to anyone who knew Rick Blak. Leaving him was the most difficult thing Chris had ever had to do in his life.

Chris was brought to the surface while the first party continued down to Rick. They emerged hours later with the unsurprising news that Rick had died. With considerable grief, they all realized they faced the monumental task of bringing out the dead man's body.

By now Clair had established a remarkable base camp just outside the cave entrance with 15 personal tents, two large sleeping tents, a cook tent, a propane-heated drying tent and a large heated staff tent. Jim Taylor, an RCMP communication specialist, provided a reliable communication link from the cave to Robson base with a portable repeater. Before coming back to the surface, the first team had succeeded in getting Rick's body past the unpleasant Refresher pitch so that future rescue teams need not get soaked so far down the cave. The tedious process of hauling the loaded stretcher started at 8:00 a.m. Sunday morning. Everyone worked in harmony to bring the body to the surface the following day. Twenty minutes later, the first flight to evacuate the camp came in, and the extraordinary team was dismantled that night. This was followed by a night in Valemount, reviewing the operation and lamenting the passing of a fine man. The next day most of the personnel returned to the Robson Base Camp for a critique and the sorting of equipment. The operation melded many disparate groups who left egos at the tent flap and united to retrieve the body of a friend.

When Clair ran the rescue operation at Arctomys Cave, he did so as the Western Region public safety specialist. Peter Fuhrmann, the last alpine specialist, retired that spring, signifying the end of era. Both he and Willi had been brought in from outside the Warden Service to teach the outfit how to run their own rescues, and they did that with unmitigated success. In 1991 the job was accepted by the men who had grown up and learned in their shadow. It was time to make the job their own.

8

The Volunteers

IN MANY PARTS OF THE WORLD, rescue groups are composed of volunteers simply because there is no professional organization nearby. The National Parks in Canada did develop a professional rescue group, but only after being provoked to do so because of increased activity in risky sports that resulted in serious accidents. The Warden Service was hard pressed to respond to accidents within their own borders and were stretched to extend services beyond that. Despite this, Walter Perren felt obligated to do what he could and went out on more than one occasion to accidents outside the parks.

The rescue for Gordon Crocker in 1961 was an epic mission involving park wardens, mountain guides and Calgary Mountain Club members under Walter Perren's leadership. After the accident, Perren actively encouraged Calgary Mountain Club climbers like Don Vockeroth to form a volunteer rescue group. The young climbers listened, and the Calgary Mountain Rescue Group slowly evolved during the early 1960s. It started when a "Rescue Committee" representing both the Alpine Club of Canada (Calgary section) and the Calgary Mountain Club was formed in late 1961 to look into the matter. Well-known local climbers like Dick Lofthouse, Gordon Crocker,

Brian Greenwood, Gunti Prinz, Klaus Hahn, Brad Geisler, Don Vockeroth and a host of others attended these sessions leading to the formation of the Calgary Mountain Rescue Group, which later incorporated under the Alberta Societies Act in 1963. Their mandate was to put together an effective mountain rescue organization for the eastern slopes of the Rockies with particular emphasis put on developing recreational interest west of Calgary. Once the group was formed, Perren took an active interest and provided instruction, direction and invitations to attend national park mountaineering courses. He also encouraged the group to attend local, regional and international workshops and conferences. The Calgary Mountain Rescue Group also became a member of the International Mountain Rescue Association.

One reason that Walter encouraged the formation of a rescue group by the climbers themselves was to have a resource of good climbers able to respond to rescues. One of the focal points for potential accidents was on the steep face of Yamnuska. Many of these climbs were well beyond the ability of the wardens to climb at that time.

Soon the dedicated members of the rescue group began training together and establishing a cache of rescue equipment with financial assistance they received from the various local climbing and hiking clubs. Their first call for help surprisingly came from Mt. Logan in the Yukon. Kluane National Park was still in the conceptual stage in the summer of 1964 when a party of Japanese were reported overdue on this remote mountain. Fortunately the party was located before the group had to send anyone on this expensive jaunt.

It was not until 1967 that the Calgary Mountain Rescue Group (CMRG) actually went to a rescue. The accident, later referred to as "Stampede Monday," occurred on Mt. McGillivary in the Bow Corridor near Exshaw, Alberta. A young fellow had gone out looking for a place to take a youth group climbing and was reported to be checking out the area around Heart Mountain. When he failed to return, the CMRG was called out to look for him. The group set up base at the trailhead for Heart Creek and sent eight two-man parties out to search the surrounding area. One group was sent to cover the Yamnuska area while the rest concentrated on the terrain around Heart Mountain. Two of the groups had no radio contact, because there were only enough radios for six groups.

Gunti Prinz, the leader of one of the groups, stopped to have a smoke and to glass the area with his binoculars. As he scanned the scree slope on Mt. McGillivary across from Heart Mountain, he spotted something dark lying on the scree. It turned out to be a body. Because he had no radio, the group raced back to the rescue base to report their finding. Immediately a larger group was sent in to help. As Ken Pawson related later, "We needed an all-out team effort to get up there and back before dark. We did it—getting back well after dark. We were bloody tired but the group had had its first real tryout." The victim was reported to have a 40-metre rope with him, but it was never found, and no one was ever quite sure whether he had climbed the mountain or not. As Ken Pawson said later, "You don't like to make negative comments over some poor son-of-a-gun who's gotten the chop … it's fortunate he hadn't taken the kids up there."

It could now be said that the Calgary Mountain Rescue Group was up and running as a non-profit volunteer public service organization dedicated to search and rescue. After the early financial assistance from the various climbing and hiking groups, Alberta's Parks and Recreation became the major source of future capital. The rescue group's generic responsibilities lay along the eastern slopes of the Canadian Rockies, but they responded to incidents as far south and north as the Blairmore/Crowsnest Pass and Sundre. As caving became more popular, the group found that it was also required to spearhead rescue capabilities in this sport.

The Calgary Mountain Rescue Group members came mainly from the climbing community, drawing in some of the finest rock and ice climbers around, including an array of international-calibre mountaineers. Supporting this group were three climbing doctors and several paramedics. The CMRG's other aim was to educate both its membership and the general public in safe mountaineering practices. They did this by heightening the awareness of mountain hazards and teaching outdoor skills such as safe travel in avalanche terrain, hazard evaluation, basic mountaineering and first aid. The group held frequent rescue practices and supplemented them with related courses. To compensate members for injuries that might ensue during a rescue, the group provided basic coverage under the Workers' Compensation Board and was able to include Supplementary Liability Insurance. Most important, the group lobbied the premier of Alberta for a seat on the Kananaskis Citizens Advisory Board which reviewed suggestions prior to establishing Peter Lougheed Provincial Park and Kananaskis Country.

It was not unexpected that the group's first technical rescue would be on Yamnuska. The 1960s saw new routes being pioneered as the sport of rock climbing took off in Western Canada, and by the mid-1970s it was in high gear. The increase in climbing activity on the mountain was dramatic; in 1975 about 300 parties registered out to climb the various routes on the face, but that jumped to 1,100 parties in 1977. With this rapid increase in activity, Yamnuska became very familiar terrain for members of the Calgary CMRG. The year 1969 was particularly noteworthy for exciting rescues. Dick Lofthouse, who was most instrumental in getting the rescue group off the ground and its most long-standing member, had his own adventure on Yamnuska. As Ken Pawson put it, "If it had happened in the States, he'd have got a bloody medal for it—here he just got a beer from the rest of the gang. But we sure knew what he had accomplished."

Lofthouse was completing a route called Bottleneck with John Martin, a 22-year-old Calgary university student. John, still a formidable "rock jock" 35 years later, was no stranger to the mountain, having put up routes on Yam since 1964. He was leading the second to last pitch high up on the face when he fell off. As John dramatically put it in a recent award-winning book titled *The Yam*, "All of a sudden I was airborne. I went shooting down through space and bang I hit a ledge really hard. Saw stars. Came shooting out into the sunlight. I was tumbling, but not particularly fast, and I remember two things specifically: I remember thinking what a nice day it was, and I remember realizing that I had knocked a lens out of my glasses and being annoyed at that."

As he fell, each soft-steel piton protection placement pulled out like the snaps on a jacket. Fortunately for both of them, Dick had a bomb-proof belay anchor. As Martin relates, "When the pull came on the rope, they all came out but I didn't know that. The time dilation was such that I thought I had fallen to the end of the rope and pulled Dick off and we were both going to the bottom. So I was quite surprised when all of a sudden I stopped falling." As Martin hung there, he called up to Lofthouse, but there was no answer. In an effort to hold the fall, Dick had been yanked upward, slamming into the rock, which knocked him unconscious. But his belay plate did the job it was designed for and stopped the fall. Fortunately someone on the scree slope below had witnessed the accident and yelled up, "Do you need a rescue?" Martin responded in the affirmative and the person ran off to summon help. Because Martin was wearing a climbing helmet, he had no head injuries. His body survey revealed a broken kneecap, a broken foot and a separated shoulder. Not bad considering he had just taken a 53-metre leader fall.

More good fortune held for Martin, because there was nobody better qualified to lower him down the face than Dick Lofthouse. When he came to, he was surprisingly clear headed and with an abundance of rope rescue knowledge behind him, he gradually lowered the injured man to successively lower stances, then rappelled down to repeat the process. As Martin recalled later, it was "absolutely fantastic. There was probably no one else around who would have known what to do, or been equipped to do it." Self-rescue was basically unpractised in mountaineering in those days, but with this epic rescue Lofthouse focussed attention on this possibility. By the time they reached the bottom, the first of the CMRG arrived at the base of the cliff to bring them down.

It was amazing how many people it took sometimes to effect a rescue, or how many were willing to respond as volunteers. Many of these accidents occurred in the late sixties and early seventies before the helicopter was in use, and adequate manpower was extremely important in getting victims off the face and down the mountain. A typical rescue operation on Red Shirt in 1969 required 21 rescuers to bring the victim safely down. No one got much sleep that night and some got none at all. Most wouldn't make it to work that day. There were some big names from the mountaineering community who responded to the call, and it showed how much time and dedication were needed.

More rescues were handled by the CMRG in the mid-1970s, two of which stood out in the memories of several members for different reasons. The first was a great success and a high point for the rescue team. A Calgary caver fell 17 metres into a crevice, over 100 metres below the entrance of Yorkshire Pot in the Crowsnest Pass, and it took the great efforts of several individuals from different groups to bring the man to the surface.

The CMRG, who ran the show, arrived in the late afternoon of May 7th, 1973, after being notified by the RCMP. The volunteers first asked if they could use Jim Davies out of Banff as the rescue pilot. This was extremely astute on their part. As they put it, "They didn't want to be flopping around in the air in bad weather in difficult country with an inexperienced pilot." Davies flew down from Banff, while the first party members of the CMRG drove their own cars trying to keep up to the red lights and siren of a speeding police cruiser careening ahead of them.

After meeting the helicopter in the Crowsnest Pass and experiencing some wild-west flying in high winds and deteriorating weather conditions, members of the various groups met at the cave entrance and settled into the technical part of the rescue. As Ken Pawson relates: "Jim and his chopper were waiting, and immediately Gunti Prinz, myself and the chap who had come out of the cave for help were lifted up to the area near the cave in deteriorating weather. As we neared the ridge we had to get over, Jim the pilot suddenly called out—'We're too heavy, I haven't got enough lift!' Then he added, 'Two of you are going to have to get out!' We all thought he was kidding but when he hovered close to the ground on a high snow-covered shoulder, he leaned back, opened the back door and said: 'When I say jump, you jump!' We then knew he was damn serious. It was quite obvious which two had to jump—Gunti and myself—as the other chap was needed to show Jim where the cave was. So we leapt from the hovering helicopter, landing on the small shoulder of snow, more or less on the ridge, with a howling wind and drifting snow all around us and me thinking that this was one hell of a way to spend my 50th birthday. I remember Gunti turning to me as we watched the helicopter disappear, 'You know Ken, all our equipment is in that helicopter and if it runs into problems, we've got nothing to get off of here with!'"

Davies eventually returned, but when they got to the cave entrance, it was covered in drifting snow and completely blocked. They had to clear an entrance which would later collapse, further hampering their efforts to bring the man out. The rest of the CMRG were then brought in along with five members of the Coleman Collieries Mine Rescue Team. It would take all of them to complete this difficult rescue operation.

They had obtained all the critical information they needed from the survivors. Earlier, the four cavers from Calgary had decided to use the fixed ropes left behind by a previous expedition. When the last man began his rappel, the rope slipped off the anchor. With some difficulty he managed to re-anchor the rope and start again. But his hampered efforts were not sufficient. He was about three metres down when the rope again slipped off the belay, and he plunged 13 metres, sustaining injuries to his face, wrist and lower back.

The most time-consuming part of the evacuation was rigging the cave with ropes, anchors and pulleys for the rescue. Although most involved were accustomed to underground conditions, especially the Coleman team, there was a lot of manoeuvring in a dark, confined environment made hazardous by thin traverses over huge drops. Their task was to bring the injured man, now in a stretcher, up a vertical pitch 27 metres high to the exit passage which was a 55-degree, 100-metre long passage that was only one-half metre in width. Even when they got to the surface it didn't end.

On his last flight that evening, Jim Davies had said, "When you get him out, shine your lights directly upwards, and if I can see a light at all, I'll put her down, even in darkness, but if I can't see a light I'll have to wait until morning." When they got the victim to the surface they heard the helicopter making low passes above them, and they shone their lights upward as instructed, but the beams just disappeared into the dark void of blowing snow. They heard Jim circle a few more times and then take off for the valley. Disappointed, they returned to the chilly shelter of the cave for the night. In the glow of their headlamps, Bugs McKeith astonished everyone by producing a bottle of beer which they passed around to salute Ken Pawson's birthday. Ken said later, "I thanked them but said I hoped in future occasions it wasn't in this bloody cave."

Next morning, when the weather eased a bit, Davies was able to land and the injured man was successfully evacuated in a Stokes litter, 38 hours after he first entered the cave. The disparate groups had worked very efficiently together under the leadership of the CMRG—something they were quite happy with. The CMRG also recognized that they needed to develop a cave-rescue team. In a report following the operation, it stated, "The lack of a well-developed cave-rescue team was a reminder to all cavers in the Rockies that a bad fall deep inside a cold, wet cave could be fatal."

Some of the CMRG members, such as Garry Pilkington, and Bugs McKeith, before his death in 1978, were cavers who were also accomplished mountaineers. But the rescuers welcomed the group from the Coleman Collieries Mines Rescue Team. They knew these miners were used to being in damp, dark and confined spaces and understood rope and cable-rescue equipment and methods. The CMRG encouraged the development of a valid cave-rescue organization after this accident. Soon after, the Alberta Cave Rescue and a cave-rescue group in B.C. were formed.

A major second operation unfolded with a call from the RCMP. The call, however, came too late for success. The RCMP reported that two young boys appeared to be in desperate straits, clinging to a small ledge in the middle of a cliff on Goat Mountain near Blairmore, Alberta. They could

move neither up nor down as they perched there, paralysed by fear, waiting for help. They were part of a family outing that had started earlier that day. After a few hours of climbing up the mountain, the family headed back the way they had come. But the energetic young boys opted to take the steeper route to the bottom, possibly thinking to beat the others. The inexperienced family saw no immediate danger in the terrain that looked deceptively easy from above.

The members of the CMRG could sense the urgency surrounding the situation. Their anxiety was amplified by the gripping ride from Calgary in the back of two police cruisers as they navigated the road south. Dick Lofthouse, Glen Boles, Gunti Prinz and Ken Pawson were all in one vehicle. Pawson later said, "I well recall that the road was icy in places, and I was thinking that anything we do on the cliff tonight can't be worse than this drive at this speed."

Things weren't going well on Goat Mountain. One of the boys had slipped from his perch and fallen to his death in full view of the second boy who was now gripped by terror. It was a grim situation when the rescue team arrived at the base of the cliff. They had little chance to reassure him as they hurriedly put on their climbing harnesses and roped up. He was about a rope length above them and around the corner of a large rock outcrop some 30 metres up. Just as they started climbing someone managed to yell: "Just take it easy, we're coming to get you." Tragically, even before Lofthouse made his first move in the dark, the second boy fell from the ledge and landed with a thud only metres from their feet on the scree slope.

There wasn't much left to be said or done at this point; it was such a shattering experience. But the rescuers tried to keep a glimmer of hope as they put on a valiant effort to save him, administering CPR over the remaining distance to the highway. When they reached the bottom they realized their effort was for naught, for it was obvious the boy was dead. Words couldn't describe how defeated the group felt. Pawson later said, "Members of our group have witnessed unhappy and unpleasant sights in the mountains over the years, but I have never seen our team so affected while under the stress of failure to save someone as we all were that night. Everyone had done the right thing, but it wasn't enough. It affected us so deeply because it was a kid you know and that's really difficult."

By the latter half of the 1970s, the group was at its zenith. But they always needed money. In a brief presented to the Alberta Provincial Government on November 21st, 1977, the CMRG's president, Lyn Michaud, tried to gain more support from the Province of Alberta by making them aware of the need for such a service. He states: "The CMRG would like to stress our willingness to carry on with a service we feel is essential. We hope the will recognize the independent nature of the sport of climbing and realize the climbing community wishes to monitor their own activities and accept responsibility for those who became involved in climbing related mishaps. As mentioned, in order to fulfill this commitment we request government support in resolving the issues presented. First, the issue of rescue support clarification, secondly, increased financial assistance, then finally, the possibility of input to the regulatory process as it affects climbing related matters. We believe the benefits to Alberta citizens and guests will far outweigh the small effect in time and money necessary to prepare ourselves fully in advance of need."

Though the plea was taken seriously, it did not ultimately benefit the CMRG. In 1979, the Alberta government hired Lloyd (Kiwi) Gallagher to establish a public safety capacity for the provincial rangers in anticipation of the establishment of Kananaskis Country. For the CMRG it was a relief in some ways, since training took up much of the time they could otherwise use recreationally. Gallagher, however, wanted the CMRG to stay committed to mountain rescue for as long as possible, giving him time to train the inexperienced rangers. To help keep them active, Lloyd extended training opportunities and offered some financial assistance.

Lloyd felt the volunteers were a very important resource when he first arrived in Kananaskis. He reflects: "The Calgary Mountain Rescue was very much a part of our initial resource. When I first came to Kananaskis Country, Ken Pawson and all the CMRG was very much a big part of everything, and they of course had many, many rescues under their belt before I arrived on the scene. The CMRG was really good for me because when I first arrived in Canada in 1965 I joined up and we practised a lot up here, not realizing that 15 years later I would become Mr. Mountain Rescue. I knew everyone so of course I would always call them when I had a rescue in Kananaskis. That went on for two or three years until they realized that I had it under control. Then they basically said, 'Well, it looks like you've got it under wraps here now, so we'll slowly fall back.'" He goes on to say, "They were a major force in this whole thing long before we came into the picture. There's a big story just tied up with those guys and a lot of them were mountain guides as well. It was ideal for me not only having the Warden Service, but also the CMRG. They also knew all the routes on Yam."

By the late 1970s, the group had started to address the issue of being trained for helicopter slinging, referred to as the Helicopter Flight Rescue System or HFRS. They attended a course put on by Peter Fuhrmann in Banff that also included members of the Kananaskis Country rangers. It was held over several days near Tunnel Mountain in Banff, and everyone there got to sling under the helicopter. For the Calgary Mountain Rescue Group, though, it was hard to find the funds to support the training. So although members had slung, they continued to rely on rope and cable rescue techniques. What developed for Yamnuska was a three-tiered response system. If slinging was possible, Kananaskis rangers or Banff park wardens would carry out the rescue. If it was a rope and/or cable rescue then a combined team of rangers and CMRG members would respond. During the early days of sling rescue, many locations on the face of Yamnuska were too steep to access by helicopter, so the CMRG continued to be a backup for some time.

By the early 1980s, with the establishment of a first-class mountain rescue capability in Kananaskis, the close proximity of another in Banff National Park and the refinements in the vertical sling rescue capabilities of helicopters, the group's days were numbered. Finally by 1984, they ceased being active in mountain rescue operations. Its members still responded to large search operations that plagued Kananaskis Country in the eighties, but they no longer trained in specialized mountain rescue.

As early as 1981 there had been talk that the CMRG was looking at disbanding, leaving their equipment available for redistribution to other volunteer rescue organizations. Arnor Larson, who was the mountain rescue co-ordinator for the East Kootenay Mountain Rescue, which operated under the umbrella of B.C.'s Provincial Emergency Program (PEP) was more than happy to gain this windfall. This sister group on the far side of the Rockies had been created to meet the rescue demands in southeastern B.C. Though younger, it was growing quickly and could use the equipment.

In a letter to Rosemary Gascoyne, who was writing a story about the Yorkshire Pot rescue and the tragedy on Goat Mountain in late 1994, Ken

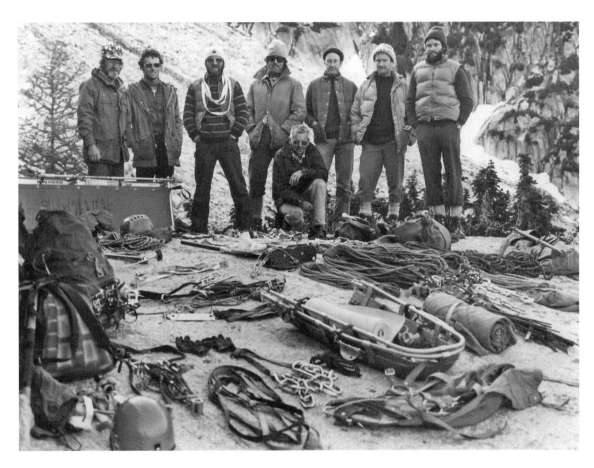

Calgary Mountain Club training. KEN PAWSON COLLECTION

219

Pawson wrote: "The Calgary Mountain Rescue Group now exists only as a backup search team and as an excuse for about 15 of us old-timers to get together over a glass of beer and tell yarns about the old days—and we never let the truth get in the way of a good story." He goes on to further reflect: "You see, when there is a search that is written up in the papers, or reported on TV and radio, there are always lots of volunteers. Some of them are useful and experienced in bush craft, but many are simply keen with no skills in the backcountry, and this can lead to further problems if they are just turned loose with no supervision. In such situations our members might still do a useful job taking care of a small group of such volunteers and doing some safe and useful searching." The Calgary Mountain Rescue Group faded into the twilight of mountain rescue history, but their

legacy lives on. Park wardens and park rangers are happy to pay homage to the group for the early role they played in bridging the years that it took to establish the professional rescue service now provided by rangers and wardens.

WHEN ARNOR LARSON WROTE to the CMRG to accept the generous donation of equipment they had on offer, he did so as a representative of the East Kootenay Mountain Rescue (EKMR), operating under the larger umbrella of PEP. The Provincial Emergency Program is the government body based in Victoria that provides direction and funding for local search-and-rescue groups across the province. The Provincial Emergency Program evolved out of civil defence and a disaster relief program set up shortly after the war to deal with issues like nuclear attack, flooding,

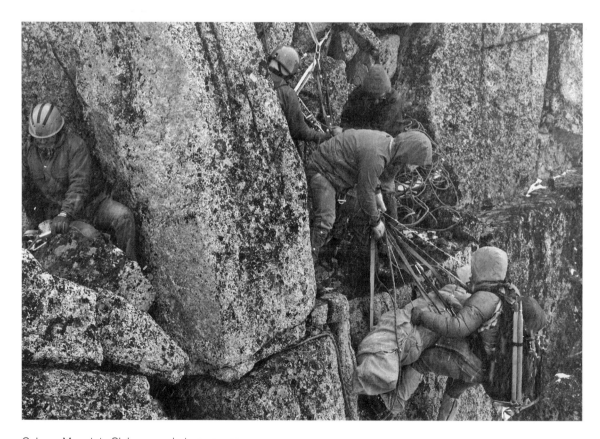

Calgary Mountain Club group shot. KEN PAWSON COLLECTION

earthquakes and other catastrophic events. But like elsewhere in Canada, the local RCMP detachment commander is initially responsible for all accidents.

It was incumbent on the local PEP co-ordinators to established their presence if they wanted to be called to a rescue situation. Six regional PEP districts were set up across the province to co-ordinate the individual field groups, all volunteer, that respond to RCMP requests for assistance.

Throughout the 1960s and '70s, some volunteer groups in British Columbia began to specialize. Most volunteer groups had only ground-search capabilities while others started to meet the need for more advanced mountain rescue. The North Shore Rescue group out of Vancouver is a good example of a group that became very successful in this area. Others like the Whistler group and the Canadian Avalanche Rescue Dog Association in B.C. specialized in responding to avalanche accidents.

The EKMR was one field unit that responded to mountain rescue for some years in southeastern B.C. Their coverage extended from the U.S. border to the Columbia River's Big Bend and from the Alberta border (continental divide) to the Columbia Mountains. They also had the training, equipment and approval to use the Helicopter Flight Rescue System for a period of years through the late seventies and early eighties. More important, there was a pilot available to them who was certified to do such missions.

Several communities had their own rescue groups that operated under the umbrella of the EKMR. The small towns of the Columbia River Valley were funded out of the Nelson regional office for the district. A main centre of activity was the Invermere Search and Rescue group, who were very active and strategically located for responding to accidents in areas such as the Purcell Wilderness, the Bugaboos and Mt. Assiniboine Provincial Park. The town of Invermere kept the necessary equipment in the local fire hall. The EKMR had an up and down relationship with

national parks over the years, as public safety wardens were often called to rescues in these regions. But as the number of rescues escalated through the eighties, Parks Canada encouraged the development of these rescue groups and even shared some joint training.

The Invermere group is a good example of how PEP works in B.C. As the mountain rescue co-ordinator of PEP's Nelson region and head of the Invermere mountain rescue team, Arnor Larson was well aware of the commitment needed to maintain a volunteer program. Motivated by disdain for the American involvement in Southeast Asia, Larson moved north to Canada in 1970 to become a wildlife photographer. He initially settled in the Black Diamond/Turner Valley area southwest of Calgary before moving to the Invermere area in 1971. That winter he began earning a living guiding people in the mountains.

As the PEP program evolved from a civil defence role to search-and-rescue, Larson saw a place for himself and joined the local mountain rescue group in 1971. Arnor excelled at cliff rescue, and over the next few years he put together small training courses geared to rope rescue at this level. In 1979, the Nelson Region of PEP started putting on week-long courses held each June in preparation for the summer rescue season, and Arnor soon found himself instructing on these courses. At the same time PEP was trying to develop solid training standards. Each spring and fall the different regions met in Victoria to standardize their training. But despite lengthy discussions, a universally accepted training standard never evolved. According to Arnor, "Everyone had their opinion, not necessarily with any facts behind it," and he found the sessions frustrating. Larson goes on: "They had a guy in the PEP office in Victoria who could see something needed to be done, and he asked me in late 1979 whether I would consider doing a course for key people from these different groups spread across B.C. who were at least doing fairly good cliff rescue at the time. Particularly North Vancouver, Squamish and in the Penticton area, where there were some active groups that had been doing some rope rescue for quite a while." Arnor was quite enthusiastic, and so every year he helped put on a rope rescue course in Penticton.

The other major development in 1979 was the use of the helicopter and the HFRS sling system, which a few select groups had authority and training to use if the conditions were warranted and if a certified pilot was available. Generally, only those groups who had access to a certified pilot received funding or training.

Getting the funds together for helicopter rental for training or rescue work was another matter. In the case of the Invermere Mountain Rescue Group, a number of stakeholders helped, including B.C. Parks and Recreation, the B.C. Forest Service, the logging and mining interests in the valley as well as PEP and the Panorama ski area. From these sources, they kept a few thousand dollars set aside so that in the spring they could conduct a heli-sling practice and rescue simulation. For several years, they managed to maintain their sling rescue capabilities and averaged one sling rescue per year. According to Larson, during this period there was a lot of vacillation within Parks Canada; one minute they were available and willing to do rescues outside the national parks and the next they weren't. Field staff in the mountain national parks were keen on helping and providing direction, but were not necessarily supported at the regional level. But it was not just the national parks; PEP in Victoria would also waver between maintaining a mountain rescue capability or getting out of it completely. This was frustrating for the different volunteer groups, particularly the North Shore group, who felt that because of their high callout statistics they needed to maintain those skills.

Parks Canada was protective of the HFRS slinging system for good reason. If untrained rescue groups began using this tool haphazardly, there was a danger that accidents would occur. The Department of Transportation had never been happy with the fixed attachment for the sling line

and wardens feared that all rescue organizations would be shut down if an accident resulted from misuse of the system.

An accident did occur when someone attached a sling line to the cargo hook after Mike Wiegele got talked into setting up his own helicopter rescue capability. Now manager and owner of the Blue River Heli-ski operation, Mike wanted to be able to rescue his clients as quickly as possible without waiting for a long-distance rescue team to arrive. Blue River is certainly remote enough to warrant this concern—and besides, he had more than enough helicopters on hand to do the job. Unfortunately, he relied on a guide fresh over from Europe to help him set things up. Mike was uneasy the minute the guide attached a rope to the cargo hook and instructed the pilot to lift off. With trepidation Mike watched as the machine and the guide—who had volunteered for this maiden flight—flew out over the clear expanse of a nearby glacier. Suddenly, to his horror the man plummeted out of the blue and disappeared from sight. They rushed over expecting the worst, but found the man alive in a wallow of powder snow. Though banged up, the man lived to return home with a different view of how to undertake helicopter rescue.

Mike went immediately to a belly band attachment system. His guides actually became quite proficient with heli-rescue but found they were coming to the aid of everyone in the area. Mike later found it was not much use in his own business and so no longer employed it. Though accidents by outside agencies were exactly what Parks feared, this incident actually served to bolster their case for the solid attachment.

Shortly after getting permission from PEP to heli-sling, the Invermere Mountain Rescue Group had an opportunity to use it. The incident took place up Toby Creek west of Invermere, where a group of young people were having such a good party that one of them fell into the canyon and drowned. Searchers located his body snagged on a small log jam in the middle of the fast-moving stream. The canyon was deep, and the pilot had to add another length of rope to the line before he could lower a rescuer to the body. They had no problem getting to the site, but once there they found the corpse was snagged on a section of the log jam and could not be freed. After a long delay, a chainsaw was brought in and used to free the body, and the helicopter made the recovery. The incident caused concern with Parks Canada's public safety personnel who were not happy about the danger of snagging the line. Also the fact they had doubled the length of the sling line did not sit well with anyone.

By 1986, Arnor Larson had formed a company called Rigging for Rescue, which was doing groundbreaking work on the strength of climbing ropes. He had a tower set up which enabled him to do drop tests using different weights and drop heights. But interest in his work was slow to develop in Canada, possibly because of the predominant use of cables rather than ropes for rescue work.

Every year during the mid- and late-1980s and early '90s, Larson would present his findings to a large and interested audience at the North American Technical Rescue Symposium down in the States. Arnor Larson and another PEP coordinator from the Columbia Valley were usually the only Canadians attending. The NSMRG came a few times, but it wasn't until the early 1990s that Parks Canada showed any interest in the symposium. Actually it was Lloyd Gallagher in Kananaskis Country who was the first professional to take what Larson was teaching seriously.

The years 1987 and 1988 were pivotal for both Larson and PEP. Arnor was now putting on Rigging for Rescue courses in the U.S. where he was receiving attention from fire and sheriff departments in the western part of the country. When Gallagher became interested in what Larson was doing in the early nineties, he invited him over to teach a week-long course in Canmore. He invited Tim Auger and Clair Israelson in Banff to attend. Clair immediately saw the value of

what Larson was teaching and encouraged other wardens in public safety to attend courses from then on.

By the end of the decade, however, support for more technical mountain rescue at the administrative level dried up. With no support, the Penticton course was cancelled, and the yearly Advanced Regional Rescue Course in Nelson was also dropped. Toward the end of the eighties, Parks Canada had the resources and range to tackle accidents outside of the parks and were less reluctant to do so. With all this happening, there was now no need to maintain a helicopter slinging capability in the East Kootenays, and the program was dropped.

Discouraged, Arnor got out of active rescue work and concentrated on running his company, teaching courses regularly in places like Sedona, Arizona and Zion National Park in Utah. Arnor maintained his guiding business, but now he spends more time on his first love, black-and-white photography. He pared down even more when he sold Rigging for Rescue in 1993 to a young mountaineer, Kirk Mauthner, who was his neighbour. He stayed on for a while as a consultant, but after nearly a decade Mauthner sold it to a company in Colorado. The company is now recognized as one of the best places to receive training in rope rescue and the dynamics of rope systems.

One very important volunteer rescue group in B.C. that seemed exempt from restrictions on mountain rescue work and heli-slinging evacuations was the North Shore Rescue Group, which has maintained this capability over the last ten years. This is because of its geographic isolation (Kootenay National Park on the Alberta border is the closest professional mountain rescue presence) and the need for that type of service in the urban density of Vancouver and the Lower Mainland which are surrounded by mountains.

ANOTHER IMPORTANT VOLUNTEER GROUP that got its start in British Columbia was the Canadian

Avalanche Rescue Dog Association. CARDA started inauspiciously enough in 1978 when two men from opposite sides of the province got together to talk about avalanche dogs. Bruce Watt from Whistler and Rod Pendlebury from Fernie both worked at their local ski area as ski patrollers, and both saw a need for an avalanche dog in their ski areas. Bruce's interest started when he lost a close friend in an explosion from a dud bomb used in avalanche control.

Rod's inspiration was less dramatic, coming from his interest in training dogs and the fact that he worked in an industry that he thought would be open to the idea of having trained avalanche dogs on-site. They realized they had much to learn about getting started. Bruce had more leverage in promoting this idea, mainly because the people at Whistler were very supportive. He had worked there since the mid-1970s and remembers it was Thanksgiving 1976 when his friend was killed in the dud recovery. As Bruce put it, "It sort of affected me, and there was no such a thing as critical incident stress counselling or debriefing in those days. They gave you a scotch and told you to forget about it." Which he tried to do.

The next winter Watt got a lot more serious about dogs when he was buried in an avalanche while showing two ski patrollers on exchange from Snowbird, Colorado, Whistler's avalanche control program. As Watt and one of the patrollers from Snowbird crossed under what they thought was a recently stabilized slope, it slid and buried both of them. As Bruce describes, "I was buried with only my hand sticking out, so they found me first. Luckily we didn't go over the big cliff below otherwise we would have been killed instantly." He was trying ineffectively to dig himself out when one of the patrollers dug down and managed to free his head. Fortunately they were all wearing rescue beacons. One of the patrollers quickly picked up the remaining signal, and they soon had the second man out.

But Watt was now fully aware of how dangerous the work was and was even more convinced a trained avalanche dog would be a very good companion. Chris Stethem, who was working there, suggested maybe he should start training a dog. Watt began by looking into the history of avalanche dogs. The RCMP recommended the German shepherd as a breed, and so he bought a black shepherd pup and named him Radar. They started training with Jim Brewin, the RCMP dog handler stationed in North Vancouver, who came up on weekends to help. Watt also trained extensively on his own.

Watt and Pendlebury found a few other people in the industry interested in training a dog. They held their first CARDA course at Red Mountain near Rossland. Dale Marino was the only RCMP dog handler in the area qualified in avalanche searching, so he taught the course. Watt and Pendlebury as well as Michael Murphy, Margie Jamieson and Jay Campbell also attended. Though Marino had no authority to certify either dog or handler, they all looked upon it as a step in the right direction. This was not good enough for the managers at Whistler, however. They wanted something in writing that said the dog was certified, since they were paying for the dog's expenses. Bruce knew Geoff Freer, a former Whistler employee now with B.C. Highways, and approached him about the matter. Jeff suggested he try taking the annual RCMP/Parks Canada dog course, and he made the arrangements for Bruce to attend.

The course was being held in Jasper, so Bruce took Radar on the train from Vancouver to the small mountain town for the course. The RCMP dog trainer was Doug Wiebe, who had sent instructions that Bruce needed to have a PEP number to attend. Somehow it never got through to Bruce. He recounts, "When I got there Doug Wiebe took me aside and asked me if I had a PEP number, and I said 'What's that?' Doug said 'I can't allow you to attend the course unless you've been sanctioned by PEP. You need to be with some recognized search-and-rescue group. It's a government course and we can't allow civilians to attend unless they're sanctioned by another organization.'" It was a big letdown. The pressure was huge for him to meet the expectations of the Whistler ski resort. It was also a waste of time and money.

The following year there was a course being held in Banff, which he planned to attend now that he had a PEP number. In the meantime, he continued to train with the RCMP dog handlers. Jim Brewin had moved to Prince Rupert; Terry Barter replaced him and the two continued training. Soon after, the volunteers from the first course had their first CARDA meeting, and elected Michael Murphy president. Bruce Watt and Michael Murphy were invited to attend the RCMP/Parks Canada dog course in Banff. It was a disappointment for Rod not to be chosen, because he and Bruce had spearheaded the organization from the start. As Watt puts it, "Rod was in the same situation I was—from a ski area, being Fernie. Because Murphy was an employee of Parks Canada, he had a little bit more pull or credibility than Rod." What really helped Watt, however, was having the ski area solidly behind him. Pendlebury was never supported that well at Fernie. It was a much smaller ski area, and he was doing most of the work on his own.

The first thing Bruce brought up when he got to the course was the need for some kind of certification if they did well. Watt approached Doug Wiebe on the matter: "I've been to a course at Rossland, I've been to Jasper and been turned away, and now I'm here. I need a paper or letter out of this course saying either I failed miserably or I am qualified to go and do an avalanche rescue." They relented and wrote him a letter validating the team's ability.

This was the first validation of a civilian avalanche search dog in Canada. This alarmed the RCMP who could see an influx of civilians clamouring to get on the course to get the same credentials for all kinds of dogs. After Bruce was certified, the RCMP said that they couldn't continue to have civilian people coming on RCMP/Parks Canada avalanche dog courses and that CARDA should de-

velop their own courses and validation. The RCMP and Parks Canada would support them and provide trainers and instruction.

CARDA held their second course in 1981 at Boulder Creek, Margie Jamieson and Art Twomey's backcountry ski lodge in the Southern Purcells. It was well attended, and the instructors under the auspices of the RCMP were Gord Burns, a dog handler from the Cranbrook RCMP Detachment, and Dale Portman, the Parks Canada dog handler from Banff. The course lasted a week and was noteworthy for its rustic surroundings and the homemade beer, which was a big hit. Twomey and Jamieson kept a running tab and were impressed by how thirsty everyone was at the end of a long day, especially in the grip of winter. Jamieson kept things organized at the lodge and well in hand while she and her dog, Moki, attended the course.

In 1983 the RCMP got together in Fernie with Pendlebury and Watt to help develop a dog training standard for PEP. The RCMP were committed to providing the training expertise while Parks Canada would provide the mountaineering training. A second Boulder Creek CARDA course was held at approximately the same time, and again it was well attended with Burns and Portman returning to instruct. At the course, the group tried to hammer out a dog training standard by adopting PEP's ground searching standards and adapting them to avalanche dogs. Eventually the PEP standards were combined with the RCMP dog training standards to form the CARDA manual.

One of the significant ways CARDA differed from the RCMP or Parks Canada was that the dogs were not required to be German shepherds. At a typical CARDA course in the late eighties, all kinds of dog breeds were represented. Some of the best dogs for this type of work were golden retrievers and border collies.

There was a period of flagging interest during the mid-1980s, but there was renewed vigour when the Whistler resort expanded and Blackcomb was developed. Anton Horvath, Pat Colter and Matt

Rogers from Whistler started training their dogs while Blackcomb had Doug Fenton and Sue Boyd. Jan Tindle soon joined the group as well. Over on the eastern side of the province, Russ Hendry and Tim Quinn started training their dogs, and Duncan Daniels joined this group from Calgary, giving CARDA an Alberta presence. Another Alberta dog actually came from Jasper when Kathy Calvert certified her dog Bear. Kathy had a considerable interest in training her own dog for avalanche work after almost being caught in an avalanche herself while travelling with a young mongrel dog she owned. After this close call she vowed her next dog would receive full avalanche training.

When Willi Schneider, of German descent, became involved, he put a more corporate stamp on the group and started to get sponsorship funding. Schneider invited some German Bergwacht avalanche dog handlers/trainers over to observe a CARDA course. Soon they were helping with the instruction as well. This led the organization to adopt a European training standard that differed from that of the RCMP. According to Burns, Schneider did a lot to bring a professional profile to CARDA and managed to get equipment and funding, but the shift in training standards proved troublesome. Finally in the late 1980s CARDA returned to the PEP/RCMP training standards. Hans Fuhrer, the public safety specialist for Kootenay National Park, became significantly involved by teaching winter mountaineering skills to the handlers.

Tim Quinn, a trapper from Blue River supported by Mike Wiegele and his heli-ski business, became the first Canadian to take his dog over to Europe and attend the annual German Bergwacht avalanche dog course. They made quite the sight, strolling down the main street of Oberstaufen, Quinn with his bushy black beard, fur cap and Indian mukluks being pulled by his giant malamute. Soon others were going over every year.

In 1991 Burns and Portman went over to get a first-hand look at the German training program

along with the CARDA dog handler Pat Colter. There were Poles, Bulgarians, Germans, Austrians and Swiss also attending. Burns and Portman left their dogs at home and concentrated on observing training techniques while Colter's small golden retriever put on a good show. It was apparent to Portman and Burns that the RCMP, Parks Canada and the German Bergwacht had high standards, with training modified to fit the unique environment each agency worked in. In 1991, Doug Fenton and Evonne Thornton went over and attended the course with their CARDA dogs.

In the 1990s CARDA blossomed under a west-coast influence. The RCMP also became much more involved during this period. Up to this point, the RCMP and Parks Canada dog handlers had been instructing only in a quasi-official capacity, but things changed when Roy Fawsett, the head of the RCMP dog training in British Columbia, joined. As Bruce Watt reflects, "We really became credible when Roy Fawcett got involved. Roy took it on himself to create courses in a very structured fashion. More of an RCMP style, and he still runs them today even in retirement. He's given us huge credibility, and he's been with us for 10 to 15 years now. We had our ATMs [Annual Training Meetings] every summer and our courses every winter and an advanced course every second year, but we never had a mentor type guy. He put our whole training program together, from puppy rearing right on up." He follows with, "Tom Howarth, who took over as head dog trainer for the RCMP and who now assists on our courses, said that he sees a time when the RCMP will come to CARDA courses to be validated." Corporal Gord Burns once said at a course, "The RCMP are not going to find a live person in an avalanche. We're too far away. It's going to be one of these people who live and work in the mountains who will do it." He followed this by saying, "The second point to all this is that the standards have to remain high."

When Dale Portman was a dog handler in Jasper, he introduced Jay Pugh and R.J. Kingston to CARDA, and helped them train their dogs Cruz

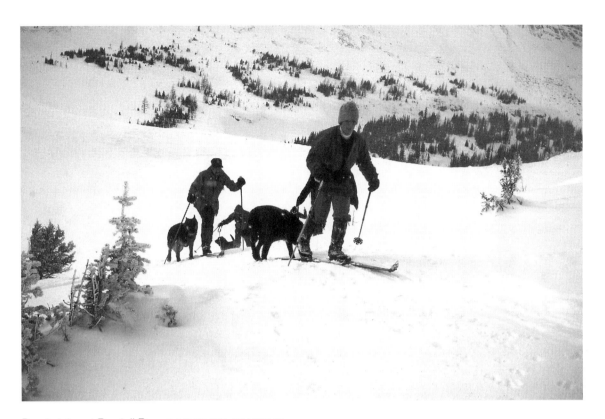

Dog training at Burstall Pass. HANS FUHRER COLLECTION

and Mia. Kathy was also now training her dog Bear with the other two at Marmot Basin ski area. Bear, a large cross between a Newfoundland and Lab, was named "the Valium search dog" by Gerry Israelson because of the dog's slow methodical way of searching. Bear never seemed to move that fast, but always came up with the buried object within the time frame required for passing the CARDA exams. Working with the dog on a Parks Canada simulation avalanche scenario, however, gave Kathy considerable insight into the pressure her husband Dale had to deal with as dog handler.

She and R.J. Kingston were invited to attend the training session at Parker's Ridge in Jasper, and each were given a selected area with two to three dummy burials to search. This was much closer to a real situation than the simulations on CARDA courses, and she felt the pressure of operating under the scrutiny of fellow wardens. Her focus must have been picked up by Bear, because they found the "buried victims" fairly quickly. It was not until later, however, that she realized how hard it must be when the dog fails to find anything.

R.J. did not have the same success that day with Mia, a high-strung German short-haired pointer. The dog was so eager, she ran quickly over the ground and had to be brought back to search more carefully. But Mia had huge potential once she settled down to work. Portman was always impressed with the dog and realized she would be a tremendous asset to the ski hill once her enthusiasm was brought under control. R.J had a couple of really good successes in body recovery with Mia outside the boundaries of Marmot Basin. His work put CARDA on the map in the Rockies.

One of the greatest challenges facing any volunteer organization is getting the opportunity to participate in actual rescues. For the most part, the professional teams will be called in first and only resort to using volunteers as a backup. But dogs need to be kept sharp by being involved with real situations. Actual cases often have high drama, generating adrenaline and fear that pushes the events to a level never matched in controlled training sessions.

Because the number of times a dog is called on a search is limited, RCMP and Parks Canada dogs are multi-faceted to keep the work load higher. This keeps them busy throughout the year, because they are able to take on police work as well as search and rescue. With real cases, the dogs become more seasoned and achieve greater searching and tracking stamina with skills honed to a level that usually can't be reached by a civilian dog.

This is not to say that volunteer groups don't possess good or even great working dogs or handlers. These are highly dedicated people, but they have regular jobs, which dictate how much time they have for actual dog work and training.

The dogs that have the greatest exposure to real rescues and good training sessions are those working at a ski hill. Here dogs and their handlers come closest to the professionals because they are using their skills at work. They also have the greatest probability of being nearby when an accident occurs. It was just such a situation at the Fernie ski area that led to the first live recovery of an avalanche victim by a dog in Canada. The ski hill was getting ready for the season, and the ski patrol, including Robin Siggers and his dog Keno, were doing some testing in a closed area. They had not gone far when they realized that a young lift operator had followed them. They quickly informed him he was skiing in a closed area and asked him to return, but the warning did not prevent the young man from being caught in a moderately sized avalanche on his way back to the ski runs. Fortunately, he had attended an avalanche training session put on by the staff the day before—he created an air pocket and stuck his hand out. The patrollers were close by, and knowing the man was not wearing a transceiver, they started probing immediately. The other good fortune for the young man was that one of the searchers was Robin's dog Keno.

Keno had not been working up to the standard Robin wanted and had earlier gone back to puppy training sessions. On this day all that training paid off. Robin was initially distracted by the probing and was not sure where the glove that Keno brought back had come from. He thought it belonged to one of the patrollers, but on receiving a negative answer, he realized it must be the victim's. Keno was more than happy to show Robin what he had found, which was, indeed, the young man. Keno had dug down far enough to uncover the extended gloved hand. By the time they dug him out, the victim had been completely buried for over 23 minutes and had lost consciousness. He revived immediately once CPR was administered. That night Keno was rewarded with more than Good Dog! Robin gave him a rather large steak for dinner.

This was an incredible success, and it more than justified the vision of the founding members of CARDA. It also fulfilled Gord Burns' prophesy that it would be a dog on scene who would have the first live recovery of an avalanche victim in Canada. CARDA now has 75 teams in the field, of which 35 are fully certified. It is not surprising that all but two of them are in British Columbia. The two active dog teams in Alberta reside in Canmore.

9

Kananaskis Country
"The Brother Next Door"

KANANASKIS COUNTRY ENCOMPASSES much of the mountainous terrain east and south of Banff National Park. When Premier Peter Lougheed announced plans for establishing the park in 1975, the province was flush with money from oil and gas revenue. Soon funds started to appear for visitor service facilities, trails and other infrastructure. A Kananaskis Country Citizen's Advisory Committee open to the public was established with a mandate to determine priorities for development.

Alpine Specialist Peter Fuhrmann had been concerned about the growing popularity of these mountains close to Calgary, feeling that the Warden Service would be pressured to provide rescue service. Knowing the wardens were already stretched to handle their own rescues, he lobbied the Alberta government to hire an alpine specialist and to set up their own rescue program.

The years 1977 to 1982 were the facility development phase for Kananaskis Country, and a five-year management plan was drawn up to outline the development of all future operations. Out of this came the realization, helped by input from Fuhrmann and indirectly from the CMRG, that public safety should be a component of this new development. Fuhrmann had the ideal candidate in mind—Lloyd Gallagher. Lloyd "Kiwi" Gallagher had ample background for the job, and he was Fuhrmann's first choice.

Lloyd was born in Leven, New Zealand, in 1939. One of his earliest memories is of his father carrying him on his back in a pack while hunting red deer and wild pig for the growing family. By the time he was ten, he was part of a local "tramping club" and by the tender age of 16 was leading two-week treks in the mountains. Part of being in a hiking club meant there was a chance of being called out for search-and-rescue work, and by the age of 14 he had been on a number of call-outs, never realizing that decades later it would become a full-time profession. At 21, he became a licenced mechanic and headed off to the South Island. For the next five years he hunted deer for the government, climbed mountains, crossed torrential streams on foot and skied on pristine slopes. But Lloyd wanted to see the world and felt Canada was a good place to start. He earned the money for a one-way ticket by working on the famous Milford Sound trail system two years prior to leaving in 1965. He told his parents he would be back in two years, then boarded a boat for a month-long voyage to Canada. After debarking in Vancouver, Gallagher had no hesitation as to where he was going. He hitched east, drawn like a magnet to the Canadian Rockies.

When he arrived in Calgary he immediately joined the Calgary Mountain Club and the Calgary Mountain Rescue Group, where he met a host of climbing partners and helped on local search-and-rescue calls. His first job was as a mechanic at the Banff Springs Hotel; this soon led to working for Hans Gmoser as a mechanic up in the Bugaboos. Hans realized Lloyd had great potential to do more than that and suggested he get his guide's licence and come to work for him in that capacity. But he was hungry to move on and see more of the world, especially the Yukon, Alaska, Greenland—and possibly Europe. He hung around long enough though to get his guide's pin, and then he headed north. To help with expenses, he did seismic work and led geologists and surveyors from the Arctic Institute of North America up Mount Logan to the research station there.

Lloyd spent the remainder of the summer and early winter on the icecap before returning to work for Gmoser at Canadian Mountain Holidays (CMH), his fledgling heli-skiing operation in the Bugaboos. Gallagher stayed with Gmoser over the rest of the 1960s and most of the seventies and as CMH grew, so did the need for new ski terrain.

Gmoser remembered the Premier Range in the Caribou Mountains northwest of Jasper, where he had skied with Mike Wiegele, and he decided to look into it as a new location for operations. Gallagher accompanied Gmoser and architect Philippe de Le Salle into the upper reaches of the timber-choked Canoe Valley. There they scouted through bush and around muskeg before finding a site for a ski lodge.

Gallagher was put in charge of construction of the lodge in 1973. As he put it, "I had built an outhouse once and it wasn't a very good attempt, so the lack of construction experience made the job challenging." He found time to get married, and he built a suite in the lodge for Fran and himself

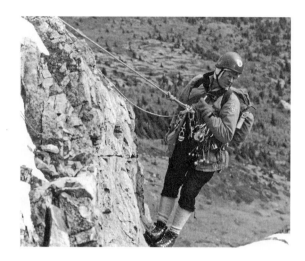

Lloyd Gallagher on rescue school. KANANASKIS COUNTRY PUBLIC SAFETY ARCHIVES

with the idea that someday they might have a family. The skiers arrived in the early winter of 1974 just as they were laying the carpet, and he quickly assumed his new responsibility as manager of the entire operation.

The planned family soon arrived, and Lloyd realized he had to consider his future with his son in mind. They needed a more stable lifestyle in a community that provided schooling. The chance to work as alpine specialist in Kananaskis Country came along quite fortuitously in 1979, and he gladly accepted it.

The challenges of Lloyd's new job were similar to the challenges faced by Walter Perren nearly a quarter of a century earlier. Many park rangers brought in from parks throughout the province had no mountain background. Some of the younger rangers had just come from college or university with little outdoor experience. With patience and understanding, Lloyd set out to mould his disparate crew into a professional mountain rescue team.

Gallagher accomplished this by exposing them to as much training as possible. It took an average of five years to bring a person up to a satisfactory level of leadership. He took them out at night on long trips in all sorts of bad weather to build up stamina. He also had to convince park managers that the schools were not a frivolous waste of time spent having fun.

Gallagher relied on the CMRG to provide seasoned mountaineers to help with rescues, especially for their ability to run complicated rope and cable rescues. There were also a number of dedicated and highly proficient cavers amongst the CMRG who could be called on to help with difficult cave rescues. To bring select managers on side, he would often invite one of them out on a week trip to one of the well-appointed park huts usually situated in some spectacular location. It made his job much easier once the managers understood what he was trying to accomplish.

In the early years he was also blessed with a generous budget. It took him a long time, though, before he was comfortable spending it. He had come from the private sector in the heli-skiing business, where accountability was paramount and funds lean, so he was careful with his spending. He admitted it took much longer to buy cable-rescue gear because the equipment was so expensive. Contrary to what some might think, doing helicopter slinging was much cheaper, because it often entailed only the helicopter, a short flight and two people.

He was a firm believer in the team approach and decided he needed to know each person very well. Gallagher's laid-back personality assisted greatly in accomplishing this. His strategy was to give everyone good basic training, then when they arrived at a rescue, decide where each person would work best. This was necessary for he didn't have the luxury of a dedicated rescue team such as Banff had. He wouldn't know who was going to show up at the staging area at any given time. As he put it, "Every rescue is like a damaged house, you need to learn to work with the pieces you have. I had to decide who I would lower over the rock face, who would be on the rope, who would operate the radios, who would be on the gear, and because we worked so well as a team, that would give me all the combinations I would need to pull off a rescue as quickly as possible."

And of course, they dealt with whatever emergency came along. He further elaborates, "In the rescue community there is a tendency to automatically think that rock rescues are the most challenging, but in fact when I look back, the biggest challenges were of course, the big searches where you have many people out there searching, especially if a child is involved or a plane is missing. There's much more work involved as the rescue coordinator. Climbing rescues are really simple things to do usually." He goes on to say, "Searches can go in a hundred different directions, and when it progresses into day three and day four, you now have the media involved. You've got the public involved and the family involved. You have everybody on top of you, and by then you're tired because you're the head honcho making all the major decisions. So searching is the most demanding and the most costly and we've had our share of big searches."

One of the reasons Kananaskis Country tends to have large searches is the added terrain of the foothills, which many mountain national parks don't have. It is easy to get lost in the featureless timber of rolling hills. The close proximity of a large city lends the country to every type of outdoor adventure from hang-gliding to horseback riding, and adventurers can access the park from many different points.

Kiwi would often invite park wardens from Banff to take part in some of their training, especially in search management, where ranger Dave Hanna was building up experience and expertise. It was an interest that would lead to consulting work when he specialized in the field. The Warden Service was actually behind in this area because they had fewer large searches. The opposite was the case in Kananaskis Country where aircraft went down, and people wandered off in the forested expanses riddled with lakes and rivers. Swift water rescue was another field that the rangers would become adept at handling.

Lloyd became quite skilful at dealing with several other agencies and jurisdictions inside and outside of Kananaskis, including many volunteer search-and-rescue organizations outside of the park. He soon developed a reciprocal arrangement with the Calgary Fire Department because of the number of water rescues the park was becoming involved in. He would go into Calgary and teach the fire department how to rappel down high-rises and office buildings. They in turn would come out and train the park rangers in water rescue. There was no cost involved; much like Parks Canada's involvement with the RCMP in training their dogs and handlers, there was only an exchange of knowledge and ideas.

Because they were part of a provincial park system in Alberta, the rangers were often called upon to respond to incidents on the eastern slopes of the mountains as far north as Hinton and as far south as the Crowsnest Pass. This involved the RCMP in several detachments scattered across the province, and Lloyd Gallagher put considerable effort into setting up policies and memorandums of understanding with them. He says, "Technically it was the RCMP's responsibility to respond to search-and-rescue operations across the country, but we were the ones being called out by them all the time. To get a large federal body like the RCMP to function at the same level of understanding with a smaller regional organization like Kananaskis Country took a lot of work. In essence K-Country was required to do the RCMP's job and to do it effectively; it took years to accomplish this with memorandums of understanding."

But things moved along swiftly: "The reason why Kananaskis came on stream so quickly was because of the co-operation between Parks Canada and K-Country." It helped that Gallagher knew Peter Fuhrmann, Willi Pfisterer and Tim Auger first-hand through guiding and Himalayan expeditions. He had climbed with a lot of different wardens over the years but especially with Tim Auger who had been on two expeditions to the Himalayas with him. He also had a sound relationship

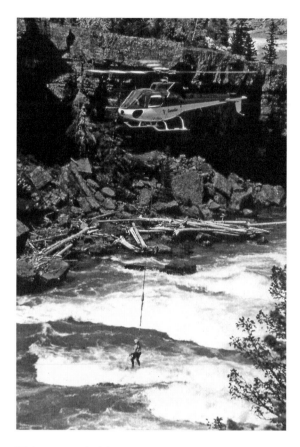

Water rescue training. KANANASKIS COUNTRY PUBLIC SAFETY ARCHIVES

with Jim Davies, the pioneering rescue pilot from Banff. They had worked together at Canadian Mountain Holidays, and they trusted each other. Gallagher also had Peter Fuhrmann's backing.

The first person Gallagher hired to help him out was Dave Smith, a fellow climber and guide. Smith had an impressive résumé that dated back to the early 1970s. He started climbing in Europe and soon found himself guiding clients for the famous British climber Dougal Haston, who had a climbing school in Switzerland. After a couple of years Smith returned to Rossland, B.C. where he opened a Nordic ski shop. By now he was married, and with one child already, he wanted steadier employment. Heli-ski guiding was an option, but it demanded being away from home for long

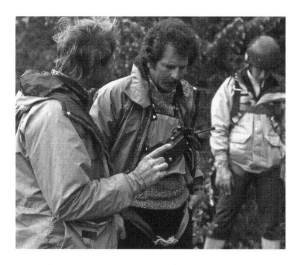

Lloyd Gallagher talking to Dave Smith. KANANASKIS
COUNTRY PUBLIC SAFETY ARCHIVES

periods of time. It was also a job that had a high casualty rate for personal relationships. Although the ski shop gave him steady work in the winter, he chaffed under the yoke of being inside all the time, running the store. Like Lloyd, he saw a great opportunity for enjoyable, steady work in Kananaskis Country.

It was only a five- or six-month job during the summer but it dovetailed well with his winter at the ski shop in Rossland. What helped get him get the job was his involvement with the Association of Canadian Mountain Guides (ACMG). At the spring and fall guide seminars held each year, Peter Fuhrmann would demonstrate some of the new rescue techniques that the Warden Service was using. They could vary from the most up-to-date cable gear to heli-slinging, and sometimes the guides would participate.

When he started working for Gallagher there was a great deal of interaction between Parks Canada and Kananaskis Country. "What I liked about Parks Canada was their willingness to share their expertise with the heli-slinging business with us." He goes on to say, "You would often get a refinement of technique when we trained together with the wardens because you had the

same people looking at the same thing at these sessions." He felt strongly that "Lloyd really had a clear vision of tapping into expertise and having working relationships with knowledgeable people so that we were not re-inventing things. We were so humble … there was so much to learn then."

Another thing that kept them humble was the lack of real rescues in the early years. Kananaskis Country was still opening up and rescues were infrequent. They did practise a lot, but it is the adrenaline rush of saving lives in high-angle situations that keeps rescue units sharp.

One of the challenges he faced was assessing what is and isn't possible in a high-angle rescue. "I found it really challenging. That really draws on your mountaineering experiences because the helicopter really distorts things. The view and perception from the helicopter, with steepness of terrain, can result in mistakes. Fortunately if you have an experienced pilot like Jim Davies or KO [Keith Ostertag] they know what is possible. Sometimes you can be fooled a little bit and it can be less steep. You are assessing whether you have to bring in more people or whether just a couple of you can pull it off. You ask: Can I keep this clean? And of course the fewer rescuers involved, the safer it is."

He remembers the first mountain rescue he went on, which involved the British Army on Wasootch Tower. "[The victim] came to rest where we could just manage to get into him with the sling setup. It was tight." The other thing Dave remembers was the injury the fellow had, which was something he would see again. It was a compound fracture of the ankle received from hitting the ground more than once on the way down, feet first. Dave remembers that the man's companions had the presence of mind to stop the bleeding and put a makeshift splint to stabilize him.

Dave relaxed once he realized the man was not dying. As he puts it, "The environment you're in, the machine, the noise and trying to keep the whole thing safe, and landing where you haven't had a chance to warm up in a normal fashion in getting up to that type of terrain or incline. It all

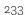

233

adds up. All of a sudden you're just there. So you have to do some quick adjustments. I felt trying to keep a level head and make sure that all the details are being looked after requires you to really have to focus when the adrenaline is flowing like that."

Water rescues were also interesting. He recalls an amusing incident that happened on an island in the middle of the Sheep River when a raft overturned. It was late in the day, and the river was still rising from the afternoon snow melt. There was little left of the island besides a few scraggly willows where the woman was stranded—but she was wearing a wet suit. Dave recalls being slung on to this "soggy little thing" and getting the woman into the sling harness. Just as they were ready to clip onto the rescue sling, she looks at him and said, "How much is this going to cost?" He was astonished and didn't know what to say to her, so he joked, "Well do you have your credit card with you?" She didn't think that was very funny at all. Later he wondered if she had seriously considered staying there because there might be a cost.

BEFORE KANANASKIS COUNTRY rangers were handed the mandate for public safety and emergency response in the park, other organizations had been responsible for rescue in the foothills. One of them was the Alberta Forest Service who, in some ways, resented the intrusion of a new rescue unit. Another was Alberta Fish and Wildlife. They had their own people who had handled emergency responses in the past and who now had their "noses out of joint." But Forestry was still an essential resource for Kananaskis, and Lloyd Gallagher was careful to avoid antagonizing easily bruised egos. Dave Smith reflects: "Lloyd was better at it than I was when it came to diplomatic skills, and we worked hard to break the ice with the Forestry people and with Fish and Wildlife."

The search for two girls lost in the Sheep River country was a good example. The Forestry Service was called out for the search, but they did not bring in the rangers until they came up empty-handed three days later. Smith found it to be quite

a delicate situation to step into. It took a while to establish who was in charge of the search while quietly slipping into the hierarchy.

He tried to review the information they had accumulated during the search without appearing critical of their efforts. He didn't particularly like what he found. As he describes it: "There's a family with two missing girls here and these guys are writing them all off as dead, and I thought this can't necessarily be the fact. It's too early in the game to be pessimistic. They are well equipped. They have camping supplies like tents and sleeping bags. We hadn't covered all the ground yet. It's day three and we've just arrived, so I asked them if I could go up [in the helicopter] and familiarize myself, and I had a hunch as to where and what area they were likely to be in, but I didn't know that yet, because I was still scratching my head trying to figure this puzzle out and not step on toes and yet get something done."

He wanted people to be spotted around the country at night to look for campfires, but the forestry personnel resisted the idea. He adds, "We had some parents who by day three, are just frantic. They are pacing back and forth, not sleeping, not eating, just filled with anxiety, and these guys are talking about the girls managing to hike out, of hitchhiking back and being picked up by a serial killer. Or they were stomped to death by a moose. All these scenarios of disasters, and I'm saying statistically it's not likely."

Finally, on an aerial survey by helicopter, Smith spotted their tent, and the search ended successfully. The girls were members of the Girl Guides, and as Smith knew, "They're trained to stay put and wait to be found and that's what they did." He was using tools that search management courses had given him.

At the end of the 1982 season, Smith quit to take on a contract with B.C. Parks in the new Valhalla Provincial Park. His kids were now school aged and he wanted to live in one place, so he returned to Rossland year round and eventually got a permanent job in the avalanche control program with

B.C. Highways. It wasn't an easy decision to leave Kananaskis Country, but he took with him some lasting experiences. "The experiences I picked up in Kananaskis carried on in other aspects of my career down the road. In B.C. they have the PEP program with lots of volunteers and there's some stiff egos there. You also run into some dedicated and capable people. I think it's a mindset. Some people haven't got their feet wet totally with this rescue business, and they don't see how demanding it can be or risky, and how depressing it can be at times. Initially they have this heroic vision of themselves, and it informs everything they do and it's awful. This is not what this is all about. It's not about them. There is almost an aura of fanaticism about rescue out there. It's almost like they live and breathe it every day. They seem to feed on disaster. On the other hand, on the good side of it, there are people who stop what they're doing and head out and deal with some things that are rather grisly and it might affect them for the rest of their lives—the things they see and the things they have dealt with, mainly fatalities. This is a lot to ask of anybody. Now maybe they didn't plan on that happening but you definitely see a change in a person's attitude once they have gone through a recovery." He concludes, "The rescue world is full of egos and egotists. You sometimes run into people who you wonder why they're even there. Lloyd is so good at doing the job but not having the big ego that goes along with it. It was quite the honour to work for him."

ONE OF THE MOST FRUSTRATING THINGS for Lloyd in the early years of running Kananaskis Country was not having the funding to hire a person in a full-time backup position. If Lloyd had been able to hire him full time, Dave is sure he would have stayed in Canmore. As it was, Dave covered for Lloyd when he was away on expeditions leading up to and including the Canadian Everest Expedition in 1982.

When Gallagher came back from that trip, he knew he had to hire a successor for the field.

By then the program had grown enough for him to split his duties. With more of his time taken up with administration, he could justify hiring someone to run the field operation. The administrative duties now brought him into the political arena. New ministers would often not see the benefit of or the program and the associated costs. This was complicated by a constant change of managers. But he was also not happy, finding he consumed more and more time dealing with fire departments, ambulance services, disaster plans, volunteer search-and-rescue groups and administration. He realized it was important to find someone who could do the field work and also help out with the administration as well.

Gallagher was called on to be an examiner on many of the yearly ACMG courses. He had noticed one man who seemed to fit what he was looking for. George Field was a level four ski instructor who had a lot of experience teaching. He was currently working his way through the gamut of guide exams to become a full guide. In the public safety program in Kananaskis, it was just as important to be a teacher as a guide, and it was this ability in George that caught Lloyd's attention. Field was hired in the spring of 1982 in a summer seasonal capacity, but this was upgraded to a full-time position with the dramatic increase in accidents soon after.

Field soon realized that on-the-job training alone was not enough to keep him fit mentally or physically for the work. He says: "There was no way any of them could keep up their skills and fitness without doing a lot of it on their own time. It was absolutely critical to any success in the future. It was a commitment and passion for a lifestyle you loved that kept you motivated through the rough going. It also allowed empathy for those who had accidents in the mountains because of minor changes in circumstance that they were not afforded but that you were. All of it couldn't be built within the framework of training alone; that feel or touch that allows you to understand how a rescue should be performed or go. Those that expect it through on-the-job training alone never rise very far above the basic level. What makes good rescue leaders, like in any other field of endeavour, is your own personal interest and passion."

What Field remembers best about starting the job was Gallagher telling him: "What I want you to do this summer is go out and hike all the trails with as many staff members as you can, and I'll see you in the fall." Field says, "It was Lloyd's philosophy that the best way to supervise people was to give them the freedom to do the job. He would give you direction and then you were on your own to solve the problem or come up with new ideas to use in the training program. It was great to have a job where you could be innovative and just go ahead and do the things needed to solve a situation." But, "Lloyd never treated me as an underling, he treated me as an equal on all of the rescues." Field's philosophy has been the same with Burke Duncan, his understudy. If he's away, Burke has complete control. As Field puts it, "We don't work on a hierarchal system, we work on a partnership that hopefully is conducive to having a happy end result for all our training and emergency missions."

After that first summer though, Gallagher started getting him involved in the dreaded paperwork. It was done slowly and incrementally, but enough to prepare George for the job after Gallagher retired.

Gallagher also had other rangers who showed promise in the rescue business. Burke Duncan was one who stayed; another was Rupert Wedgwood, newly arrived from Antarctica. During this period they spent much of their free time training together. Burke eventually became Field's right-hand man when Gallagher retired. Wedgwood moved on to the Warden Service in Jasper and then Banff and is currently the public safety specialist in Jasper National Park.

Another promising ranger at the time was Dave Smith (unrelated to the Dave Smith of Rossland) who also moved on to work in Jasper National Park in the public safety field. He worked

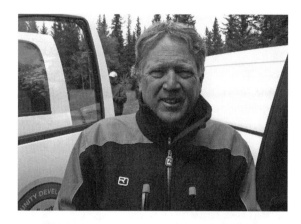

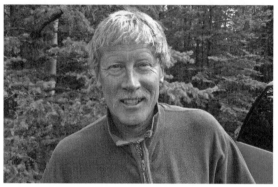

George Field (top) and Burke Duncan (bottom). GEORGE FIELD COLLECTION

in Kananaskis Country for nine years in the late 1970s and early eighties and remembers it as an interesting time of growth.

Dave's earliest recollections are of rescues on Yamnuska he was called to as a seasonal ranger assigned to Bow Valley Provincial Park. One early rescue he remembers vividly is flying with Lance Cooper and fellow ranger Mike O'Riley to the top of the mountain late in the day. It was early in Cooper's flying career, and it was completely dark when he headed back to Canmore. They were there for a young woman who had taken a leader fall near the top of one of the many challenging routes. She was in serious condition, having broken her ankle and a few ribs. With nothing but a large juniper bush for an anchor, Dave lowered O'Riley down the face to the girl. He set up a 3 to 1 raising system and soon had them both off the face. Once on top they gave her first aid, made her comfortable, and tried to keep her warm throughout the long night. At first light they heard the reassuring sound of Cooper's helicopter coming up the valley from Canmore to take them all home. The success more than justified the time they dedicated to extracurricular training.

Smith remembers another rescue on Yam later that summer that involved two inexperienced young men trying to scale the Grillmair Chimney route. It was the first year that the University of Calgary had a climbing wall where the two fellows had taken a one-day climbing course in preparation. According to Smith, "They got halfway up and then got scared. They couldn't go up or down so they stayed right there and waited for a rescue." Alex Baradoy was the public safety ranger at Bow Valley at the time, and he and Smith slung in to a nearby ledge. From there they traversed over to the stranded climbers. Smith remembers one of them used a carpenter's hammer in place of a piton hammer and the other guy had a cycling helmet for a climbing helmet. After lowering them to the base of the climb, Smith recalls, "We charged them—it was Lloyd's call. It was one of the few times he ever did that. Whether they got the money from them was anyone's guess. After that there was a huge outcry from everyone saying we shouldn't be charging people for rescues. But these guys needed to get the message."

Another dramatic rescue involved one of the longest cable rescues done at the time. Smith remembers lowering George Field to the injured party while Gallagher supervised. The accident occurred near the Red Shirt Route, one of the longer routes on the mountain. "The lower was straight vertical, almost 450 metres and they had to put extra cable on. It went smoothly because we used rollers and Teflon pads at the top and the cable never touched the rock after that, it was so steep." After the airy descent, they got the injured party to the base of the climb and carried him the rest of the way by wheeled stretcher. The man

lived to climb again after reaching the ambulance safely at 2:00 a.m.

The rangers calculated there have been on average one-and-a-half rescues per year on Yamnuska since the sixties. Because of Yam's vertical nature, the rangers usually used a rope system to get victims to a spot from which they could be slung off. They did manage some direct sling rescues in less steep locations, but they needed a very confident pilot (like Lance Cooper or Paul Kendall) for this close work. Only if the accident occurred near the top would they consider raising the person up and flying them off from there.

If rescues were in difficult terrain, and manpower at issue, they would ask Banff National Park wardens or ACMG for help, but not volunteers. Over the years, they used several guides to help out. Field says, "Some of them [were] on the route next to the accident and called us and said: 'Hey! We're here so we will do what we can.' Often by the time the rangers have got there, the guides have already brought the people to the scree slope from where they can be slung off if injured. Sometimes the guides are in the parking lot gearing up for a climb when the rangers arrive. George is quick to respond to an offer of help … they're up to date on the standard rope rescue systems so it works well."

The summer of 1986 was incredibly busy for both Kananaskis Country and the national parks. Not only did highway traffic accidents increase dramatically along the Trans-Canada Highway as a result of people driving to Vancouver for Expo 86, but also the wardens were kept hopping with big rescues. For the rangers in Kananaskis Country it was a summer defined by major searches that left emotional scars and made clear the need for sophisticated stress debriefing. Lloyd was actually a pioneer in recognizing the importance of dealing with cumulative stress and the impact it has on families.

It started on June fifth when a small plane lifted off from the Springbank Airport with the pilot and an Alberta government biologist to do a game survey for bighorn sheep and cougar. When they failed to return by 3:00 p.m. the military was notified; they immediately sent aircraft out but failed to pick up the plane's emergency locator beacon. In the meantime, friends of the two missing men began their own search by plane, leaving the Calgary International Airport at 4:40 p.m. They were never heard from again.

The operation now took on epic proportions when 19 aircraft joined the search. A team of 30 military personnel flew in from CFB Namao Airport just north of Edmonton to oversee the air search. They based their operation out of the old McCall Field, adjacent to the international airport in Calgary.

Lloyd Gallagher was contacted in Kananaskis Country to organize and direct ground searching in the area. It was a huge area to cover and he called in everyone—rangers, park employees, park wardens, volunteer search-and-rescue groups and members of the old disbanded Calgary Mountain Rescue Group. Hundreds of people showed up, many not used to rugged terrain but willing to help, either as spotters in aircraft or as searchers on the ground. Those with limited travel skills were teamed with more experienced individuals who dragged them over ridges and peaks looking for anything unusual.

It was actually the ground searchers who found the first missing plane. Dave Smith recalls: "My task was to walk Mt. Allen from Ribbon Creek to Dead Man's Flats on the Trans-Canada Highway. The fellow with me was really slow, so I decided to go down into the valley bottom. We glissaded down on our feet, and when I got to the bottom I stopped and looked back up for the volunteer, and suddenly 15 feet away I spotted an airplane tire." Sure enough aircraft debris and body parts lay scattered about. It was the third day of the search, and the first plane to be found was the one flown by the volunteers who had gone looking for the missing friends.

An unrelated plane crash on the west coast of British Columbia acted as a catalyst to find the missing men as soon as possible. The B.C. men had actually survived the crash but succumbed to their injuries after struggling through the thick bush. The fact that they had not died on impact gave everyone renewed hope that the missing men might be similarly fortunate.

Meanwhile the rangers first had to bring the bodies out from the remote crash site. Jeff Palmer, one of the rescue pilots regularly used by both Kananaskis and Banff, observed, "It looked like the plane had sheared off the peak [Mt. Lougheed] and then blew over the top into a steep long freefall. It was a real mess." Rangers had to climb up above the site and lower themselves into some very tight places to complete the recovery.

By Thursday, June 12, 350 people were taking part in the most intense phase of the eight-day search. With the army now involved as ground searchers, just assigning people to new search areas was a monumental task. The media attention was intense, making it difficult for Major Mike Barbeau, the search master, and Lloyd Gallagher, the ground search leader, to keep abreast of developments. And of course, the two men had to coordinate efforts between them. As George Field later recalled, "You put an extravagant outfit like the military together with a cost-conscious outfit like Kananaskis Country and you have a definite difference in attitude and style." He goes on to say, "It was an incredibly huge search. We had 300 volunteers in front of the emergency centre in Calgary who just wanted to come out and help, and we didn't know what their abilities were. I had done lots of smaller searches with groups of people and that wasn't a problem, but this opened up a whole new search management arena for many of us in the business. We were going, Holy Mackerel, this is a big one. Then before it was over another aircraft went down."

The day after the men were found beneath Mt. Lougheed, the air search was called off because of high winds. When the winds calmed the day after, Major Barbeau addressed the media saying, "I have a good feeling. There are a lot of people out and the weather is good." The fateful words were spoken too soon. A military Twin Otter with three airmen and five volunteers from the Civil Air Rescue Emergency Services (CARES) went down near the top of Cox Hill in the foothills. Soldiers searching nearby had no problem finding the wreckage.

One of the first soldiers on scene was quoted by the media as saying: "When I arrived, the plane was just a great ball of flame and debris scattered all over the place. To me it seemed the plane had tried to turn between three mountains and just hit the top of one of them." Someone had managed to survive the crash and subsequent explosion. "He was the only one who suffered. You could see the marks where he tried to drag himself out of the burning plane." The soldier then said. "How many more people have to die before the search is called off?"

According to the *Calgary Herald*, it was a stunned and very weary Armed Forces spokesman, Major Wally West, who broke the news to the reporters. "There were no survivors." It was the members of CARES who were stunned and horrified the most by the crash, but they vowed to continue the search. It was also the first time in their 10-year history that they had lost a worker. Suddenly they had lost five.

Fortunately, two days later the first missing aircraft was found. It had just been a routine work day for pilot Jim Lapinski as he flew a small Initial Attack fire crew to their work site. Thirteen days after the first plane went missing Lapinski finally spotted it. Jim Davies flew RCMP constable Jim Krug and public safety specialist George Field to the site. Now they understood why it had taken so long to find the missing plane below Mt. Kidd. Later Field and the coroner would have to rappel 45 metres down a cliff to get to the site, and everything would have to be airlifted out. One of the largest air searches was over, after an appalling toll of 13 deaths. The standard search procedure used successfully by the military on flat ground in the north or in prairie regions was definitely not as effective when employed in the

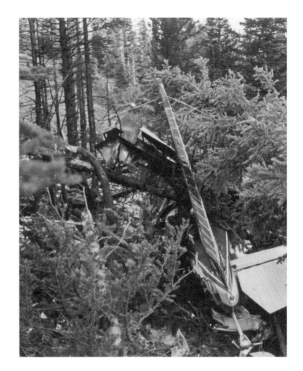

Downed plane rescue in Kananaskis. KANANASKIS COUNTRY PUBLIC SAFETY ARCHIVES

mountains. Two of the crash sites were located by ground searchers, and only one was found from the air by a pilot on a routine mission. Ground searching using professionals and volunteers, in the end, was the most effective tool used. But the summer was not yet over for the park rangers.

Immediately on the heels of the plane disasters, the rangers were called out to search for two missing children. Though it was a search that resulted from a homicide, it brought to light many important issues that aided in future searches. It also added to the cumulative stress individuals were dealing with, lending greater credence for critical incident stress debriefing. The Dolejs case haunts dog handlers, ground searchers, park rangers and RCMP members even to this day for the diabolical nature of the crime and how it unfolded.

Dolejs was estranged from his wife and two kids after going through a messy divorce. But he still had partial custody of his children, and he

239

arranged to take them fishing for the day. When he did not return that evening, the frantic wife notified the authorities, sparking the second largest search that summer for Lloyd Gallagher and his Kananaskis rangers. Dolejs was found minus the children at his vehicle in the McLean Creek area west of Bragg Creek shortly thereafter.

Despite intense interrogation sessions, Dolejs said nothing, and a massive search effort was launched to find them. Two Parks Canada dog handlers were called in to assist Gary McCormick the RCMP dog handler from Cochrane. It was a large search and the three dogs had no end of territory to cover. Again the main effort for the ground searching came from the rangers, but there were many volunteers and RCMP members involved as well. As one of the Parks Canada dog handlers pointed out, "There was an urgency about it. We felt we needed to find the children before they both expired from the elements or starvation, maybe animals or dehydration. It was all so immediate, and yet in the back of your mind you were saying, 'He's done them in.'"

The RCMP questioned Dolejs over the next few days, trying to get some idea of where to look for the children. Though Dolejs finally admitted killing them, it was a year and a half before the bodies were found in shallow graves. Until then, the dog handlers and searchers were left with a sense of not having done enough to find the children. As one of them pointed out, "We knew that when and if the bodies were found, we would all have some concern about where that was … and we hoped they wouldn't be found in our search area." In the end it was tragic for all who took part. It involved two small children and a mother left with guilt and grief. Dolejs only gave up the secret on the condition he be moved from where he was imprisoned, because he was getting beaten up regularly by the other inmates.

Shortly after the Dolejs case, one of the park rangers from Kananaskis Country went missing from the Lake Minnewanka area in Banff park. A brief search turned up a dinghy in the lake with its skin punctured by what looked like a knife. His body was never found, leaving a troubling end to a difficult summer.

Gallagher felt no doubt that his staff had started to feel the effects of dealing with so much trauma after this hard summer. He was already holding critiques after each rescue, but now he began to think about bringing professional people in for critical stress debriefing. As he put it, "We put ourselves through things like picking up parts of bodies or young children who are hurt and that is something above and beyond what the average person would do. We all need support for that, and if we don't get it we end up carrying this baggage around in our minds forever and it affects our families, our marriages, our home life and our friends around us." But first, Gallagher did his own research. He talked to people such as the Calgary Fire Department with similar stress situations. "We set up a network of key people [who] got to know the type of work the rangers were doing … In this way they could actually do a better job debriefing the group." Gallagher was well ahead of his counterparts in the more conservative Parks Canada.

He realized that many psychologists had no understanding of public safety or of the stress incurred in mountain rescue. Finally he found a couple of people who were doing this type of debriefing full-time for the Alberta government. He regularly invited them to rescue debriefings to let them see what the team dealt with and at the same time let the team get comfortable talking about issues that bothered them.

George Field had certainly felt the effects of the searches that fateful summer. As he put it, "That summer was exceedingly difficult for me. Thirteen bodies in the air crashes, and a staff member had gone missing, and it's assumed he might have committed suicide in Lake Minnewanka, the Dolejs kids … " Gallagher took notice and suggested he take a couple of weeks off. Field reflected, "I took two weeks off and sort of talked to myself and got myself organized. In the middle of the two weeks I was walking across the street in downtown Canmore and got to the centre line and looked up and saw the Three Sisters [a mountain with three peaks that overlooks the town] and the beautiful sunlight and just stood there in the middle of the street, and all the weight came off my shoulders then. I took the other week off and got myself organized and back on the job again. That was early in my career."

Burke Duncan also appreciated Lloyd's efforts to help those who needed it. "Lloyd instigated an in-house program. We put money aside, and we still do, to get psychological help outside the government system. If the government takes too long to get involved, we'll go to the private psychologists and have them do an immediate evaluation of things should someone desire help … It affects their sleep. It affects the way they work and it's something you have to deal with." He goes on to say, "We do make a difference, and if you let these things undermine your ability to do the job, you alone will be the loser.

Gallagher has a very human approach to things; he is extremely personable and that allows people to readily communicate their concerns. Soon he found that wives, girlfriends and families of the staff felt comfortable opening up to him. This was fine by him, as he considered all these people to be part of a larger family. He also felt it was important to foster social contact amongst the group to develop a bond of reliance and compatibility needed on dangerous and difficult jobs. When the search or the rescue or the recovery was over, Gallagher not only thanked the rangers but also their wives, families and girlfriends. Lloyd also realized how critical families were in recognizing stress and in dealing with it. For this reason, families were always considered in debriefing situations and in the healing process. It would be almost 12 years before Parks Canada adopted this practice.

THE FOLLOWING WINTER the rangers were rewarded with the successful recovery of an avalanche victim on Mt. Joffre, south of South Kananaskis Pass. The two men from Calgary had left from Kananaskis Lakes on March 29, 1987, intending to climb the north face of Mt. Joffre. Though they did a cursory check of the snowpack, they failed to get a current avalanche update from the rangers. If they had done so they would have found out that the avalanche hazard was high, which might have deterred them. They eventually reached a wind-scoured slope above treeline, where they stopped to test the snowpack again with their ski poles. Below them was a series of rock ledges culminating in a cliff almost 40 metres high. As reported in the *Calgary Herald*, the two men decided to ski across the slope one at a time. Only two metres from the safety of the rocks on the far side, the slope broke. The lead man felt the snow slab push against his ankles then he saw a fracture above him. At that point he yelled "Avalanche" to his partner who had just started to cross the slope. The wall of snow hit the second man, knocking him to his knees, but he managed to scramble to the safety of the rocks.

When the avalanche hit the victim, he dove into the snow head first. He reasoned this would put him in a better position to grab a rock or tree and pull himself out of harm's way. It was the wrong move, for as he bounced over a ledge headfirst, his face was slammed into the rocks. His jaw and nose were shattered, and several teeth were knocked out. The impact flipped him onto his back, leaving him speeding downhill head first when he became airborne. He landed on his back cushioned by his backpack only to be swamped by the avalanching snow. Backstroking wildly to try to keep near the surface, he yelled and spit to keep his airways clear. When he came to rest in the fast-setting snow, only his head and arm were free. His partner viewed it all from above and was convinced his friend was dead.

Though it looked bad, he found his friend alive but covered in blood and sporting two badly sprained ankles. Unable to travel, the victim had no choice but to wait for his partner to bring help. Amazingly the rangers arrived in only three hours.

They had grabbed their first party packs and skis, notifying Alpine Helicopters in Canmore, and were soon on their way. The survivor had provided them with an accurate description of where to go, and they had reasonable weather. The two men did a number of things correctly, and they had luck on their side, but more important, there was a professional organization in place to respond quickly. Not all accidents turn out as well.

The autumn of 1988 wrapped up with another downed aircraft in Kananaskis Country. The aircraft had filed a flight plan from Calgary to Fairmont in British Columbia, which took them over the middle of the Kananaskis area. When the plane failed to reach Fairmont, the military were automatically called in to conduct the search, as downed aircraft fall under their mandate. Much like the RCMP, they are structured with a rigid chain of command and are at times reluctant to turn to outside help. They didn't notify the Kananaskis Country rangers for two days. When they were finally contacted, the rangers quickly found the aircraft using a ground search. They were helped in this case by two Calgarians out on a multi-day horseback trip. The riders saw a fire in the area where the plane went down and notified the park. They also noticed a concentration of aircraft that seemed to be searching for something. Also, a hiker came forward to tell the rangers that he had seen an aircraft flying around Tombstone Mountain on the day it went missing. The rangers concentrated on this location, and four hours after leaving the highway by horseback they found the wreckage at treeline on nearby Elpoca Mountain. During the search, the military had up to 11 aircraft involved plus a civilian volunteer group of 50 to 60 ground searchers who did not know the country as well as the rangers did. Kananaskis Country alone covers over 4,000 square kilometres, a fact which Gallagher pointed out in a Draft News Release following the search.

Lloyd was upset that Kananaskis Country had been overlooked in the early phase of the search and was quick to point out that "Early notification of an air search would allow ground personnel to start gathering vital information which would aid the air searches. A communications centre can be established, patrols started in high probability areas, local helicopter companies can be contacted about sightings or Emergency Locator Transmitter signals, interviews can be carried out with visitors and other government agencies about sightings, vehicle licence numbers in parking lots can be recorded to make contacts about possible sightings. All of this could be done without in any way taking responsibility away from the Department of National Defence for the search or its coordination."

Gallagher went on to express concern about the 44 hours which had elapsed before Kananaskis Country ground personnel were asked to join the search. According to the Calgary Herald, a military spokesperson defended the department's decision. "The general rule of thumb is you exhaust your air search capacity first before opening an unknown area to hundreds of people to aimlessly conduct a ground search."

However, it led to some positive action. A memorandum of understanding was produced for future air searches that occurred in Kananaskis Country. Overall authority of the search, both ground and air, would be with the Department of National Defence, while Kananaskis Country's expertise in ground searching would be fully utilized and under their own direction.

THE BANFF WARDENS had watched Kananaskis Country develop into a first-class professional rescue service from its inception in the early eighties. By the beginning of the 1990s the rangers felt they were drawing abreast of their neighbouring counterparts. George Field feels comfortable reflecting that: "Well, the little brother down the road is slowly growing up." He goes on to say, "I think over time we have established ourselves as an equal rescue group between us ... it takes a long time to convince a warden that we are as good as they are, because they have a long history of it and rightfully so."

By 1990, the year of the Healy Creek avalanche, they had grown up. They were called in by the Banff Warden Service to help in the search, much like the Banff wardens were called in back in 1986 for the downed aircraft search. The Kananaskis rangers came in with a large number of staff and were totally self-contained with their own rescue gear, snowmobiles and proper clothes for the minus 30 degree Celsius weather. Dale Portman vividly recalls their distinctive presence saying, "It was the first time I'd seen them in their new protective clothing. They had really well-fashioned yellow anoraks with flashes and stylish ski pants, and they looked pretty spiffy in their uniform. I remember Bruno Engler being there taking pictures and saying, 'Boy those guys look good, I'm going to take their picture ... How come you guys don't have outfits like that?'"

For the Banff rescue leader it was relatively easy to integrate them into the overall search, because the two organizations had worked together in the past. But as Field pointed out, it was more than that. "It had a lot to do with the guides' association where the basic training is similar between the two staff ... In Kananaskis Country we base our climbing and all our rope work upon the guide standards, which is what the wardens do as well. We use the same organized rope systems. We use the same helicopter sling rescue system. So all things being equal, even though we don't train much together, our background, philosophies and where we're going is very similar. We have meetings when techniques change so we know what the other guy is doing."

They needed this vote of confidence, because 1991 proved to be a busy year for Kananaskis Country. It started with a mid-winter avalanche at Rummel Lake. Two men following ski tracks put in place earlier in the day crossed high up on a basin north of the lake and were caught in a large class three avalanche. A party of four down in the valley witnessed the event. They too had momentarily considered skiing the slope, but had decided against it. Instead they watched the

two skiers get carried through a small clump of trees. One of the skiers managed to stay on the surface, but the other was carried into a gully where he was completely buried. The observing group below was now only 200 metres from the deposit and quickly went to their aid. The wife of the victim, travelling 30 minutes behind, joined in the search. Neither men were carrying rescue transceivers otherwise the victim would have been found within five minutes.

As one of the rescuers put it later, "We just shook our heads when we saw those skiers out there. It was really crazy. I'd pulled my camera out and was going to take a picture to show people what not to do." Then the avalanche occurred. After a hasty search for the buried man, one of the rescuers skied out to report the accident. In the meantime the rest continued to probe. A helicopter was dispatched immediately with a first party on board and Ward and Smoky on the way. In all 40 people were involved with the search. Two hours after the avalanche happened, the victim was found buried under 50 centimetres of snow. There was no evidence of a struggle and there was no ice mask around the victim's mouth. He most likely was knocked unconscious on the way down and succumbed rather quickly with snow blocking his airway.

Shortly after this accident, four men stopped their truck in an avalanche area not far from a sign that warned people not to stop. They were outside the vehicle when they heard the roar of the avalanche. They sprinted for their lives, leaving the truck idling in the middle of the road. Once clear of the path, they looked back to see their truck disappear in a wall of billowing snow. They made the front page of the local newspaper the next day and, after assessing the damage to their buried truck, probably reflected on how lucky they were to be alive.

That same day a hunter and his dog went missing in the Ware Creek area near Turner Valley. On February 9, his vehicle was spotted parked near the area by a rancher who was checking on

243

his cattle. He reported to the RCMP in Turner Valley, and they started to investigate. They ran the plates and found that the last contact the registered owner had with friends and co-workers was on February 4. No one knew he planned an extended mid-winter stay in the Ware Creek area. Although a cougar study team remembered seeing his vehicle parked there February 5, it wasn't until February 11 that the RCMP actively started looking for him. By then, he had been missing for 5 days. They made preliminary search flights over the area, but when they failed to turn up anything, they notified the Kananaskis Country rangers. In the meantime some of the missing man's friends started searching for him.

Things were pretty muddy for ranger Dave Hanna when he took over the operation on February 12. Now eight days had transpired since the man was last heard from, and the area was badly contaminated. The missing person's friends, who had mounted their own search, left cigarette butts, candy wrappers and footprints throughout the snow-covered heavily timbered area. When trained rangers finally tried to sort things out, everything they found was eventually traced back to the missing person's friends. Search dogs were brought in on the initial stage of the search but had no success in finding the man's track. All they could do was send in teams to randomly search trails and cutlines. The 32-square-kilometre area was then divided into several segments and each segment was carefully grid-searched by experienced searchers using map and compass.

All of this was helped along by a software program that Doug Hanna had designed to establish the probabilities and percentages of success. Grid searching, which requires individuals to be carefully spaced over an area, involved considerable manpower and time. Using factors such as type of terrain, steepness, cover and the number of searchers, Doug was able to calculate the possibility of detecting a missing person in any segment covered. He stated as an example that it took nine people eight hours to search a square kilometre

to arrive at a 50 percent probability of detection. But in the end, the only thing they found that belonged to the missing person was a hunting arrow embedded in a tree. It was broken and badly weathered. The arrowhead was marked with his wildlife certificate number, and it turned out to be an arrow he had used in some earlier fall hunting excursion. Aside from the vehicle and the arrow, no one turned up any evidence that the man or his dog had ever been there. To this date, neither man nor dog has been found.

While this was going on, a skier went missing for three days and was finally spotted from the air when he signalled the helicopter using a flare. When he had left the Burstall Pass trailhead Sunday morning, he had no plans to spend any nights out. After skiing up onto the French Glacier and then over onto the Haig Glacier, he became disorientated, made a wrong turn and skied down into the creek drainage that wandered into the wilds of B.C. His trials were further complicated when he broke a ski binding. He stopped to make the necessary repairs, then settled under a big spruce tree for his first night out. Fortunately he had brought along a light sleeping bag, and that night he stayed relatively dry.

On the second day he tried to retrace his route by following his old ski tracks back up onto the glacier but soon found them obliterated by wind and snow. That night he dug out a snow cave below a big rock and put in a long, very uncomfortable night in a sleeping bag that was now wet. When morning came he was not only cold but damp. He had packed trail mix, beef jerky and crackers, so he had food which he carefully rationed. By now he knew without a doubt that he was lost. Drinking water became a problem without a stove, because as soon as he built a fire, it would smoulder out as it melted down into the 1.5 metre snowpack. He had brought a map of the area, but without a compass he was still confused as to where he was. When he hadn't returned from the weekend outing on Tuesday morning, his sister reported him missing. His vehicle was located by the rangers at the trailhead, and because it was parked there, they felt he was camped close by. When they investigated further, they found a guidebook inside the vehicle with a pack of matches marking the description for the French Glacier area. Soon they were in a helicopter and in the air. They followed his route over from the French onto the Haig Glacier where they spotted a flare.

He had shot a flare on Sunday when he heard a light plane fly over but nothing came of it. When the helicopter flew by on Tuesday, he felt unbelievably fortunate, because the rescuers spotted the last flare he had. His only injuries were some frostbitten toes. More important, he had learned a couple of big lessons: Don't ski alone and always let someone know your plans. He was pleased, though, that he went out for the day relatively prepared and did all the right things once he got lost.

The 1992 season started dramatically in early May when rescuers from several locations scrambled to get to the top of Yamnuska before dark after being called out for an accident on Red Shirt. The climber was only 30 metres from the top, leading out on the eighth and final pitch when he disappeared from sight. His three climbing buddies thought nothing of it until they suddenly heard a scream. As one of them put it, "I heard him scream and it actually sounded almost comical at first, like he was fooling around. Then it began to sound more desperate … he had lots of time to scream." They watched as he appeared above them, smashing into the rock face as he fell. He pulled three piton placements out, but the fourth piton, the one above the belay station occupied by his climbing partner held. His belayer held him and stopped the fall. But in the sudden arrest, the leader pendulumed against the rock face, breaking his right wrist, ripping his right ear off and smashing the back of his skull.

The eerie silence that followed left the two climbers above wondering what had occurred. When they heard the sound of gurgled breathing they knew. They found the victim dangling from the rope, barely conscious and incoherent. There was little the rope team could do but secure him to the belay ledge and climb out for help. His partner stayed there to help if the man regained consciousness.

They didn't know that two hikers had witnessed the dramatic fall and called for help on a programmable radio they carried. Lloyd Gallagher immediately had Lance Cooper on the radio. Cooper had just finished a rescue at Lake Louise and fortuitously had Gord Irwin and Mark Ledwidge on board when he rerouted for the mountain. Tim Auger got the call at home in Canmore and jumped in his own vehicle. Altogether nine other rangers were dispatched to the scene. The two climbers who had just completed their route were also recruited. They met at the base of the mountain and at 9:25 p.m. Cooper lifted off with three rescuers for the top. He returned for four more, and on his final flight bordering on darkness, he slung up a load of rescue gear and equipment. With that he headed back to Canmore.

In total darkness, with only the beams of their headlamps dancing about, the team of rangers, guides and park wardens set up the anchors to lower Jock Richardson to the injured party. By now the victim was in and out of consciousness and suffering from hypothermia. Richardson secured the victim on his back, piggy-back fashion and the crew at the top brought them up. Amazingly, only four hours after his fall, both men were off the face and on the summit. But it wasn't over yet.

At the top, the team determined that the victim's head injuries were so bad that they couldn't chance waiting until morning for the helicopter. Eight men immediately headed up the mountain with a wheeled, detachable stretcher. When three paramedics arrived in the ambulance, they followed behind Gallagher and a few other rangers to meet the party. Up top, the victim was placed on a spine board, which in turn was secured to a sled then carefully moved down the mountain. The injured man was now conscious but wanted to sleep.

Because of the nature of his head injury he was intentionally kept awake by a steady stream of verbal and physical prodding on the way down. The eight rangers met the summit party 500 metres above the staging area and transferred the victim to the wheeled stretcher they had brought.

At 2:00 a.m. they met the paramedics on their way up, who tried to stabilize the victim, now combative, a sure sign that his condition had deteriorated. They also had heat packs to counteract the hypothermia while they continued to progress tediously down the mountain. They reached the ambulance at 4:30 a.m., nine hours after the accident happened and four-and-a-half hours after starting from the top. He was rushed to the Foothills Hospital in Calgary where they successfully reattached his ear. One week later he was released from hospital. As Tim Auger reflected later to the *Calgary Herald*, "What was so interesting about this one was that it was so close to dusk, we really had to scramble to get to the top of the mountain as fast as we could. Cooper did some nice flying."

THE KANANASKIS COUNTRY rangers often travelled to different parts of the province to answer calls for their assistance. Most of these were for missing persons or drownings. On several occasions they teamed up with volunteer groups such as the Turner Valley Search and Rescue or Rocky Mountain House Search and Rescue. One interesting search was for a girl who went missing from the Ram Falls campground, 68 kilometres southwest of Rocky Mountain House. Ram Falls is the major attraction in the area with a campground nearby. A fourteen-year-old girl and her small dog went missing on Tuesday, July 6th, 1993, and by Friday were presumed dead.

It began at 4:30 p.m. when she left her parents' campsite, deciding to take her black poodle Cookie to see the spectacular Ram Falls, only a few hundred metres away. She was following the wrong path, however, and was soon deep in the woods. Though she suspected she was going in the wrong direction, she continued on confused,

hoping the trail would eventually lead back to the falls. She kept on walking until it got dark. Realizing she had to spend the night out, the lightly clad girl settled under some fallen timber, with only her dog for warmth. Throughout the night the poodle never once left her side.

She found a cutline to follow the next morning but now it started to rain. When the cutline led nowhere, she began to seriously look for shelter to survive the second night. With deadfall lying all about, she built the frame for a lean-to and covered it with brush. This was remarkably resourceful, considering she had never camped out before.

Meanwhile a large ground search was underway involving several volunteer groups, the RCMP and Gallagher with his rangers. The search also included three RCMP dog teams. That evening they checked out a trapper's cabin on Lynx Creek, hoping she might have holed up there, but it was empty. The next morning she left her lean-to and continued to search for any sign of habitation through the continuous rain. To her great relief she stumbled upon the Lynx Creek Cabin and its welcome sign. Inside, she found a foam pad and a pillow and some dry instant soup. She shared the dry soup with her steady companion then tried unsuccessfully to build a fire with the wet wood. But despite the lack of fire, she wisely got out of her wet clothes and hung them up to dry in the confines of the cabin.

Back at the campsite, her parents' only consolation was knowing that their daughter was bright, resourceful and level-headed and that her dog was with her. The rescuers kept all the options open, but it became increasingly difficult not to think she had drowned in the falls or the river. By Friday, the search was stepped up when they asked for increased help from the military.

The young girl realized people were searching for her when she heard helicopters overhead, and she decided to remain at the cabin. There were now 150 people out looking for her, but they concentrated on the South Ram River. By mid-Friday, family and searchers who had scoured

35 square kilometres of bush several times, did not think she could survive the steady rain and cool temperatures with no food, shelter or adequate clothing. As experts knew, after 48 hours, missing persons are usually found dead. For the parents it was nearly unbearable. There was also the possibility that it could be an abduction. Throughout the ordeal, the parents could not eat and barely slept, and when they did they were plagued by nightmares.

It was purely by chance that things changed dramatically on that same day. Three horseback riders, totally unconnected to the search team had wandered off their chosen path and were surprised to see the cabin. When one of them whimsically called out: "Is there anybody there?" they were shocked to hear a young girl's voice reply. The child was thrilled to see them. They put the girl, clutching her dog, up on a horse and rode for several kilometres before finally running into a member of the search party. It was an RCMP dog handler who had a radio, and he immediately called for a helicopter. Soon she and the dog were peering out a window, flying over the timber-covered foothills to the hospital in Rocky Mountain House.

To the overwhelming relief of her parents, the girl was in good condition and not even hypothermic. To this she could thank the stalwart dog that never left her side. The media had carried the story of the search for days, and now the girl was greeted by congratulations signs that blossomed everywhere.

BY THE MID-NINETIES, the Kananaskis rangers had developed the same smooth proficiency and professionalism as the Warden Service. Now they encountered a rash of climbing accidents on the mountains behind the town of Canmore. One of the adjustments that rescuers had had to make in this climbing playground was the quick transition from flat ground to steep rock when slung there instantly by helicopter. George Field says, "There's a transition or acclimatization when you're climbing that allows you to adjust to the circumstance. For a guide, slinging under a helicopter can be rather dramatic."

As an example, Field talked about a peaceful day off in Canmore, working inside his garage when he noticed through his open garage door a helicopter flying high up on the east end of Mt. Rundle. He thought something was going on up there; then the phone rang. It was Gallagher saying, "Can you get up here? There's been a climbing accident." Field quickly jumped into his truck and drove to the staging area just as the helicopter returned from the accident site. He had his slinging harness with him, and in a flash he was flying through the sky. It took less than fifteen minutes from the time he left home to be in the middle of a mountain face, on a ledge, dealing with a severely injured climber. The transition had been quite stunning. When he was flying back down, he saw his house nestled in the valley and realized that he had left his garage door open in his haste. All his toys were sitting there, open for anyone to view and possibly steal.

Burke Duncan used another example to make a similar point about leaving the backyard, "hoping in your haste, that you've taken everything you'll need." His example described another accident on the same face. He got slung to the site in failing light. Rangers had gotten two of the climbers off the mountain, but Duncan and the third uninjured climber spent the night out high up on the side of Rundle. "You leave the comfort of the flat terrain and you have to make sure that you have the appropriate equipment along in case something goes wrong or it doesn't work out. Maybe you don't get off that night. You have to have the ability to survive the night and wait for the helicopter in the morning or walk out. Whatever needs to be done."

WHILE THERE WAS PLENTY OF MONEY around in the early years of Kananaskis Country, nearly two decades later all the programs with Alberta's Parks and Recreation were suffering financial strangulation. Though it was nice to have a flagship provincial park, the reality was that it would require major funding down the road to maintain the infrastructure of roads, campgrounds, trails and bridges. The politicians didn't have the vision for this. As well, the staff went through a period when they were hampered by a series of poor ministers. The public safety program survived in spite of the politicians, but it mirrored similar developments in the national parks. For Kananaskis Country had been well funded up until the 1988 Calgary Winter Olympics, but once the events were over, a lot of funding went with it.

Lean years followed, and money for training, staff and equipment began to dry up. One young trainee, Sharon Irwin, recalled that she received some of her best training in public safety during the first year she worked for the Alberta government as a ranger. But that changed well before she left to work for Parks Canada as a park warden. She laughs ruefully, recalling a training day in which "They didn't have enough money for a helicopter so we used one of the fire towers instead. The instructors had a rope set up through a pulley at the top, and the oval ring was lowered down to the rescuer. Then a bunch of guys ran like crazy once you had hooked on and pulled you into the air. I think someone else was standing close by making noises like a helicopter—you know, whop, whop, whop, whop …" It became difficult to hang on to good people, and with limited hiring, the staffing situation began to be problematic. The park was now run by an aging staff due for retirement with few people to replace them.

But like the wardens, the rangers had streamlined into a small response crew that could operate on a smaller budget. Still, they always seemed to get big searches and sometimes water rescues. They certainly showed up for the flooding of the Oldman River in 1995. Nothing showed the Kananaskis Country rangers' versatility better than this near disaster. Duncan and Field had gone down to the Oldman River on three separate occasions to sling people stranded in their homes surrounded by rising water. It was a real eye-opener for the local ranchers and farmers who had never seen a flying circus like this before.

Lance Cooper flew them to many of the houses scattered about with nice white picket fences, but dangerous with telephone wires that had to be avoided. They would sling in and then go inside the house. "And there would be Ma and Pa and a couple of kids." The rescue harnesses were designed for adults so they had to be improvised for the kids. As Field explained, "We put two kids in the rescue bag [Baumann] and then in a scoop stretcher. We thought maybe the two kids would panic, but they had a great time. They thought it was a great ride."

They evacuated people from several houses, but recalls one stubborn fellow who did not want to leave. He was an ostrich farmer and he was going to stay behind. If the farm got swamped or flooded out, he wanted to stay with his ostriches. As Field put it, "He didn't want to go out at all but finally decided his mother should go out and meet his brother who was on dry land. She was about to be picked up when he came outside with a big Solomon [ski] boot bag and said, 'Could she take this out with her?' Inside were six ostrich chicks." In case the farm got inundated, they would be the only animals saved. But at least his mother would have some ostrich chicks, and his brother could continue farming ostriches.

Duncan recalls: "We were totally used to the mountains, and when we got down there we had a whole bunch of urban hazards we had to think about." The first rescue they did was a fellow on a tractor stuck in the middle of the river. The water had come up around him while he was trying to cross. The water was up to the seat, and they plucked him from his perch and dropped him off on shore.

Eavestroughs blown off by the down-wash from the helicopter's rotors were a new concern to them. Duncan notes: "It was totally different for him [the pilot] too. Lance was about as excited as he can get, which isn't a lot." Fortunately everything went well and it was a successful operation.

They got good press coverage from the media, and when floods hit the Calgary area in June of 2005, they were ready to go again. On this occasion they evacuated many people from flooded campsites who wanted to watch the water rise. As one ranger said, "One thing you can't do in the rescue business is protect people from their own stupidity."

Later that summer in September, 1995, they were back to familiar ground with another climbing accident on Yamnuska that, had the weather cooperated, would have been a routine sling operation. The lead climber was on the final pitch of Forbidden Corner and was just about to clip into his protection (piton) when the rock he was standing on broke away under his weight and he fell. He bounced a few times on the way down before the rope came taut and his partner held him. With injuries to his wrist, arm and hip, he was unable to continue. His partner got him onto a nearby ledge and into a large rope bag where they spent the night huddled together. It was a cold night for the month of September, and with precipitation in the form of snow, it was very uncomfortable. Unfortunately, they had signed out to climb the Direttissima route, so the Kananaskis rangers were unsure of where to look first. They were finally able to make voice contact with them, but it wasn't until 4:00 a.m. that they could pinpoint their exact location on the face of the mountain. Field accomplished this by using a megaphone and having the men shout answers down from above.

Field had to call in a team of twenty-five to try and pull off the rescue the next morning, for it was too foggy and snowy for the helicopter to fly. The rescue teams climbed up in groups of four. The first crew carried little, as they quickly moved out to make contact with the stranded climbers. They needed to get there fast, assess their injuries and start warming them up. The second group carried ropes and first-aid equipment. The third brought the stretcher and other gear. The fourth and fifth groups didn't start until later, when it was determined that the helicopter would be grounded because of the weather.

The first party made contact at 9:30 a.m. and determined that only one of the climbers was injured. Anchors were set up on the snow-covered summit and a rescuer was lowered to the stranded party 100 metres below. Eventually both climbers were brought up to share the drafty summit and swirling snow with the rescuers. Considering the two had spent the night out just below the summit in the inclement weather, they were in good shape. As Field put it, "They were very lucky," helped along by the fact they were "very strong and very fit."

All through the day they worked at getting the injured party down under very slippery conditions with the fresh snow. Finally at 5:00 p.m., they got the victim to the hogback where the actual trail started. Just then they had a small break in the weather, and the helicopter managed to get in and sling the person down to the waiting ambulance. It had taken twenty-five men all day and most of the night to get the injured climber off the most difficult part of the mountain and five minutes to get him down the remaining 500 metres. Throughout the rescue there was concern for the freezing conditions they were all working under and the threat of frostbite to both hands and feet. Hands especially because they were handling wet ropes and snow-covered gear, but also feet because they had to stand around a lot while each task slowly and haltingly unfolded.

One of the most dangerous operations during that period was a helicopter sling rescue that involved a woman lost on Fortress Mountain in the cold weather of late October. A woman from Calgary wanted to go for a scramble up on Fortress Mountain and was joined by a lady from Scotland. The Calgarian chose the standard route up the west ridge of the mountain. But when they got to the summit, the clouds closed in and they got lost on the way down. After wandering into steep terrain, the Calgarian slipped and hurt herself badly enough that she could no longer travel. Fortunately they had descended below the worst of the weather, and visibility was better. She marked where she thought they were on a map and sent her companion for help. Unfortunately the woman left without the map.

She reached the car and drove to Canmore but had no idea who to contact. Desperate, she stopped at a video store and just turned to the woman standing next to her and said, "I have a friend that's stuck up on a mountain. Do you know who I should call?" It just so happened that the woman with her husband managed the Assiniboine Lodge, a popular backcountry lodge on the B.C./Alberta border and knew about the resources available for Kananaskis Country. She said, "Yeah, you need to call George Field."

Field soon had a team organized but had no idea where the stranded woman was. With no map, the Scottish lady only had a vague idea of where they had gone. The weather was cold with blowing snow, not unusual for late October. The group searched most of the night, concentrating on the Chester Lake and Headwall Loop areas, which are approaches to the mountain from the west. Spreading out, they hiked along, regularly calling out but getting no reply.

The woman could see some lights dancing in the distance for a while, and then they disappeared. She was looking down into the headwall area as the searchers came up the valley, but they turned around when the snow got too deep. The searchers returned to their vehicles at 3:00 a.m., thinking it didn't look good for the benighted woman. Burke Duncan remembers trying to finally get a drink from his water bottle when they returned to the trailhead and finding it frozen.

In the early morning light Kathy Moore, one of Alpine Helicopter's rescue pilots, arrived. The rescuers put teams out in different locations using the helicopter and continued to search the area. They called in Scott Ward, and had him searching with his dog Data. The winds were now gusting over a hundred kilometres an hour, and it was tricky flying. Field flew with Moore that morning and recounts, "We at times were caught in extreme downdrafts which caused Kathy to have to veer off to maintain her air speed, otherwise we were going to get pushed into the ground. She did an incredible job with the gusts and strong winds lining the helicopter properly … I'm not one to push a pilot, but I said to her, 'You know that col we have to get to is 90 degrees to our left at nine o'clock.' And she very sternly said to me, 'I know that but I need to get facing the wind here.' In other words, 'Don't bother me George, I'm doing my job and I know what I have to do.'" And rightfully so. "It was very, very difficult flying. She did an incredible job of getting our people onto the mountain."

It was now around ten or eleven in the morning; the woman had been out since the previous day. It was a small miracle she was still alive. Fortunately she had a couple of plastic garbage bags with her that she had crawled into for the night. The next morning though, she got out of one of the bags to get a bite to eat, and the wind blew it away. This certainly put her at a disadvantage in dealing with the elements she so far had survived.

Scott Ward was the first to find the woman. He remembers: "I found the victim when I noticed the dog's ears perk up. I glassed the slope below me and saw her sitting there." It was a similar situation to Sam indicating the lost hikers in Jasper a few years earlier. The rescuers were able to fly a team in close to her location. From there they slung in two rescuers with a Baumann Bag, which would completely cover her while she was being flown to the staging area nearby. Burke Duncan flew out with her.

When it was all over, he reflected back on how dangerous the slinging was. "The big thing was the wind; it was extremely windy hanging under the helicopter. She was in a Baumann Bag, and she wasn't very keen on flying out in this manner. I'm quite sure she would rather have been inside the helicopter. I was just trying to reassure and talk to her, so that she knew I was there outside but beside the bag on the flight out. She had to have her face covered because of the wind, so she couldn't see anything which was probably good considering our circumstance. It was tremendously noisy. Every little loose thing that had any slack was flapping and snapping in the wind. Even the taunt straps holding us were hammering and buzzing." The wind got under his coat and then under his pants and eventually it pulled his wind pants down over his harness. He remembers looking down and across the valley at one point and realizing they were hardly moving at all. They just hung there suspended in the wind. It seemed they were fighting for every bit of ground.

Once they got around the corner of the mountain and lower down it got less windy and much quieter, and Duncan got a chance to survey his own situation. For the longest time he wasn't sure whether the ripping noise he was hearing was his warm-up pants or his sling harness. Luckily, it had been his pants that were ripping apart in the wind. It had been a long dangerous flight under the helicopter, but around three o'clock they touched down safely at the hospital landing pad.

Lloyd Gallagher provides some insight in understanding the relationship between the helicopter pilot and the rescuer: "In many of these operations, the trust that builds up between us, being together, training together, working together, responding to rescues together, whether the pilot was Jim Davis, Kathy Moore or Jeff Palmer, we just felt more comfortable with each other. So when we get hooked up [under the helicopter], I know the pilot is the best pilot we've got at this stage of our career. They know I'm not going to do anything crazy with the sling gear and he/she can do the best to put me as close to the patient as possible, under the conditions. And I'm going to do my best to make sure that I don't put him/her into some sort of hazardous scenario. That comes from time together. It comes from time and patience and having respect for each other in our profession."

Helicopter sling rescue capabilities made life much easier for a mountain rescue operation, but they were of small use inside a cave. But cave rescues were something that the Kananaskis rangers found themselves responding to on numerous occasions. Gallagher: "Cave rescue is far more complicated than rock rescue in general.

Everything has to come out of the system. The area you work in is cramped and tight and you can only get one or two people in there to do the pushing and pulling. There's no chance of having eight or ten people to help. It's dark, muddy and the victims usually are hypothermic while your rescuers are slowly getting that way. Overall it's just that much more complicated than anything above ground.

"One that comes to mind is Grotto [Mountain] where the man had a broken back. The rope had broken and the person had slipped down. We ended up having a lot of people in there trying to pull him out, but I remember it being a lot of hard work, a lot of time, a lot of manpower, and it was much more difficult than any climbing rescue that we were ever on." Asked if any cave rescue people were able to lend a hand, he replied, "No! but the Calgary Mountain Rescue Group was very much a part of our initial response back then … When I first came to K-Country, Ken Pawson and all the CMRG was very much a big part of things, and they had conducted many, many rescues before I arrived on the scene."

BANFF AND KANANASKIS COUNTRY share an eastern boundary along three wilderness areas, the White Goat, the Siffleur and the Ghost River

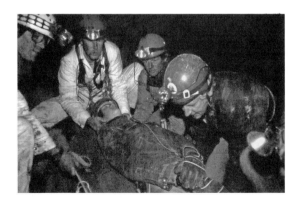

Burke Duncan, George Field and Lloyd Gallagher on cave rescue practice. KANANASKIS COUNTRY PUBLIC SAFETY ARCHIVES

251

where responses to accidents sometimes overlap. The Ghost River Wilderness Area is a good example. It borders on Banff National Park and there have been people, who not knowing where they are, call the Banff Warden Service. Banff in turn will immediately call Kananaskis Country's office in Canmore and ask, "Do you want us to do it or do you want to do it?" As Field points out; "There's no border conflicts because we sat down with the Banff guys, Tim Auger in particular, and if they get a call and come into the Ghost which is our responsibility and they save a life, great. If we get called out because people think they're in the Ghost and it happens to be Banff and we do it, Tim is going to say—Great. It's got nothing to do with borders, it's got to do with saving lives and that's the bottom line." In reality, there is more concern in Banff amongst the public safety wardens over jurisdiction with Jasper National Park than there is with K-Country.

Outside of Kananaskis Country and the Warden Service in the mountain national parks, recognition for what the rangers do can be skimpy even within the Alberta government itself. Some years ago, Gallagher made a video for the National Search & Rescue Secretariat. He later had occasion to talk to the Minister in charge of the program and was shocked to discover the minister knew nothing about the rescue work. One of the reasons for this lack of recognition is that those involved keep a low profile on what they do and sometimes that works to their advantage. In a sense it's easier for them to get the job done. There's no false media hype about individuals being heroes while doing their job. "Its not in our make-up to thump on our chest, or go to the public relations people or show the minister some gross pictures or tell them a story about how we deal with things," says Field. As Duncan further states, "Or maybe we have to be proactive and go to the media and give them the information. That's not really something which we want to do, but maybe it's something we need to do. Let them know that there is a provincial search-and-rescue organization out there doing the equivalent of what the Banff wardens do. Maybe that will help our funding shortfalls. The park wardens have been doing it for twice as long so everybody right away thinks, oh it must have been Banff who did the rescue. It's the same thing with the Starrs Ambulance Service. Starrs is always mentioned as the helicopter that rescues everybody, but outside of the City of Calgary or a highway surface, 99 percent of the time it's Alpine Helicopters that has done all the really hard rescue work, put their neck on the line, trained with us and felt confident with us. The [rescue pilots] at Alpine have done incredible flying to save people's lives and never get mentioned."

In 1997, Lloyd Gallagher retired from his responsibilities with the Alberta government. He passed the torch to George Field, his chosen successor, who had come up through the ranks and been with the outfit nearly as long as Kiwi. Field's challenges today are based on funding and trying to maintain a public safety program and capacity second to none in North America. Burke Duncan, his second in command, carries the technical and practical elements of the job to the field level. Gallagher, who remains nearby in Canmore, continues to stay busy guiding clients up mountains and along trails in the summer and then enthusiastically switches to skis and a toque during the winter. He also keeps in close touch with the men and women in the field who know they can come to him if they need help in any way. He is aware that the rangers in the public safety field face the same challenges as the wardens in Banff. They have an aging staff with few young people in training. They have a limited budget and a low public profile and do not always garner the support from management that they need. Despite this, George Field and Duncan Burke would not trade the work for anything less.

10 A Younger Crowd

BY THE 1990S PARKS CANADA could justifiably claim that they had established a unified and professional mountain rescue organization with many significant missions to their credit. The eighties are remembered with fondness, and not a few think that the program reached a pinnacle during this period for a number of reasons. Throughout the decade, a large budget bought the training and equipment for an expanding program; the two alpine specialists maintained good political representation at the regional level, and the avalanche control program resided firmly with the Warden Service.

Developments in rope and cable rescue and newer, more powerful helicopters expanded the domain of the rescuers while improving the safety margin. It was a time most veterans look back on (sometimes nostalgically) as an exciting and formative period in the advancement of the public safety program.

The emergence of the Public Safety Advisory Committee was also proving significant as it gained clout. Clair Israelson remembers it started as a means of introducing Mike Schintz, the new operations manager, to the wardens working in public safety. The meeting amongst the six mountain parks to review significant rescue events,

discuss the latest technical developments and consider the training program for the year was so successful it was decided to continue it annually. It was a place to air concerns and reinforce working relationships. Throughout this period, both Peter Fuhrmann and Willi Pfisterer reported to regional office, giving the program stability and representation.

As the guiding program took on greater significance, the committee provided a forum to determine likely candidates for training. During this period, public safety training positions (as a stepping stone to the guide program) were established in Banff and Jasper. The smaller parks, with considerably fewer serious rescues, did not require wardens with full guide status to run the program, though a strong climbing/skiing background was still essential.

The Association of Canadian Mountain Guides (ACMG) was now part of the international guiding community, giving even greater credence to the standards they embraced. Throughout the 1980s Tim Auger and Clair Israelson, who had their guide status, encouraged younger wardens with potential to pursue this course if they wished to specialize in the public safety program. It was apparent that to maintain a professional rescue organization, it was necessary to keep abreast of the climbing and guiding standards set by the mountaineering world—and that could only be done by getting advanced training outside the Warden Service. Since the job did not provide sufficient opportunity to maintain this standard, only those who were serious about climbing recreationally as well as professionally were considered for additional training. Several young wardens had this potential though not all wanted to obtain full guide status. These talented people were soon able to find a niche in smaller parks like Waterton and Glacier.

One of these was Eric Dafoe, who started in the Warden Service in Banff in 1981. He brought with him a background in skiing and avalanche work obtained while he worked as a ranger in Kokanee Provincial Park. He had also developed an interest in climbing, and his natural ability made him a good fit for the public safety program. His winter skills grew after working at Sunshine with warden Tim Laboucane, with whom he would work later in Glacier National Park. The years at Sunshine made it easy to qualify for a job in this park when an opening came up in 1983. However, for a person interested in public safety, it was not considered the best park to go to. If fact, it was a real backwater, almost overlooked by the climbing and skiing community. When he got there, management support for the public safety program was practically non-existent. The wardens found themselves tied to the highway doing traffic control during avalanche shoots. Highway accidents also kept them hopping, particularly in the winter.

Though there were experienced wardens in the park—some of whom were excellent skiers—few were motivated climbers. Many looked at public safety as a necessary part of the job rather than a choice of careers, and Eric had his hands full to turn it into the job he wanted. First he needed management to recognize the function as an essential part of the warden duties and to put him in charge of it. Once that was accomplished he was able to put out a training program for the wardens in the park. He scheduled extended trips into the backcountry and led by example. He climbed and he got others to go with him. Slowly Eric brought a credibility and recognition to Revelstoke/Glacier as a place that could look after itself without being propped up by the larger parks. He continued to attend the advanced climbing schools and maintain a steady presence at the Public Safety Advisory Committee meetings each fall.

One of the climbs he went on that was high on the list of warden achievement was the advanced school on Mt. Alberta. Tim Auger led the party of five wardens consisting of Pat Sheehan, Darro Stinson, Ken Schroeder, Dianne Volkers and Eric up the formidable mountain considered to be one of the most significant challenges in the Canadian Rockies. But on a fine day with dry rock, it turned out to be a stellar trip that was one of the highlights of Dianne Volker's climbing career, and it set a high standard for a warden training school.

Though Eric provided as much training as he could for the warden staff in Glacier, he was quite happy when Tim Laboucane came from Banff in the late eighties to help him out in this task. Tim had a natural ability and keenness and did well on all the regional schools he was sent on. In 1980 he had progressed to full-time warden in Banff, working for Tim Auger at Sunshine ski hill in the winter and as rotational backcountry public safety warden in the summer.

WATERTON LAKES NATIONAL PARK also gained a young warden keen on climbing during the eighties. Brent Kosechenko started out with the Warden Service in Nahanni but gained his enthusiasm for climbing when Willi Pfisterer arrived in 1981 for a training school. Though the biggest public safety problem in the park was the notorious South Nahanni River, the park also housed a world-class climbing area in the Cirque of the Unclimbables. Willi always came up a couple of times a year to teach basic mountaineering and ski touring saying, "Look at all these

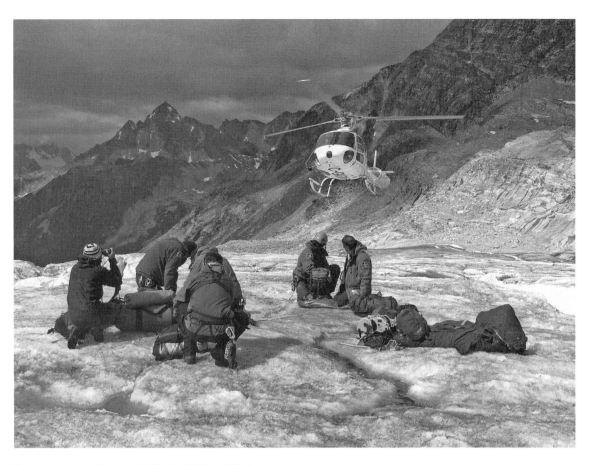

Crevasse rescue training in Glacier National Park. SYLVIA FOREST COLLECTION

mountains! Learn how to operate in this environment because sooner or later you will have to." Willi loved this park where he could travel in wild, open spaces and Brent responded to his enthusiasm. He learned how to walk with skill and respect through the rugged land and even how to climb. Brent later went to Kluane National Park, where his mentorship with Willi continued. Willi always responded to enthusiasm, and when it became known that management in Waterton was looking for a person strong in this field, he recommended Brent for the position. Max Winkler was still CPW in Waterton, and he respected Willi's opinion enough to agree to the transfer. Derek Tilson had been in the role for years but wanted to move on to other work in the Warden Service. Larry Harbridge filled the position for a few interim years, but when he moved on, Brent was offered the job. It was a big leap, but he had Derek who was still very active and capable as backup while he learned both the job and the park.

After Willi retired in 1987, Brent found himself taking direction from Peter Fuhrmann. Though Peter's style was different, Brent appreciated the scenarios Peter had them work through. The only drawback of the smaller more isolated southern park was the lack of good climbing and a ready supply of climbing partners. He did get out with the wardens he was now helping to train, but did the best climbing either with friends or with Derek Tilson.

In 1991, Edwin Knox became a seasonal warden in the park and added to the pool of wardens interested in mountain rescue. Edwin, who was originally from Prince Edward Island, came out to see the mountains in 1977 and stayed to make them part of his life. He became a good skier and general mountaineer who developed strong travel skills and an ability to fit in with the team. Brent was pleased with this added depth and put Edwin's tall frame and considerable strength to good use on several rescues and search incidents. His skills were such that Brent could leave him to run rescues in his absence even on more technical terrain like the Bear's Hump behind Waterton townsite.

Edwin recalls with satisfaction one particular rescue of a stranded climber on the Bear's Hump that required technical skill and a thorough knowledge of improvised rope rescue. They had to climb up to a ledge above the young man, place a bolt belay and set up a rope lowering system to reach him. Edwin went down, secured the panicky chap and continued with the lower until they reached the bottom of the cliff, completing the rescue with confidence.

The two other small parks, Yoho and Kootenay, were also going through a period of transition, with opportunities opening up for younger staff who were keen on climbing and public safety. Kathy Calvert, who had been in an acting position in the public safety program in Yoho, went to Jasper with husband Dale Portman when he became dog handler there in 1987. The position was quickly filled at the GT3 level by Terry Willis, a seasonal warden from Jasper. Terry had joined the Warden Service in 1980 with few climbing skills but a strong background in skiing. Although he started skiing at Whistler near his home town of Vancouver, he accelerated these skills when he got a job on the ski patrol at the Marmot Basin in Jasper. Here he developed a long lasting interest in public safety watching and helping the wardens in the avalanche program. His first posting was in Elk Island, but he soon transferred to the Sunwapta

Warden Station in Jasper where he received plenty of exposure to both climbing and rescues.

Throughout this time Kootenay was well looked after by Hans Fuhrer, who was more than capable of minding his own shop. He provided excellent climbing opportunities to anyone who wanted to get out, and his ability to impart the best skiing instruction was unassailable. The park was utterly fortunate to have him in the public safety position for as many years as it did, but finally, in 1995, he retired to Edgewater with his long-time climbing partner and wife Lilo.

The park administration had foreseen his retirement, and had geared up for his replacement by securing the talents of Reg Bunyan. Reg was a gifted young climber who definitely had an interest in the sport long before he joined the Warden Service. He actually started climbing in Europe in his youth but also spent time climbing in England where the rock climbing standards are high. He started working at Sunshine Ski Resort in Banff in 1981 (with a brief move to Pacific Rim National Park), where he was earmarked for the public safety program working with Tim Auger.

While the small parks were absorbing talented people who were not enrolled in the guide program, both Banff and Jasper sought candidates for that training. But grooming people for the demanding job of running the public safety program in the intense climbing centres of Banff, Lake Louise or Jasper took years. Knowing it was important to plan ahead, the Public Safety Advisory Committee began to council management to develop training programs focussed on creating either full or assistant guides to fill future positions. With more and more attention being paid to rescues by the media, and sharpened attention to the consequence of liability, it was felt that obtaining six full guides between the two parks was a reasonable goal.

But the guide program was becoming more and more difficult to complete and costs were rising. The time commitment was also expanding with each new course tacked on. With this in mind, the committee felt it was necessary to establish a specific training position rather than just wait for the individual to start the process on their own. In 1984/85, Mark Ledwidge and Pat Sheehan were the first candidates in these positions identified respectively in Banff and Jasper.

This move could not have come at a more propitious time, as trained guides would be needed in the next decade. It was always intended that the wardens would assume full responsibility for the program, which was essentially the case when Peter Fuhrmann retired in 1991. Even during the last half of the 1980s, Peter's role had slowly changed, allowing the Wardens to absorb more and more of the field work. During his last years in office, his work became more administrative than field oriented. Much to Willi's chagrin, he found he was spending more and more time in the regional office himself as Peter's time was taken up with several commitments.

Despite the increasing bureaucratic demands of the office, Peter continued to run many of the regional schools. The "Fuhrmann Sanctions" affected those who attended in different ways. His tendency to get late alpine starts did not sit well with everyone, but there was some tolerance. Cliff White recalled one school in particular where a late approach resulted in an exciting climb. The climb was up the East Ridge of Mt. Temple, and with a choice of two different approaches Peter separated the wardens into two teams. Gord Irwin and Brad White took their team up the rock ridge proper over the quartz steps to the bivouac at the base of the black towers, while Cliff and Peter's group tackled the Aemmer Couloir leading to the same spot. With spectacular weather and excellent climbing conditions, the first group reached the bivouac site early that afternoon. After settling in they called Peter's group to see how they were doing. To Brad's amazement the reply was something like, "Fine! Just coming up to the route now." Peter's group had not even left the parking lot.

Cliff relates: "Some people were just getting off the couloir when the six of us started up about 2:30 or 3:00 p.m. You had to believe in Peter's lucky stars, which I did." Cliff had been on many of Peter's schools and things had always worked out even if it didn't look like they would. He and Doug Martin were in the lead that began to lengthen as Peter cheerfully told stories on the way up the now sloppy snow. Both advanced climbers listened with half an ear as they kept a concerned eye out for rock fall. Cliff does not recall who first saw the large boulder "the size of a deep-freeze" as it noiselessly soared down from above, but fortunately it was a long way up when they spotted it and they had time to move. Peter was about nine metres behind, when Cliff—now that they were well out of the way—turned to say in a calm voice: "Rock!" Peter looked up, "and his eyes got big as saucers" just before he and the other two rope teams leapt for safety. With a wicked sense of humour Cliff relates: "It was really fun to watch these guys leaping out of the way. Doug and I had a good laugh." They arrived intact at the bivouac for a fine night and finished the climb off in good style the next day. It was one of Cliff's finest climbs in the Rockies, and he remembers it fondly.

But such episodes had others questioning the wisdom of late starts. Cliff pointed out the difference between Peter and Willi: "You would know what you were going to be doing with Willi at least a week in advance. With Peter you didn't know until nine o'clock that morning. Even if it was on the sheet he would change his mind and reorganize the groceries." Often they would set off in "the most God awful weather" only to have it clear up just enough to get through the school. Ironically for Cliff, Willi seemed to have the opposite luck. Willi would have everything calculated to the nth degree, but often "The weather was just so bad that no amount of planning helped." Despite the grumbling, a lot of wardens found the spontaneity of Peter's trips had merit, because they were expected to do rescues at the drop of a hat and the off balance approach was realistic. It required a rethinking of new problems that many benefited from.

By 1991 an opportunity to take a reasonable government buyout came available to senior employees, and Mike Schintz, who took advantage of this, suggested Peter do so as well. Peter's life had recently been complicated by his daughter's struggle with cancer, and it was a good time to pass on the alpine specialist mantle. When she lost the battle, Peter was ready to go. By 1991 both Peter and Willi were retired, spelling the end of the era of alpine specialist. In the end, both men left a legacy that cannot be replaced or diminished. They nurtured the Warden Service through incredible years of growth and maturation, enabling the inheritors to bring full professionalism to the rescue organization.

GOOD THINGS DON'T LAST FOREVER, though, and the winds of change blew strongly with the onset of the next decade. The public safety program—now in the hands of the young Canadians Willi and Peter had so assiduously moulded—would face serious challenges and losses under a new political climate. Whereas the eighties were a period of spending excess, the nineties were typified by funding cutbacks and intense scrutiny of former programs. The national parks in the west were turned upside down with a new Organizational Review headed by two fierce women sent out from Ottawa. Their task was to downsize and cut costs where possible, which ultimately meant the elimination of key positions in Western Regional Office. One of the positions was the warden coordinator, which was never filled after the retirement of Mike Schintz. With the loss of both alpine specialists and the warden coordinator, there was solid concern for the possible fragmentation of the public safety program amongst the parks. This was forestalled by creating one position to maintain a unified program. The new position was intended to be filled successively by senior personnel on a rotational basis. It fell initially to Clair Israelson with the intent that Tim Auger would continue after a year or two. Though the job was not that attractive to active field men,

Clair knew it was important and did not hesitate to assume the role, thinking it to be temporary.

Minor changes in public safety positions were put in place to adjust to the new roles. Gord Irwin, who had been in charge of the backcountry in Banff, moved to Lake Louise to be in charge of public safety in Clair's absence. Gerry Israelson was already running the program in Jasper after Darro Stinson left to work for a short while in the regional office.

Just prior to these changes, other young candidates for future public safety positions were gaining experience, and this included women. Kathy Calvert and Dianne Volkers had made inroads in the field, but this would be taken to a new level by two other talented and ambitious young women.

The next woman to show interest in public safety was Sylvia Forest, Kathy's younger sister. Kathy had introduced Sylvia to the Warden Service at the youthful age of 15, when she took her on a whirlwind trip through the backcountry of Banff. It must have left an indelible impression, as she later doggedly set about becoming a warden herself with a very intense focus on public safety. By the time Sylvia applied to the Warden Service in 1989, climbing was familiar as old boots, having started the sport early in her life (at 12 years old) with her father Don Forest. Before joining the service, Sylvia worked as an apprentice guide at the Banff Cadet Camp, which enabled her to fully appreciate the responsibilities of the job she hoped to get.

Lisa Paulson was introduced to the possibilities of the Warden Service and the role of public safety through Clair Israelson a few years later, while working as a ski patroller at Lake Louise. As patroller, she was able to work in the avalanche control area and subsequently took up climbing with friends in the summer. The Warden Service intrigued her as a real challenge, and she too set about taking steps to qualify for the job. She was hired on as a term warden at Saskatchewan River Crossing where she met Pat Sheehan in 1991. The rapport between the two was established early

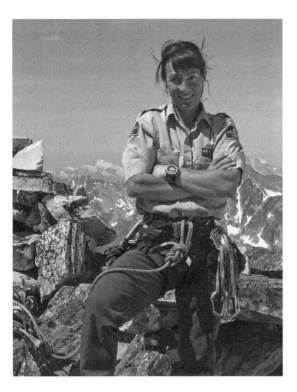

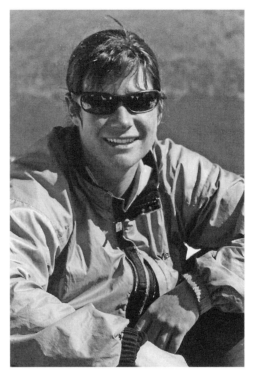

Sylvia Forest. SYLVIA FOREST COLLECTION

Lisa Paulson. SYLVIA FOREST COLLECTION

after she attended a climbing school he ran that summer, enhancing her desire to carry on in that field. She and Sylvia soon became fast friends, which led to a good climbing partnership.

During the late eighties and early nineties the last major wave of new talent entered the Warden Service to form the next generation of public safety. Percy Woods joined the Warden Service a year before Sylvia, with less of a climbing background, but with the necessary aptitude and interest. He too focussed on entering the public safety field and took up climbing and skiing with a vengeance. His biggest obstacle was learning how to ski; moulding his tall lanky body to the grace of a downhill skier did not come easily and to this day he admits he lacks style but can get the job done. He put his name forward to the advisory committee early in his career and was subsequently put in the training program in Banff.

Steve Blake gained his skills in the mid-eighties when he joined the ski patrol at Lake Louise in 1986. He skied and climbed in the area until 1991 when he briefly worked for Kananaskis Country while pursuing a degree in Environmental Science and Geography. This led directly to the Warden Service in Jasper later the same year. He established good relationships with all the wardens working in the public safety field and was recognized as a good candidate for a position in Jasper. As such, he too was put in the public safety training program sponsored by Jasper National Park.

Rupert Wedgwood was the other new talent on the horizon. His eclectic background opened the door to a term job in 1991, initially in resource management and ultimately in public safety through winter work at Rogers Pass. Rupert picked up the more advanced skills quickly while climbing with friends and undertaking the

259

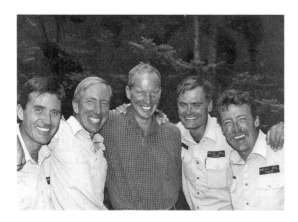

Mark Ledwidge, Gord Irwin, Percy Woods, Rupert Wedgwood and Brad White. MARK LEDWIDGE COLLECTION

arduous task of becoming a proficient downhill skier. Like Percy, he became a competent skier, but the grace one achieves from learning the sport early in life still eludes him. The one area he did excel in, however, was the ever-expanding world of ice climbing, where his tall frame gave him a natural advantage.

IT WAS ALSO ABOUT THIS TIME that the Warden Service involvement at the ski hills came to an end, though it would dwindle painfully out for another year or so. But technically by 1990 the avalanche control program was now conducted mainly by the pro-patrol hired by the ski hills. The amount of devolvement differed with each hill, but by 1993 the wardens were gone completely.

Despite park monitoring, Clair Israelson had grave safety concerns about the control program under the new management at Lake Louise. This was resolved when they hired Will Devlin that winter. Will was a dynamic young man who had spent considerable time in the public safety program in the north. He had helped get the new Auyuittuq National Park on its feet for the inevitable mountaineering problems faced by climbers attracted to its wild granite walls. He then went to Kluane in the recently vacated public safety position. He had

also worked many years for Clair at Lake Louise and was more than qualified for the job.

Will did not change the method of avalanche control from that developed by the wardens immediately, despite the different approach management eagerly sought. He continued to keep areas closed when the hazard got high then stabilize the slopes with the traditional bombing or ski cutting. Eventually, however, he began to keep the ski runs open through skier activity. It proved cost effective for the managers despite the increase in personnel, as it reduced the amount of bombing needed. The other ski areas employed the same approach. Parks Canada can be given credit for this, because they withdrew from the program slowly, ensuring that the new management would hire the trained people they needed.

But the withdrawal from the ski hills still left a great hole in the Warden Service public safety training program. To keep from losing the skills completely, more effort was put into the highway avalanche control program, particularly on the Sunshine road, the Trans-Canada Highway and Icefield Parkway around the Columbia Icefield. During the late eighties and early nineties the control program at Sunwapta Warden Station got a big boost. There was much work to be done here and wardens Evan Manners and Pat Sheehan (who had been offered full-time positions at the station in 1988) found opportunities to increase their understanding of how avalanches are triggered and propagated. Evan thought the effort compensated for some of the lost training at the ski hill; one big change was in the diligence employed in taking weather readings at the snow plots.

Gerry Israelson made it his goal to improve the forecasting and control program for the Columbia Icefield despite the low volume of traffic. Even Yoho received a boost when Terry Willis finally brought in a bombing program for the glacier on Mt. Stephen. Kathy Calvert had tried on several occasions to convince management that a bombing program for the glacier that hung over the Trans-Canada Highway on the Field Hill would be successful, but to no avail. Finally after both a large transport truck and a freight train were hit by an avalanche off Mt. Steven (causing huge damage), the idea went ahead.

As the eighties merged into the nineties, the regional and local schools that formerly saw large numbers of wardens participating from other functions began to dwindle. This was due to many reasons and was not just a reflection on budgetary cuts. The Warden Service, on average, was aging and specializing. A hiring freeze during the early nineties had left a dearth of young staff to backfill the roles left by older wardens who had moved on in the service or who had retired. Fire management, resource management and law enforcement all tended toward specialization as did public safety. In addition to this, there was a new favourite kid on the block. As the Warden Service matured, so did the focus and direction of Parks, and the emphasis was swinging solidly toward resource management administered by people with advanced degrees in science. When the freeze was lifted, the new people brought on were often older, having spent their youth obtaining the much coveted master's degrees in science. They also brought fewer outdoor skills to the service.

But although public safety received less money for training, it also required fewer people for rescues and did not need the all-inclusive schools of the past, particularly at the basic level. As Clair noted, "There was not much incentive for the wardens [not in the public safety function] to go on schools because they were never used on rescues anyway." The older fellows did not really mind; at ages now approaching 40 to 45 years and with young families, they did not want to freeze on a glacier or maintain a high standard of fitness required for former "sanctions." Now schools were often vehicles for public safety trainees to practise their skills on those who still enjoyed climbing. Dianne Volkers, an avid climber, noticed the leadership role she had enjoyed in the past was supplanted by having to play "client" for the new trainee. Functionally this made a lot of sense,

but it did little to engender blanket enthusiasm for those who saw a dwindling future in the program.

But some good schools did continue, and they still produced the camaraderie of old. Tim Auger tackled the classic north face of Edith Cavell with Reg Bunyan, Steve Blake and Percy Woods. It was a great climb for Steve who felt it was a marvellous opportunity to climb with more experienced mountaineers. Reg Bunyan also remembers a climb on Mt. Brussels with Tim under less than stellar conditions. He recalls sitting out in the rain, looking up at the formidable rock ahead wondering if they were going, when Tim gloomily glanced out at the valley below then said stoically, "Well, this is an advanced school so I guess we'd better go."

Accidents also continued unabated, occasionally reminding the wardens of the hazards of their occupation. One of the greatest dangers was actually from the frequent use of helicopters. Helicopter pilots did not have a long life expectancy, especially in the early years, and the added danger of slinging on a rope further reduced those chances. Although many wardens had some uneasy moments flying in bad conditions, there were remarkably few really close calls. But there were some. A warden named Al Bjorn (B.J.) recalls one incident during a heli-sling training session when he was sure his days were over. They were several hundred feet up when he overheard the pilot say "Mayday! Mayday! Fire in the cockpit!" Sure that the helicopter was about to explode in the air, B.J. said his farewells to the world, but fortunately nothing happened. After landing, he found out the smoke was due to a short in the battery—which was serious enough, but it had not prevented the pilot from landing safely.

Another incident that added to the growing number of grey hairs of dog handler Dale Portman occurred on a rather remarkable rescue dubbed Ferris Bueller's Day Off. The search for an older man on the Crowfoot Glacier began on the afternoon of the day he was reported missing by a friend from Calgary. The friend was very surprised that his trekking buddy would have gone even an hour on his own, characterizing him as the sort of man who did nothing alone, least of all venture out on a glacier without an experienced companion. The friend was thoroughly alarmed when he was not found by the following day, and he arrived from Calgary to help with the search.

Dale flew down from Jasper with Todd McCready, where he met the other dog handlers Scott Ward and Gord Peyto and the search team headed by Clair Israelson. The dog handlers spent most of the day searching more unlikely areas in the subalpine regions while rescue teams of two combed the upper glacier and surrounding rock terrain. Clair also had the aid of two helicopters for moving the crews around as sections of the search area were eliminated by different teams. But the weather, which had been good for the past several days, began to worry the searchers, who received an ominous forecast of a drastic change. A large system was due in late that afternoon bringing snow and almost blizzard-like conditions for the high mountain areas.

Since the man had already spent two nights out, a third night in a storm would not bode well for survival, especially at his age. The day wore on without success. The buddy, confined to the moraine areas around the hut, continued to dog their footsteps, wandering as far as he was allowed, blowing a whistle to distraction. The searchers could hear this forlorn whistle from time to time as they combed the area above large, open crevasses that should have alarmed any lone hiker. At one point, Dianne Volkers and Dave Norcross thought they heard a faint whistle in the distance, but when they looked up and saw the despondent companion wandering on the rocks above, they ascribed it to his sad bleats.

Finally, time and weather began to run out. Clair held a short debriefing to see where they stood and to examine what had been searched and what needed to be looked at again. Tim and Dianne had seen no tracks leading to the larger crevasses, but the team thought there was a remote possibility he had wandered that far. Tim went up to search them again with the helicopter, hoping they could get close enough to see more than earlier flights had revealed. But Todd was now alarmed at the approaching weather system and indicated it was time to head back. Just as the helicopter banked to the side, a last ray of light pierced the colliding clouds, illuminating a small hole in a depressed snow trough. To Tim's amazement he found himself gazing briefly at a small dot of colour that feebly waved at the retreating team. Realizing they had found the man and that he was still alive, Todd flew back for a team to bring the him up. Fortunately he had landed on a snow bridge and was not wedged in, making the extraction fairly simple. With the storm clipping the tail rotor, Todd soon had the team and victim back at the base rescue headquarters at the lodge, where the frozen soul was returned to the land of the living. The storm that had held off just long enough to complete the rescue, hit with a vengeance, covering the crevasses with enough snow to bury them for weeks to come. There is no doubt in Clair's mind that had they not spotted him at the last minute, his fate would have been sealed in the icy tomb.

Earlier that afternoon, Dale Portman had been convinced *he* was leaving the land of the living. Dale had just been picked up from the upper slopes of Bow Canyon and was still high above the canyon when the pilot from Banff, in a voice he tried to keep cool, called out: "Mayday, Mayday … Engine flare out, helicopter going down!" The engine had quit. With no place to land and the canyon below, all Dale could see was a wall of rock rushing up at him like a freight train—but his communication over the headset had been cut off by the pilot who needed no distractions from a frightened passenger. With eyes as wide as saucers and hands now turned to claws on the door handle, all Dale could do was think briefly "I'm going to die!" when suddenly the skids skimmed over the blackness bringing the machine to a safe landing on the large alluvial channel beyond the rocks. Shaking, he looked over at the man he thought he was spending his last seconds with, who turned to him, now perfectly calm, and said: "Oh? I forgot to tell you … I flared out [auto-rotated] over the rock and got the engine back."

The nineties were scarred by many personal challenges, mishaps and losses; the first was a frightening incident on Mt. Lefroy in 1992. Dianne Volkers and Christine Aikins were climbing with two friends when they ran into icy conditions forcing them off the normal route in search of good snow. But when the snow ran out they moved back over the ice to rock bands above. Christine was leading on Dianne's rope when she dislodged a large rock that plummeted between them. It did not hit either of the girls, but it did plunge through the joining rope which jerked Christine backwards off her stance. They had been moving together short-roped, and there was no protection in place. When Christine fell, Dianne was unable to absorb the shock, and they were both swept downward on the icy slope below. Dianne's efforts at self-arrest as they picked up speed were ineffective, and finally even the axe was flung from her wrist. Then they were sliding, bouncing off the ice runnels on the ever-steepening slope as the now useless crampons jolted them further with each contact with the ice. Miraculously, they finally stopped just before hitting a huge boulder field that Dianne feels "would have killed them." As it was, they were severely banged up; Christine had a broken ankle and injured shoulder while Dianne had broken ribs and a punctured lung. Both suffered from deep abrasions and shock, but they were alive. Unfortunately they did not have a radio, and it was not until around 1:00 p.m. that help was summoned when other climbers with a cell phone showed up.

The reaction at the Banff warden office was one of frenetic activity, with typically worsening weather threatening the rescue operation. The girls were now very cold even though their fellow partner, Jim Baker, had descended to the Abbot Hut for blankets and sleeping bags. Fortunately Lance Cooper was flying, and he chanced the bad weather to bring them out. Both girls recovered to continue their careers, but this near loss cast a pall over the Warden Service.

The next serious accident followed quickly. By 1992, Pat Sheehan had only one course to complete to become a full guide, and he was getting as much climbing in as he could in preparation. Luckily for him, he had found a willing and able partner in Lisa Paulson, the pretty young seasonal warden stationed at Saskatchewan River Crossing, close to the Sunwapta Warden Station. In fact, they were very much in love, and Pat often stated he had never been happier. As for Lisa, she would have married him on the spot if he'd asked.

The handsome young man was usually the life of any party. His penchant for cooking spaghetti into a solid mass at summer wind-up parties (while singing) was often joked about and always permitted. His twinkling blue eyes and Irish charm gave him a larger than life quality

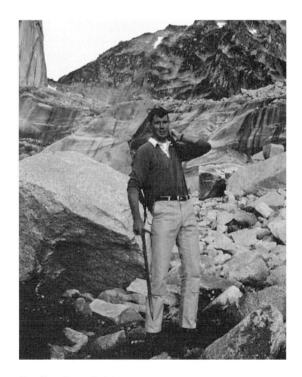

Pat Sheehan climbing. MARK LEDWIDGE COLLECTION

that averted close scrutiny of his bad jokes; he had the ability to lighten the day, even when the climbing or rescue work was serious. Lisa was thrilled to share his love of climbing, and trusted him as a teacher and mentor for her own growing ambitions. Without much thought other than the joy of being together and the beauty of the warm day, they set off on November 26 to introduce Lisa to her first ice climb.

Pat spent 20 minutes at the base of the route showing her basic ice climbing techniques for the fairly easy short climb north of Curtain Call on Tangle Peak near the Columbia Icefield Visitor Centre. It was around noon when they set out, delayed by a discussion of whether or not to take a radio. Eventually they decided in favour of the extra weight. The ice was in superb condition, and Pat climbed with confidence, sinking the axe solidly into the soft ice and placing ice screws for protection every 10 metres. Lisa had no problem following and they ascended the climb in good form.

Gerry Israelson was also having a nice, if less ambitious day, with Bill Hunt, the new public safety trainee. Bill had taken Pat's place in the program when he moved on as permanent warden at the Sunwapta station and was now working closely with Gerry. They were driving to the rescue room when a measured call came in from Lisa at 3:45 p.m. saying that Pat had fallen. Gerry thought this was terrifically funny and anticipated the ribbing he would give his young protégé when he talked to him about the climb later that day. The smile faded on both men's faces, however, as the second and third report ominously conveyed the seriousness of the situation. Minutes later Lisa called again to say that Pat had a broken femur, broken wrist and was bleeding from the head. The report that he had difficulty breathing galvanized everyone into action. Within minutes the helicopters from both Valemount and Banff were enroute, with Todd McCready flying for Jasper and Tim and Clair flying with Lance Cooper from Banff. Jim Bertwhistle and Terry Damm were

the closest wardens stationed at Sunwapta and at Saskatchewan River Crossing respectively, and were the first to reach the trail access. The next half hour seemed interminable to Terry as he slogged through the deep snow and willows that tangled around his legs, keeping him from reaching the base of the icefall.

They arrived to find Lisa trying to give Pat CPR. She was a skilled medic and had reacted with a coolness that amazed Terry.

After they had reached the top of the climb, Pat had placed two solid ice screws as a belay anchor to lower her off the climb to speed up the descent. He explained he would then rappel from another pre-established station at the top of the waterfall. This seemed to take a long time, but finally she saw the rope snake out over the ice as he began his descent.

She saw him begin the descent smoothly, but suddenly the rope seemed to pop and he was falling, airborne. He dropped about three metres, then bounced, hitting once, giving a gasp before sliding to an arrest on the slope below. She called out to reassure him as she worked down the ice steps to his body, which was face down on the ice in a crumpled position. Though he was conscious when she reached him and able to respond verbally, it was with a sinking heart that she saw his right leg and wrist were badly deformed and his breath was short and raspy. She extracted the radio from his pack—so grateful they had brought it—and called in the accident.

Pat's confusion was almost reassuring, as he tried repeatedly to get up, unaware of the seriousness of his injuries. When she asked where he was hurt he replied that he thought his arm might be broken and that his leg hurt. She tried desperately to keep him with her mentally as she thought about moving to a better location, but then realized that he was having difficulty breathing. There was a pocket of blood under his right eye, and the blood coming out of his left ear and nose indicated a skull fracture. Finally she settled for reorienting his body with his head uphill to ease his breathing and maintain his airway. She caringly placed her toque on his head hoping that shock was all she had to worry about. Then during one of her transmissions to the rescue party, Pat lost consciousness. His breathing stopped, so she initiated artificial respiration which generated a weak pulse for a few moments. But his condition was deteriorating; the skin became yellow and cold, the eyes dilated, and air became entrapped in the tissue surrounding his face and neck.

Todd arrived and slung Gerry in even though it was now dark. They swiftly transported Pat to the waiting ambulance and lowered him directly onto the outstretched gurney. But Gerry knew he was dead. His heart had stopped in cardiac arrest that no amount of CPR could reverse, even though he was not pronounced dead until his arrival at the hospital.

Just prior to this, the Banff helicopter had been told to step down, which was a relief since they were already flying in the dark. But Clair Israelson and Diny Harrison, a close friend of Lisa's, were brought down by truck to the staging area on the Beauty Creek highway flats, and they greeted her when she finally stumbled out from the base of the fall. She distinctly recalls Clair gave her the only comfort that helped by saying she had done everything humanly possible to save Pat. Even if he had landed on a hospital gurney, no doctor could have done more.

The loss was enormous to everyone, possibly most of all to Gerry as he had mentored Pat carefully through the guide and public safety programs and valued him as a friend. The rescue crew retired that night to the Sunwapta Warden Station where they attempted to absorb the abrupt change in their lives. Everyone was deeply shaken. Pat was the first warden to die climbing in the Warden Service—though he was climbing on his own time—and it seemed unthinkable. The protective shield was shattered and the idea that wardens were somehow invulnerable was gone forever. Wardens and guides *could* die climbing

despite the training, the knowledge and the care.

It also became obvious soon after, that Pat's death had consequences beyond great personal loss, as difficult as that was. The movement to specialization, the hiring freeze and the budgetary restrictions compounded by an aging Warden Service left the middle ranks of public safety personnel diminished, and there was no one in the wings to take Pat's place. Gerry felt they needed someone of Pat's calibre at Sunwapta station to handle some of the most serious accidents in the park. After Pat died, the public safety staff realized they did not even have a warden enrolled in the guide program. The young people with the most potential had not yet even begun to train in this field.

After Pat's funeral, Clair, now nominally head of the public safety program, paid attention to a name that cropped up repeatedly. This was Brad White, Cliff White's younger brother. Brad, who had actually joined the Warden Service as a young man in the early eighties, had the same natural climbing aptitude as Cliff when he started as a seasonal warden. But where Cliff eventually became interested in fire, Brad remained focussed on the public safety program. Though he was committed to becoming a guide, he was not given support from Parks Canada to enter the program. At that time, financing was given to those in full-time positions, because the future of a seasonal warden was always questionable. With the hiring freeze looming, Brad's chances of getting a full-time position were limited, and he was bluntly told that becoming a guide would not make any difference. Despite this, it was the career he wanted, and when he became a full guide at age 29, he jumped at the chance to become assistant manager for CMH when Hans Gmoser offered him the job.

But life as a guide, though exciting for an unattached young man, is hard for those who eventually settle down with a family, as Brad did a few years later. With his wife Donna following a productive career in Banff, the visits were beginning to seem a little too infrequent (six days a month).

265

Still, it was with mixed thoughts that he considered Clair's offer of Pat's job. He knew there were hard feelings about bringing someone in who was not a warden when jobs were scarce. He had also gotten to know Pat well, having climbed with him on many occasions.

One trip with Willi Pfisterer on a centennial climb celebrating 100 years since the inception of national parks was particularly memorable. Willi wanted to celebrate the event by setting off fireworks from the summit of Mt. Edith Cavell on the first of January of that year. He had flown some old tires and some wood and the precious fireworks to the summit. He then amalgamated a team of climbers that included his daughter Suzie, Brad, and wardens Pat Sheehan, Gerry Israelson, Frank Staples, Jeff Weir and Evan Manners. Brad recalls it was devastatingly cold for such an adventure, but they were prepared for the minus 35 degree Celsius temperatures that day. The townsite wardens towed them to the base of the climb with skidoos. There they encountered a solo climber returning from an aborted attempt of the East Ridge (of Edith Cavell) after freezing his feet. He was amazed to see the wardens out and assumed they were there to get him. To his dismay, he found out they were ferrying in the climbing team, and he was quite indignant when he realized they intended to drop the team off first before returning for him. The protest brought a classic response from Willi who replied: "Well you already *focked* them, so three hours won't make any difference!" Willi saw no reason to sacrifice the climb at this stage.

They made the summit where the temperature plummeted to 44 below zero and built snow caves—with some difficulty—for the coming night. When all were cosily ensconced in their shelters, Gerry opened up a celebratory bottle of champagne which froze the instant the cork was popped. They then lit the fire and enjoyed the pyrotechnics as best they could, ducking one errant rocket that blew up in front of them when the escalating wind hurled it back in their direction. Unfortunately, it was also minus 44 in the town of Jasper, and few of the townsfolk ventured out to witness the magnificent effort (even if it could have been seen at that distance). The next day the wind was so strong, they literally had to crawl down the descent route.

Despite the possibility of hard feelings, Brad accepted the position once he was assured it would be full-time work. This was a godsend for Gerry, for whom Brad truly enjoyed working. He was also a ray of light to the wardens at Sunwapta. It is unlikely anyone else could have filled Pat's shoes as competently. In fact, Sunwapta experienced a minor renaissance when the next crop of eager young wardens committed their time to the program. And this time, management came forth with support, realizing that getting well-trained quality individuals was a long-term commitment that required some planning.

DAVE SMITH HAD GONE TO WORK at Sunwapta in 1991 after learning many of his public safety skills while working at Kananaskis Country for Lloyd Gallagher. Dave took the 10-month public safety training position, but would later run the station, eventually staying a total of nine years. The other arrivals at the station in the mid-nineties were Sylvia Forest, Lisa Paulson and Rupert Wedgwood. Lisa had come through her ordeal, surviving Pat's death with strength and solidity, and her commitment to climbing, if anything, had deepened. Steve Blake also entered the public safety arena and went to Jasper townsite in the public safety training position in 1993. For a few stellar years, Jasper was replete with talented people enrolled in the guide training program hoping to find a future in the Parks public safety program. Steve began his first course in 1993, while Sylvia and Rupert started in 1994. With Percy Woods in Banff starting his guide's courses in 1996 and Lisa in 1998, the continued stream of new people coming on board began to fill the gaps after Pat's death.

But the losses and changes in the public safety program did not change people's actions in the

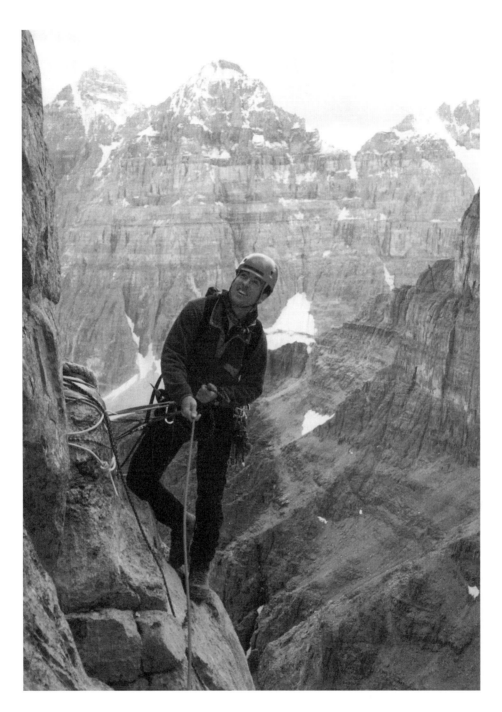

Steve Blake. GORD IRWIN COLLECTION

mountains, and 1993–94 continued with a steady stream of accidents. There was also an increase in popularity of some climbs such as Slipstream that posed high objective hazards to both climber and the rescuer. Wardens were called in repeatedly over the years to collect bodies swept by avalanches off this climb, often at great peril to their own safety.

Rescue work in other parks also stayed high. Waterton did not experience a significant increase in numbers, but those rescues they did seemed to be more complex. The majority of incidents were searches rather than rescues on technical climbs. Most people are found within the first or second day, but on June 23rd, Derek Tilson found himself back in the role of rescue leader for a major search. Though Derek was not the designated public safety warden, he was on call when a young man from San Antonio, Texas, was reported missing on the Carthew Summit trail which angles up through open talus slopes over 2,440 metres. The terrible weather was a contributing factor. The temperature plummeted during the night, decreasing the poorly equipped, inexperienced man's chances of survival even more.

The call had come in, typically late in the day, leaving little chance of finding him that night, but when they had no success late the following day, Derek elevated the search. Accordingly, he notified the backup in Banff who responded with helicopter support, additional personnel and three search dogs. Both Tim Auger and Clair Israelson arrived to oversee the operation, allowing Derek to concentrate on the search using his local knowledge of the terrain. One of the first responses was to employ the method of "purposeful wandering" using a few highly skilled individuals to search areas they knew well and could travel through easily. They also put in containment along the trails, leaving lookouts to check areas where an individual could emerge and be accounted for.

On the night of the 24th, the man was still missing, but they knew from relations and friends that he was lightly clad with only a lunch and a rain poncho in a small day pack. Derek also had concerns about the possibility of him running into bears—for which Waterton is almost notorious. The terrain itself did not offer any significant cliff bands to wander over, but the country was rough, offering more than one opportunity to come to grief. Still, Derek thought there was a good chance that he had wandered into what he called a "sucker basin" and picked up a lower trail leading out. In the end, this is precisely what had occurred. A trail crew had been sent to the cabin on Boundary Trail for the night specifically to watch out for him, and at 6:45 the following morning, they received a call that the missing person had "just wandered in."

The search wound down successfully, but the searchers had employed all their training, local knowledge and search techniques before it was over. The search critique reinforced the need to consider the individual's mental state, because the young man was very confused. The aunt and uncle who had initiated the search said he had the mental capacity of a seventeen-year-old, but later corrected that age to much younger. He had become confused when he tried to read the signs at Carthew Summit, and did not respond to the search efforts going on around him. Certainly he made no real attempt to be seen when searchers passed over him by helicopter.

But the summer was not over in Waterton. One rescue gave Brent an occasion to star in the drama of pulling a stranded climber off a cliff on the Bear's Hump, just outside of town. A young man decided to solo one of the many popular routes on the only real good rock in Waterton, but was not quite up to the task. He began late enough, at around three-thirty in the afternoon, progressing through broken rock bands until he encountered an overhang that was beyond his ability. He was not initially convinced he could not climb the projection, and made two almost fatal attempts before deciding to stay put and call for help. Brent immediately assembled a rescue team and in the fine warm light of an early summer evening, set off to bring the man down with a straightforward rope lower. From a well-anchored location about 23 metres above the stranded climber, Brent descended to the hapless victim, at one point using a directional pulley to keep the correct approach. Once there, he was able to provide the fellow with some of the essentials he had left without: a jacket, a helmet and a climbing harness, before lowering him to the ground. Edwin Knox remembers the incident with humour as it was much appreciated by the local residents (and a few tourists) who got out their chairs and ordered pizza for the event.

One of the last incidents of the summer in Banff did not end so happily. Again the climb was on a route becoming increasingly popular, but which had high objective hazards. This rescue required little of the Warden Service but highlighted the increasing need to find a way to inform climbers of local hazards. The Aemmer Couloir on Mt. Temple, where the accident occurred, is easily seen from the Trans-Canada Highway, and almost acts like a magnet to climbers who are attracted by the visually clean line. Unfortunately, it is prone to cornice and snow buildup near the exit on the east ridge, a condition compounded that summer by wet cool weather.

The people involved were a husband and wife team (experienced climbing guides) from Utah, who had climbed extensively throughout the world and were now enjoying the sport in the Lake Louise area. But they failed to inform themselves of the local conditions when they signed out at the warden office. They were only reported missing by campground staff after they failed to return by the evening of the following day.

Alarm for the missing people reached the warden office at midnight of the 10th, but no one knew exactly where they had gone, making it difficult to establish an overdue time. The following day, an aerial search was underway when the husband reached Lake Annette and alerted hikers to the accident. The clouds were down to around 2,100 metres, but now at least, they knew where

to look. Tim Auger took the time to record the sequence of events with a measure of detail and sympathy not often found in a rescue report.

The couple had taken the precaution of starting early, indicating they knew the value of catching early snow conditions, which allowed them to climb quickly while the route was still in good shape. But the warm dry spell they were taking advantage of meant that the freezing level remained high on the mountain, and sloughing activity, usually expected later in the day, started far too early for their careful plans. The first serious rock outcrop forced them into the avalanche trough in the main gully, which they did not exit, feeling that they were making good time there. But an avalanche trough is probably not the best place to be no matter what time of day. The early morning sun did not need much power to activate the semi-frozen mushy snow on the steep rock on both sides of the gully and a heavy wet avalanche punctuated with rocks hit the trough with a force that swept the two climbers to the bottom.

Both husband and wife were knocked unconscious, but upon recovering—and probably astounded to be alive—they assessed their predicament. The husband had chest pains and lacerations to his face, but was otherwise ambulatory. His wife had broken her femur and could not move at all. It was imperative that they get help, so with a farewell to his wife, the husband set off, somewhat like the deluded lover in *The English Patient*, telling her he would be back shortly with help. Two days later he was found by hikers as he tried painfully to make his way across the rock field above Lake Annette. On later reflection, he realized that he could have only gone another 45 or so metres before passing out. He had spent two nights out, as had his wife, through unstable weather with cool temperatures and periods of rain. Unfortunately, she was not able to move, and she succumbed to hypothermia.

Tim flew directly to the base of the couloir, where they spotted the missing woman with little difficulty. It was obvious she had died some time ago, but rather than take her back right away, they returned for the husband, who was still badly in need of care. The last and most difficult part of the rescue remained when they had to inform the family of the outcome.

S‌ylvia F‌orest b‌egan w‌orking earnestly in public safety when she moved to Sunwapta in 1994. During these years, she would encounter some of her most traumatic rescue situations as well as some of the highlights of her career. Most significant, she entered the guide program along with Rupert Wedgwood. Warden Garth Lemke was actually the park candidate in the training position, and as such, received the financial and training benefits that went with that situation. Sylvia, therefore, did not expect any financial compensation but was determined to become a guide anyway. She was taking a big bite out of a very tough pie.

Sylvia had to overcome two things she could not change. She was small at five foot one, even for a woman, and she was rather old at age 33 to be starting the program. On average, most candidates were ten years younger than she was. She had actually taken a rope handling and general mountaineering course (non-certification) the summer before to see if she was ready to go on the certification courses required for full guide status. She did not receive much encouragement either, when a fellow warden who had worked in the program for several years told her it was very competitive and she had little chance of getting in. Although she had to swallow the $4,000 price tag, Gerry recognized her dedication, and he gave her support by giving her time off for training.

She got an early initiation into rescue work on a difficult rescue at the toe of the Athabasca Glacier on the Columbia Icefield soon after arriving to work at Sunwapta. It actually started as a typical situation, all too common at the toe of the glacier so accessible to visitors with no experience with crevasses. The receding glacier was particularly broken during those years, leaving a network of snow covered deep crevasses. The wardens had responded on numerous occasions to people slipping into the shallower slots, often just plucking them out, but often the result was more serious. The major problem was that people would rather walk on snow, which covered the crevasses, than on ice. To partially alleviate this problem, the wardens encouraged independent guides like Peter Lemieux to take people on glacier walking tours.

On July 13, Peter, who ran Athabasca Glacier Icewalks, was finishing a tour when his attention was arrested by a number of people shouting near the top of the main glacier tourist trail. When informed that a man was in a crevasse, Peter radioed the park and was told a rescue team was coming. Being familiar with crevasse rescue, he proceeded to the accident site to see if there was anything he could do. The victim in the crevasse was a doctor from Germany who had been taking a picture when he stepped back onto the snow-covered surface. The snow bridge gave way and he fell through, leaving only a hole at the lip. The man was over seven metres down, but he could still be heard when he replied to their calls.

Peter relayed the details of the accident to the approaching rescue team, then set about seeing what could be done. He first tried to lower a rope with a loop in the end to the victim. When it failed to reach him, Peter set up an ice anchor with several ice screws to give himself a belay to the edge of the crevasse to get a better idea of the situation. Because of the heavy snow cover, Peter could not determine exactly where the doctor was, so he attempted to reach him by entering the crevasse off to one side. In the process, however, he dislodged more snow that ended up on top of the victim. When he reached the doctor, all he could see were feet sticking out of the snow. Peter could no longer hear him but periodically the man's feet would flail when Peter tried to dig him out. But the confined area was now clogged by snow, making it difficult to free him.

Sylvia was the first person down after Peter had removed much of the snow. In fact the warden response was remarkable. Cliff White and two other wardens were doing a helicopter forest survey in a nearby valley when they got a call to fly directly to the glacier. The Sunwapta wardens had responded in record time, arriving 15 to 20 minutes after they got the call. Backup teams continued to arrive to relieve the digging effort but the doctor's body had already melted the ice about him which then began to freeze solidly to his body as his core temperature dropped. Sylvia went down to chip for 45 minutes until hypothermia started to deplete her reserves. She was relieved successively by other wardens slim enough to get down to him, but ultimately, being the smallest person around, she went down again for another hour after much of the doctor's body had been freed. They were greatly aided by the arrival of a power chipper, but it was clear that time was running out. It had taken them some hours to free him to the point of being able to get a raising system attached to bring him up, but the stress of moving can be fatal to a hypothermic body. Movement promotes increased circulation, drawing the colder blood from the extremities to the internal organs and causing them to go into shock. Sylvia was hopeful, however, when they were finally able to raise the doctor with her aid toward the lip of the crevasse. Then to her horror, as she held him, he looked at her briefly then died. The hours of toil brought her nothing but a haunting memory of that bleak face for years to come.

Two other fatal accidents occurred that summer. The next victim was dear to the hearts of many in the Warden Service, as he had the potential to be a vital member of the rescue service. His name was Simon Parboosingh—a young man, only 23 years old, who had just recently joined the Warden Service and was working in Lake Louise while taking his summer assistant guide exam. Though Simon had not been a member of the Warden Service for long, he had already made good friends. He was known for his generous good nature and sense of humour as well as his extraordinary talent as a climber. He was climb-

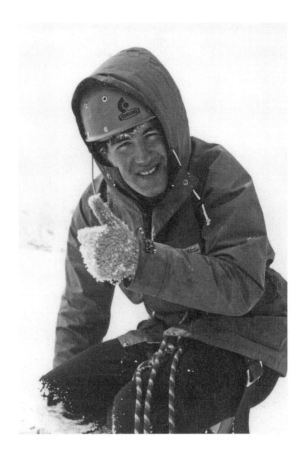

Simon Parboosingh. PERCY WOODS COLLECTION

ing at a standard rarely seen in the service, quickly making a name for himself on the extreme rock climbs being pioneered in the Rockies. Percy Woods, soon to enrol in the guide courses, knew him well and often joked they would be the next generation to replace the likes of Tim and Clair when they retired.

The tragedy of this accident was that it happened while Simon was on his summer assistant guide course. The guide and trainees were descending the upper slopes of Mt. Athabasca—making their way down the Silverhorn Route from the summit as part of the exam—when the accident occurred. The examining guide and the candidates he was roped to had already crossed a small soft snow slab, likely deposited by recent wind action, which may have destabilized the slope. When Simon

271

and his climbing partner Tim Pouchy crossed the slab, it released, hurtling the pair over the cliffs below. The lead guide fortunately had a radio with him and immediately had rescue warden Evan Manners and a party on the way. Tim amazingly survived the enormous fall over rock bands with only a thoracic injury to the chest, a broken shoulder blade and a fractured ankle. The rescue team found him on the surface, buried up to his shoulders, semi-conscious and incoherent. It took 10 more minutes to find Simon, who was completely buried. Evan later stated to the press: "Trying to find signs of life in a fellow warden was especially difficult … that made it so hard for us." Both men were immediately evacuated to the waiting ambulance below, but Simon was pronounced dead at 8:07 that night.

The accident underlined the difficult nature of assessing avalanche hazards, even for veterans in the field. The loss to the public safety training program was enormous. Many had counted on Simon being a strong member of a future public safety staff that would definitely be needed in the coming years.

The last accident of the summer was equally tragic, and one that stands out because of the difficulty of the dangerous mission. On September 1st, a young British couple set out to climb the standard ridge route on Mt. Victoria from Abbots Pass hut on an intermittently stormy day. The hut custodian was away that day and did not realize until the following morning that the couple had not returned. Another climber set off up the ridge to see if he could find signs of them but returned with no news. The alarmed custodian immediately descended to Lake O'Hara for help. Tim Auger responded quickly, conducting an aerial search of the face that evening, but high winds and low clouds restricted their effectiveness and they found nothing. The next morning, following some strange tracks seen the evening before over snow ledges well below the ridge on the east face, they found the young woman's body on the lower Victoria glacier at the foot of the face.

Finding her husband became much more difficult as the persistently bad weather closed ferociously in about the peak, limiting all flying and aborting an effort to sling a ground team onto the summit ridge. The following day the weather was worse. Still, they were able to drop off a party on the west approach route to the Abbot Hut from where they would try to continue up the ridge. This approach was the least favoured of all the options, however, because the ridge was in poor condition, being iced up and now cloud-covered and buffeted by severe winds. It would be a nasty, dangerous climb. The ground team succeeded in reaching the hut and even proceeded up to just short of the South Peak, but finally turned around when conditions became too dangerous to proceed safely.

On the morning of the fourth day, the weather cleared and the forecast was good for the day. Tim was finally able to put a team on the main summit to check the register and look for evidence of the climbers back along the ridge. Another party was slung onto the glacier at the base of the east face to search the crevasses below the cliffs, but when neither party found anything, the aerial search was resumed. With the much improved light, however, close examination of the face revealed an old sliding mark from the ridge below The Sickle, a particularly tricky, exposed section of the ridge between the south and main summits of the mountain. On a closer flight, they spotted something dark on the lower lip of a small crevasse on the east face. It turned out to be the end of a climbing rope that disappeared deep in the crevasse and led to the missing husband.

With the bright light of a slanted fall sun casting shadows across the face, Tim was able to piece together the tragedy of the climb. He wrote: "We'll never know exactly why they fell. They were wearing crampons. In any case, a bad slip here exposes climbers immediately to the steep smooth east face.

"The untied end of the rope suggests that the pair did slip here, one probably pulling the other off of an insecure belay, causing them to fall the length of the face until they were stopped by the crevasse, now the tomb of the husband. After the fall, [the woman] found herself below the ice cliff, and in the direction she searched, she probably could see no way to return to the summit ridge, so she began her treacherous descent. She apparently lost her footing immediately on entering the final slope. She was still wearing crampons, but it appears she had lost her ice axe and mitts some time earlier.

"This horrendous chain of events was initially triggered by a simple slip and failure to immediately self-arrest. [The husband] was probably killed in the crevasse fall (broken neck). It is understandable why [the woman] chose to descend rather than regain the ridge. In the end she was close to making it to safety; however, she must have been exhausted and without her ice axe to steady herself, the final slope amounted to a trap. This was an especially tragic story. She was five months pregnant." In a later interview, Mark Ledwidge pointed out that she had managed to descend over 300 metres, much of it difficult, before falling just short of reaching easier ground. She might have made it if she had had her ice axe to stop a slip.

OTHER CHANGES AT HIGHER LEVELS that year would have long-reaching consequences for the public safety program. Parks Canada had been slowly moving toward Agency status within the government, independent of direct fiscal control of department heads. It would be run as a business and expected to fund operations by recovering money from services provided. A new Director General took over to implement cost recovery, and it was a mandate she took seriously, especially in the field of public safety. This meant the cost of each rescue had to be fully recovered, or if possible, the rescue had to make money.

Turning this concept into reality became Clair's problem as current head of the public safety program in Western Canada. This was an enormous dilemma that other branches of search and rescue in Canada, such as the coast guard and military, had washed their hands of, realizing that in the huge expanses of Canada's lightly populated wilderness, it was totally impractical. When it came to the public safety program, the managers in Western Canada felt that while literature and signage and any preventative information served the public as a whole, specific rescues served only the individual. Therefore, the cost of each rescue must be recovered from that person in whatever manner possible.

Clair must have felt it was his karma to be faced with a problem he had already butted up against in the 1983 "Issue Analysis: Mountain Search and Rescue in the National Parks." At the time, the Public Safety Advisory Committee concluded Parks Canada Policy provided "no clear direction on what levels of mountain search-and-rescue service should be provided to the public." There was also no direction on what "objectives, responsibilities and levels of service should exist" for the delivery of a rescue service. The paper did point out that one subsection of the Policy Directive states that parks must "search for and provide aid to all visitors who are feared to be in distress or potential danger." It even goes so far as to say they should respond with aid for persons in distress outside of the park if called upon to do so. But it defined no realistic limits to the development of public safety services. Clair later pointed out that he felt that Parks had no "legislated mandate" to provide a rescue service. Without this mandate, there was no one responsible to see that the service had funds to sustain a certain standard of practice. Thus, when Agency status came about, those responsible for identifying where the money would come from were forced to say it must be generated by the program itself.

Clair knew that asking people to pay for their own rescues was going to create problems. So at the first meeting he said, "Put it into the gate fee structure." It was the most practical and realistic solution possible, but it contravened the desire to not shift "real costs to non-beneficiaries." Besides, by the time Clair was given this problem, other parks functions had already staked out much of those funds. It was a nightmare he would tackle with the aid of Dan Vedova, a park warden from Pacific Rim National Park, and with Jenny Sparks, on assignment from Ottawa to work on this and future risk management policy. Other people were involved during the process and at other levels, but most of the work was done out of Banff over a two-year period.

One of the first tasks was to assess the cost of rescues and decide what generated expenses. From there, they could determine possible ways to recoup monies. They investigated several avenues, the most onerous one involving insurance agencies to collect the money, leaving them the purse holders for the public safety program. This option worried Jenny, who saw the potential for a degradation of the public safety program if the insurance companies failed to distribute the necessary funds needed to employ trained personnel or supply adequate equipment. They were, after all, in the game to make money, meaning much of the profit would be pocketed by private industry. But without an insurance policy, the cost of a rescue was prohibitive.

At one point during the early eighties when the possibility of parks charging people for rescues was first hinted to the public, it engendered some strangely furtive behaviour. On one occasion Willi searched for two days looking for a couple of climbers overdue on Mt. Columbia. He did not find them, because they were hiding in a snow cave. They were convinced they would be charged for the rescue and hoped to sneak down the Saskatchewan Glacier rather than pay for the helicopter.

But one of the results of the cost assessment was uncovering where the real cost lay. Very little of the money needed for the program went toward risky, technical rescues. The majority of the funds actually went toward training and maintaining staff and equipment. It also turned out that the majority of responses to accidents occurred in the frontcountry, rather than with risk takers. Since the rescue team was maintained to deal with rescues, most of which occurred in high visitor use areas, it was logical to view all park visitors as having the potential for needing a rescue. The logical source of money, if this argument was embraced, was from the gate fees.

But the road to cost recovery through the gate fees meant dealing with what Dan felt was an entrenched ideology maintained by bureaucrats who were convinced that "low-risk people were indemnifying the high-risk user. " And that was not fair. It took days of detailed examination of statistics and cost analysis to dispel this concept, but before that was accomplished, there seemed to be a genuine move to enroll private insurance companies to take over the job.

This alarmed Jenny so much that she felt it was necessary to research the consequence of this action. Her feeling was that if private insurance companies became involved in recovering the cost of rescue, they would also have a controlling say in how the public safety program was run. They would look for ways to cut costs—which meant dictating the level of service available to the public. She felt this jeopardized the level of service no matter what money was brought in—it was just a question of time. She brought this to the attention of her manager at Pacific Yukon and to the risk management branch of the B.C. government and asked if she could do a risk assessment on this option of cost recovery. There were a number of elements to possible levels of risk—not only to the public but also to the wardens, who would have to work under possibly reduced safety margins. The resultant report, presented to park managers, indicated that this was a poor option that would put both government and the public at an unacceptable risk.

The outcome was very much a double-edged solution. The cost recovery efforts were dropped, but shortly after, so were the employees who were tasked with the solution. When the end of the year came around, their names were no longer associated with the positions they had held prior to this work. In fact, the positions themselves were eliminated.

Before this occurred, however, Clair was embroiled in two other controversial issues. The first of these was the Five Mountain Park Avalanche Plan instigated in 1993. Reg Bunyan was actually seconded from Kootenay National Park to work with Clair on this after parks were no longer involved with ski hills. The plan was intended to be a solution to the training dilemma forced on the wardens in public safety when the source of training at the ski hills dried up, but it was also tied into the cost-effective mentality of management at the time. It was also, in Reg's words, "a way to level the playing field—make things uniform, so that parks were doing the same thing and not off on their own wavelength."

Clair felt that it would be cost effective for all the parks to have a similar approach to avalanche control and forecasting that could be managed with an integrated avalanche control program. It would also ensure training opportunities for younger staff through reciprocal training programs with the Snow Research and Avalanche Warning Section people at Rogers Pass. It was a big step, but potentially had great returns. To help propel the concept, Clair hired Chris Stethem, now well established as a private avalanche consultant with a fairly significant reputation. Clair's objectives for Chris were to find a way to maintain expertise in avalanche control and forecasting as well as outline a cost effective way to unify the parks in their individual control programs. Problematically, this also included Glacier National Park, whose own unique and independent program was well established long before it became an issue for other parks.

With the advantage of being completely independent of Parks, Chris set about the task with an objective mind. He immediately recommended eliminating the park boundaries altogether, administratively and functionally, as a way to integrate the avalanche control program. The program could then be tied together with remote control weather stations and a computer that would manage the data and be linked to synchronized forecasting. A standardized avalanche control program could best be accomplished by adopting a 106 mm recoilless rifle mounted on a moveable trailer capable of being positioned in strategic locations throughout the five parks. Since there was a fire sale going on down in the United States just then, these rifles could be picked up at next to nothing along with the surplus ammunition. Cost wise, it was hard to pass up. Management could barely contain themselves, and they gave Clair the go-ahead to buy all he could.

Training wise, Chris suggested that the SRAWS folks at Rogers Pass adopt a few seasonal wardens for a couple of years and send some of their people to different parks to work directly with those operating in the field. In the end both Rupert Wedgwood and Lisa Paulson went to the pass for a couple of seasons, but that was as far as it went. What looked good on paper had little application in reality. As Reg would later reflect: "It was an interesting idea but was fundamentally flawed." Though the cost-cutting initiatives were seen as just "good sense" at the regional level in a government era of reduced dollar accountability, they were strongly resisted in the field. Even the idea of reciprocal training was fought by both the SRAWS personnel in Rogers Pass and the national parks in Alberta. Clair was alarmed at the growing animosity between the two levels of operation, but nothing prepared him for the "fire storm" over the 106 mm rifle.

The gun had many advantages beyond that of providing uniformity among parks. It was affordable and could be moved easily among target zones, giving it an all-weather operational capacity. Once an individual was trained in its use, he could go to any park and be familiar with the program. But the people in Rogers Pass had used the howitzer manned by the army since the inception of the gun controlled avalanche program and saw no reason to change. One of the disadvantages of the new gun was the type of ammunition it used. The shells used in the recoilless rifle are detonated upon impact with a hard surface, as the firepower is located at the base rather than in the nose. The howitzer shell, on the other hand, detonates even in soft snow as the firepower is in the nose. Because hard wind slabs rarely form in Roger Pass, the 106 mm increased the chance of rounds not exploding.

One advantage that Clair saw, however, was the opportunity to speed up the avalanche shoots. A growing problem at Rogers Pass was the limited highway space to park steadily increasing traffic flow during the period avalanches are shot down and the road cleared. Installing more than one gun at various target sites to bring down avalanches simultaneously could have alleviated this developing problem.

Despite some obvious advantages with the new ideas, the resistance to the Five Mountain Park Avalanche Plan was deeply entrenched and led to bitter confrontations. Before the new plan could be put into effect, it was defeated by a singular event in the United States. During an avalanche shoot in California, a 106 mm recoilless gun blew up, killing two forecasters, effectively ending its use there.

To give the field personnel in Rogers Pass credit, they did try to operate the gun, which now required a protective shield. But they had to string a long cord from behind the shield to the gun trigger. This was not rigged properly and when the gun was being raised to the correct setting for the high target, the cord was pulled too soon. The shell exploded on the other side of the highway instead of up on the mountain. This was the final demise of the whole controversial issue, and with much relief, everyone returned to the comfortable, time-worn system that had worked in each park since the inception of avalanche control in the early sixties.

The second controversial issue to land on Clair's plate during these years was one that the public safety wardens had hoped to avoid for all eternity. The Department of Transport had never been happy with the solid non-releasable sling hookup to the rescue helicopter. When the rescue helicopters in the U.S. and Europe moved over to a dual release (jettisonable) arrangement, the pressure to convert to this system in Parks Canada mounted steadily. In fact, by not using an jettisonable system, Parks Canada was the anomaly. Even the North Shore Rescue Group in Vancouver had a jettisonable system.

Added to this change, Transport Canada was also looking seriously at requiring a twin-engine helicopter for rescue work. But in this instance, the implacable bureaucracy steamrollered over the objections raised by both the wardens and helicopter pilots, and the dual release mechanism was adopted almost as a concession for not having to be saddled with twin-engine helicopters. Although the mechanism was hugely more expensive than the simple bolts used previously, it was far more affordable than twin-engine helicopters. With much grumbling (fixing what didn't need fixing), everyone was forced to adapt to the new method. The downside was that only qualified rescue leaders could attach the complicated device to the helicopter, meaning someone with this capability had to be on call at all time. Mark Ledwidge feared there might be a shortfall in qualified people available to attach the sling rope if rescue pressure continued to mount.

The looming threat of being required to use twin-engine helicopters for all rescue work was much more serious. In addition to going far beyond the small budget of Parks Canada, the helicopters were unsuitable to the work and added no measurable safety margin. Indeed, they were almost be a liability for their limited ability to hover in close quarters. An accident in the United States demonstrated their restricted ability in a tragic accident on Mt. Hood in Oregon. A twin-engine military helicopter was called in to rescue a group of students caught out overnight in a vicious storm. When the helicopter tried to hover long enough in the poor conditions to evacuate them, it crashed, leading to several deaths. Ironically, a single engine news helicopter hovered right above the scene, filming the whole sad event without a problem.

There were significant changes in "upgrading" other equipment as well. The winches for the cable rescue were becoming much more sophisticated, now having an automatic raising capability (power sourced) that reduced the number of men needed to effect a cable rescue. In one case, Percy Woods and Gord Irwin were able to do a two-man operation to bring an injured man up from the face of Mt. Edith by themselves. It was a hair-raising mission that Gord does not recommend, but they were still successful in getting the man off.

But it was during the early nineties that Tim and Clair decided to check the safety of the cables they were using—largely because Lloyd Gallagher had been working with Arnor Larson, who always stressed the importance of testing the systems he worked with. The concern over the cable harkened back to an incident that occurred much earlier in Glacier National Park, when Willi had one break during a rescue practice. At the time, the wardens thought it had happened because they were using a light cable. Willi immediately had all the rescue gear X-rayed for abrasions and found a surprising number of hidden flaws. Consequently, Tim and Clair decided to test the breaking strength of the cable at a rock quarry east of Banff. They loaded a weight similar to that of a victim and rescuer on the end and dropped the load over a sheer drop at various heights. To their horror it broke quite easily without much of a drop. This presented the cable in a new light. They quickly checked out the possibilities of putting more reliance on rope over the cable.

By 1995 the schism between The Regional Office in Calgary and the field staff in the parks was causing serious credibility problems. Many chief park wardens felt that the cost cutting should be extended to middle management rather than rest exclusively within the parks, but despite this, good people were still lost at the field level.

One of the first persons to leave the program that year was Gerry Israelson. Over the years Gerry, along with other leading members of the public safety program, had found himself at odds with the proposed changes coming out of Regional Office that his brother Clair was burdened with espousing. As the tension escalated between the two camps, it became more and more difficult for him to resolve his own beliefs and the responsibility he felt to the park. It finally came to a point where Gerry did not feel he could contribute effectively to the program. So when the opportunity arose to mentor young wardens through another aspect of work, he took it gladly and headed up the backcountry program in Jasper. He sincerely felt that leaving the battle to an uncompromised younger generation was the realistic thing to do, so that spring he graciously traded a rope for a horse. Fortunately, he was a gifted athlete and had no trouble picking up riding skills. The devious road to understanding horse mentality, however, took a little longer.

The people Gerry had worked with found his loss hard to take. He had set an example of leadership, courage, and friendship that would be difficult to replace from so limited a field. But public safety is the kind of work that attracts Type A personalities, and Gerry knew that the people he had been mentoring were up to the task. One of the more capable people was Steve Blake, who had started as a term warden in Jasper in 1992. His career in public safety was given a huge impetus that summer when he had the opportunity to climb extensively with Pat Sheehan as well as Gerry. He was already an accomplished rock climber but was keen to learn much as he could from the two veterans about the wilder world of high-end mountaineering. The following year he moved to Sunwapta for the summer (following Pat's death) where he literally plunged into the rescue world.

Steve's admiration for Gerry's ability in this field escalated after two significant rescues that required careful thought and a bit of daring. The incident on Mt. Andromeda began when two young, relatively inexperienced Parks Canada staff working at the Columbia Icefield Centre decided to test their ability by tackling Skyladder near the north face. The climb would have been successful had they not talked a young girl into going with them. They didn't encounter any real problem, however, until they came to the descent route. The girl took one look at the rotten bands of steep rock plunging into the abyss and the narrow exposed rock crest that had to be crossed and declared she was not going any farther with them. She had lost all confidence in their ability to get her down safely. They argued for hours as the weather slowly drifted in, making the last option to descend the way they had come up a poor choice as well. But now she was entrenched and refused to budge from where she thought she was safe—the summit of a high peak in the middle of the Columbia Icefield with a storm approaching.

With little choice, the boys left her on the summit and slowly negotiated the descent, finally reaching a radio at the upper parking lot at 1:00 a.m. Steve was woken to a broken message from the two saying they were safely down. This seemed like good news to Steve, who sleepily told them to give him a phone call in the morning if they wanted to chat. The next part of the message, however, got his attention. "Yah, well we left one member of our party on the mountain." With a brand new spin on the situation, he told them to get to a phone and relay the whole story. After weeding out the repeated apologies for leaving the girl on the mountain, he called Gerry to instigate a rescue.

By that time the upper part of the mountain was completely socked in. With a formidable forecast for the next few days, Gerry decided that they would have to climb in, expedition style, to set up fixed lines for the descent. They both anticipated finding a distraught, hypothermic woman unable to down climb the route that had so terrified her. He knew Steve was a strong and capable climber, and he was his first choice as rope partner to climb the route. A second warden team of Dave Smith and Terry Winkler were also brought in to help set a static line from the AA Col to the glacier below. With full loads the two wardens climbed the route thinking that the woman could quite well be dead. Steve was therefore surprised to see a head pop out of a mound of snow saying, "Boy am I glad to see you guys! What took so long?"

Relieved to find the feisty creature alive and coherent on the fog-bound summit, they set up the small tent and fortified her with hot tea before telling her she was about to be "guided" down the route she'd balked at the day before. Meanwhile, Steve thought he had time to fix his crampons that fitted poorly after being set for his ski boots and immediately started readjusting them while she pondered her fate. But the weather is a fickle mistress, and no sooner were his hands full of nuts and bolts, than the clouds parted, revealing the parking lot far below. Steve barely had time to cram the handful of nuts and bolts into his mouth before Todd McCready was on his way. There was no time to bring in a rescue harness, they decided. She would have to go off alone in the harness she climbed in.

The poor woman had little time to absorb the new development, which was probably just as well. She might have balked at swinging out over the north face of Andromeda, if she'd had time to think it over. As it was, the rescue line came in and she could only wail: "You're going to fly me out on just one carabiner?" As she departed from the summit rocks she had so adamantly refused to leave, Gerry's parting words were: "Yeah! And don't touch a fucking thing!"

With a few minutes to reflect on their next course of action—while Steve recovered his items of hardware glad he had not swallowed anything critical—they thought about getting a ride off themselves. Todd was up for the effort, but this time he would have to pick up two men and a load of gear. At over 3,000 metres with the less powerful 206 Jet Ranger and strange cross winds, the boys trusted Todd to make the call. When the rope came in and they clipped on, they were surprised to find themselves being dragged toward the sweeping chasm of the vertical north face. Todd could not lift the weight and knew the only solution was to gain air speed through a vertical drop. Steve looked over at Gerry, trying to say "It's okay! I can stay here and set up the tent for the night. You can come back and get me tomorrow!" But all he saw were eyes as big as saucers as they pendulumed out over the void in a giant arc, dropping like a stone as the helicopter sought denser air to power them forward. But Steve was into the process now, and just before they landed, he experienced a moment of elation thinking, "This is really good." He was also significantly impressed with Todd, but had to ask if he was having a bit of a problem with the weight. In classically laconic Todd style, he replied: "Yeah, I didn't have enough onions to get you guys up." The phrase still comes to Steve's mind with little bidding as he chuckles, "Yah. Onions!"

The denouement of the story came from the young woman herself, as they approached the parking lot. Brad White who had arrived in time to greet the lady recalls: "She was still in the air when she yelled 'I don't care how much this costs! I still wouldn't go down with those guys. They could have killed me!'"

The second rescue that increased Steve's appreciation of Gerry's skill as a rescue leader occurred on Mt. Robson. The warden office received the call from a couple of guides from Yamnuska Mountain Adventures who were climbing up toward The Dome. It was a fine warm day—hot almost—when they heard cries for help from above. When they got to the individuals in distress, they found one fellow barely holding his partner who had fallen in a large crevasse. The two guides worked their way to the survivor on the uphill slope where they set up a solid ice belay to bring the man up. At that point, they ran into trouble when they could not get him over the lip of the crevasse.

Steve recalls they arrived to find the three men struggling valiantly to get the fellow to safety. At this point the lightly clad man had been down for several hours and was showing the strain. He was also still wearing a large pack which aggravated the problem. Gerry quickly pointed out that the raising system was set up on the wrong side of the crevasse, and immediately had everyone working on a second raising system on the lower side where there was no overhanging lip to contend with. Steve was sent into the crevasse on the downhill side where he was able to reach the victim and attach him to the second anchor. Once this was accomplished, it was slick work to bring the two men to the surface. Steve took the exercise to heart, realizing immediately the value of the lesson and appreciative of the experience saying: "So this was a good one for me … just to see him working in the rescue business and assessing the site within two seconds."

It was fortunate that Steve had had the opportunity to be involved in technical rescues as well as some demanding warden climbing schools. The mentorship he received aided greatly in his progress toward full guide status, all of which he would need when Gerry left in 1995. Steve moved into an acting supervising position as field rescue leader in Jasper. He worked for Will Devlin, who replaced Gerry as head of public safety in that park. Will had come to Jasper as the dog handler when Dale Portman vacated the position in 1993 and was the only permanent warden in public safety available to fill the position. Everyone else with any degree of climbing experience was still working at the seasonal level. Realistically, Brad White was the logical choice to replace Gerry, but he had moved back to Banff that year to be with his family. The long-term separation was too much of a strain on this arrangement and it was with reluctance that he passed on the opportunity.

WHILE JASPER WAS ABOUT TO UNDERGO a period of instability following Pat's death, Banff fared better with Tim Auger at the helm. Tim had an uncanny ability to survive several near-death experiences as well as a challenging career in the volatile public safety arena. When Clair asked him if he wanted to take a turn at running the position in the Regional Office in Calgary, he discreetly refused. He had no longing to jump into that head-slashing environment. He was happy with the situation in Banff and the people working there. Mark Ledwidge split his time between Lake Louise and Banff, working with both Tim and Gord Irwin, now looking after public safety in that field unit. Gord also had Percy Woods working for him in a training position after he started his guide courses in 1995.

By 1996 the survival of the middle management positions in Regional Office was looking doubtful. The cost recovery efforts in rescues and the avalanche plan not only failed but also created an atmosphere of suspicion and dissent that eroded field support for Clair's position. It was still a surprise for him, however, when the job was eliminated in the spring of that year. Clair was asked to take over front-country management in Banff, while Dan Vedova went back to Pacific Rim. Jenny Sparks, also a casualty of the cost recovery program, was offered work in the Department of Fisheries and Oceans. The alpine specialist position that formerly united all the parks was gone, apparently for good, and the only unifying element left was the still operational Public Safety Advisory Committee.

The move to frontcountry had the predictable effect on Clair that surprised no one. It was not his field nor remotely in the realm of his interest. Finally on one rainy afternoon while out for a bicycle ride he gave himself a chance to think things over. Auspiciously the sun broke through the clouds, highlighting the beauty of the mountains, offering a glimmering insight into what he should do next. It was working as a rescuer in the mountains that had brought him to Parks Canada, and if that was no longer possible, there were other opportunities. He was still a full

guide and that opened up many different fields. For a brief time he worked in his own business aiding others to access helicopter sling systems, but not long after he was offered the executive director position for the Canadian Avalanche Association. It was eminently suited to him and without a look back, he gladly took the job.

OPERATIONALLY, FOR THOSE LEFT running the public safety program, nothing really changed. The availability and quality of the rescue service to the public continued with the same excellence. If anything, the service was more efficient than ever and the training, though less frequent and not mandatory for all wardens, continued at a high standard. But the atmosphere had changed. There was more competition for the few public safety jobs available and two in-house deaths lent a greater seriousness to the work. Much of the carefree feeling of the seventies or the spontaneity of the eighties was lost in an atmosphere of a new mindfulness. The training schools were not characterized by hilarious star-filled nights on remote glaciers, where tension was relieved with rum and snowball fights. The days when large numbers of wardens sharing these experiences from parks far and sundry were over, and only those with useful public safety skills or those marked for advancement attended.

Not all the parks had the luxury of having highly trained personnel for rescue work to the degree Banff did, however. The smaller parks still had to make do with no qualified guides and a staff that was trained mostly in-house. Even Jasper had no fully certified guide on staff after Brad and Gerry left. But the park was still well staffed with talented people, having both Steve and Sylvia working toward full guide status, and already possessing excellent ability and experience. Lisa Paulson, now running Sunwapta Warden Station, also had excellent climbing and skiing skills that had given her reason to consider the guide course. By this time, Rupert Wedgwood was pursuing what would be a chequered course on his road to full guide. Will Devlin, himself no slouch in public safety, had excellent management skills and was not too concerned about the guideless status of the park. There were many other wardens in Jasper who had been around for years and could still play a critical role in a rescue situation. People like Greg Horne, Rick Ralf, Evan Manners and Murray Hindle provided a much-needed backup and were often called for rescues. Another staff member, Randy Fingland, was also working at Sunwapta and through close association with Sylvia had honed his climbing skills to an above-average standard.

With this array of capable people, Will felt he had a strong core of wardens to respond to rescues. Sylvia moved into the public safety training position in Jasper townsite, where she worked closely with Steve and Will in responding to rescues, many of which were on the Columbia Icefield. Will remembers well one of the successful rescues he attended with Gerry before he left.

A group of friends were returning from a climbing trip on the Columbia Icefield but were not experienced enough to ski roped together through the crevasses. They kept falling over trying to cope with the rope in the uneven snow. Rather than ski at an equal pace, one person after another untied, leaving the leader to ski on ahead trailing the rope.

When they all grouped together on the second icefall beneath the summit cliffs of the Snow Dome, they realized the last person was missing. Nor could they see her anywhere above. They quickly retraced their tracks, and found she had fallen into a crevasse. They decided to send the second girl down for help while the two men remained behind to raise her out. Once again inexperience was a problem. One man went down to attach her to the rope leaving only one person on top to bring her up. Unfortunately, he did not know the mechanism of the pulley system for crevasse rescue, and when he tried to pull her up with a direct pull, he only succeeded in raising her above the snow she had landed on. But he could

not lower her either. The rope had frozen into the overhanging lip of the crevasse, holding her fast in her harness beneath the dripping walls. He could not raise the second man either, and by the time the wardens got there, they had to deal with two people in the hole.

The rescuers first had to find a safe place to establish a camp and set up an anchor. The place was riddled with crevasses, and they had only a small working area of two metres or so. It was amazing that the whole party hadn't fallen in, and it seemed a miracle that the lone woman sent out for help had even made it to the highway. Sylvia was sent down to bring up the now very hypothermic young woman. The girl was soaked to the skin and almost paralyzed from hanging in the restrictive webbing of the harness for several hours.

It was good they had sufficient manpower, because the rope sent down to raise the woman inadvertently got crossed with the rope the second man was hanging on. Suddenly, when the additional weight came on the line, the anchor began to pull. Steve Blake, who was field rescue leader, quickly had Randy sit on the buried skis until everyone was safely out of the crevasse. Once on the surface the woman was momentarily exposed to a fierce wind. But the tent they had set up for her was right on the edge of the crevasse, and she was bundled up immediately in down jackets and sleeping bags. Though the tents were ringed with crevasses, it was the exposure to the icefall above the Snow Dome cliffs that worried them. The five rescuers and one skier crammed into the one tent got little sleep as they warmed bags of Magic Pantry and water bottles to hand to Randy and Will who were in the other tent with the woman and the other skier.

All hope of getting her out that night was gone, but that may have saved her life. She was in extreme pain from hanging in the harness as long as she had and was so badly hypothermic that any attempt to move her further might have been fatal. With a tent, sleeping bags, dry clothing and food waiting, she was bundled up next to warm, supporting bodies. Unfortunately, one of the would-be supporting bodies was that of her party leader, who had formed an unreciprocated attachment to the young woman. Seeing that she needed to be warmed, and without consultation with the wardens, he attempted to climb into the sleeping bag. This seemed to alarm the girl who was already stressed from the cold and the pain. Randy diplomatically persuaded the fellow to let himself and Will handle the warming through the night.

For Will, the experience was remarkable as the woman hovered between unconsciousness and semi-consciousness, able to take warm liquids intermittently but all the while moaning and groaning as she fought for her life. He was amazed at the warming process, feeling the coldness of her skin turn warm as the blood circulated through her body like a tide of cold and warm water, surfacing then submerging from the core of her being. As the blood warmed around the precious vital organs, it flowed to the limbs, only to cool there until the process was repeated, slowly raising the body temperature without sending her into fatal shock. Randy recalls that the circulation of blood seemed to be triggered by any movement she made. When she shifted her legs or moved an arm, the cold blood from the limbs would circulate to the body core and lead to unconsciousness.

By morning, she was out of danger, but Will believes even a few more minutes in the crevasse could have been disastrous. It was one of the few times that rescuers fought so hard to save another human being over a prolonged period and succeeded. Sylvia, herself, never really warmed up until she was flown out, spending a chilly night on the glacier despite having adequate gear.

She recovered to go on many more rescues, some of which she shared with Lisa Paulson. The two women thrived in the competitive, male-dominated field and formed a strong partnership that played a big part in a difficult recovery that summer. It is noteworthy for being the only all-female rescue/recovery done in the short history of mountain rescue in Canada. It involved a party of two men who were climbing the difficult Centennial route on the north face of Mount Colin. They were more than halfway up when the leader took a fatal fall. When Sylvia got the call, she was able to reach Lisa as well as Randy and Al McKeenan, a young seasonal warden with basic rock climbing skills. The winds were terrible when they arrived, so she decided to go in immediately with Lisa, as they were the most experienced technical climbers of the four. They were only able to get to a low promontory on the mountain before the winds picked up even more, preventing the pilot from bringing in the other two wardens. With conditions worsening, Sylvia decided that she and Lisa might be able to handle it by themselves. They had to climb into the location, where they bundled the body up and prepared to lower him to the base of the mountain. The descent was long and arduous, with Sylvia guiding the cumbersome form over cliff bands as Lisa lowered her from anchor to anchor until they reached the bottom. They had to wrestle him a considerable distance from the rock face before it was safe enough for the helicopter to reach them through the gale-like winds. Sylvia now reflects on the effort with some pride but ruefully notes: "It would have been very difficult if he were alive and hurt."

Steve Blake had his hands full with another big rescue on Mt. Robson that required using multiple rescue skills. Five people in two parties had set out to climb the Kain Face in whiteout conditions, and had wound up establishing their bivouac camp below The Dome in a highly crevassed, avalanche prone area. During the night, a falling serac triggered a large avalanche that swept the upper party of two men down the slope where one fell into a deep crevasse. The other three with the survivor searched for this missing man an hour and a half before going for help.

When Steve got the call, he realized he would need experienced people to operate safely in that location. It was initially reported as an avalanche incident, so he brought in both Will Devlin and a CARDA dog handler to search the debris. With better light during the day, it did not take long for the search to turn into a crevasse rescue. They were working in a dangerous location requiring spotters to watch for collapsing seracs and avalanche activity. It was imperative to reduce their exposure to the dangers, so once the body was brought to the surface, Steve left it there to evacuate the rescue team. Then he returned by sling to retrieve the body. The rescue was done as quickly as possible and everyone returned safely. This made Steve happy; he was particularly satisfied with the way the team had worked in the difficult terrain, feeling they had come a long way in their ability to respond to the multi-task rescues on the always dangerous Mt. Robson.

RIVER RESCUES ALSO CONTINUED to crop up often enough to remind wardens that water was still a dangerous element. In fact, Tim always thought this type of rescue was most likely to include an element of surprise. In July, Tim was called to a canoe wreck in the Bow River in the middle part of Hoodoos Trouble Channel not far from the Banff townsite. There was a root ball in the middle of the channel that had initiated the accident with the first party, but canoe mayhem suddenly multiplied as party after party dumped in the same stretch of river. As they were picking up two stranded paddlers on an island, another canoe tipped in the troublesome water even before the first group were taken to safety. The people were all picked up by the jet boat, leaving the wardens to salvage the canoes and gear now blocking the channel. While clearing the waterway the next day, two more canoes wiped out at the same location. One was spotted floating by without the occupants, leaving yet more people to pick up. Aside from the unusual volume of work here, Tim was amazed at the strength of the current, and the force the water exacted when they were trying to recover the canoes.

Water recoveries were probably more common in Waterton, which is peppered with accessible waterfalls, the most well known being Cameron Falls near the townsite. A tourist happened to notice some young people trying to cross a log above the fall. She decided to notify the RCMP thinking it was dangerous, but even as she reported their behaviour, a man fell in. Within minutes the wardens were on scene to conduct a hasty search where the man was last spotted. By now a sizable rescue force had been assembled, consisting of wardens, RCMP officers and civilian volunteers. They even had a scuba diver who searched the bottom of the falls.

But almost as soon as a wallet was been recovered, giving the RCMP the victim's name, the man's fiancé and a friend arrived to relate the sequence of events that led to his fall. They had all been outside the protective fence above the falls when the man slipped and fell in. The difficult part for the family and witnesses was watching the man struggle to reach safety before succumbing to the force of the water. He had been carried over the first series of falls to a bench that breaks up the drop to the lower falls. He stopped momentarily here and could be seen standing, but when he tried to get out, he was caught by the current and swept over the main falls. By the time Derek Tilson got there, the people were in hysterics, thinking the man could still be saved.

After the initial search, they realized that the man must be trapped behind the lower fall. A closer look revealed a rock fissure, much like a crevasse, that was his likely resting place. The following morning, armed with a meat hook secured to a long pitch pole, they went back and continued probing. They managed to hook the body and hoped to pull it free with eight people on the end of a rope attached to the probe. The force of the pull only succeeded in launching the pole vertically out of the crack at great force. Repeated attempts throughout the day produced nothing, indicating the body was wedged in and held by the unrelenting force of the falling water. They shut down the efforts once again, hoping the family would appreciate their efforts.

283

Consultation with other agencies did not lead to anything workable but something had to be done. They bit the bullet and decided to lower a man into a position giving them leverage to yank the body free. They approached the family and asked if they had any objections to this drastic recovery action. The family was more than pleased that an effort was still under consideration and agreed readily.

The next day, Derek went down to attempt the unpleasant task and succeeded in setting the hook, although he did not know precisely where. The ropes were attached to a pulley system set up at the far side of the falls to provide added leverage, but this time, the hook was set deep between the bones and held. The men began pulling, stretching the rope tighter and tighter until "it was thin as a dime." Derek remembers that "The body just fired out of there … it went right across the whole Cameron Falls pool. That is one memory I will always have. The body just suddenly sprung … spooosh! Completely across the pool!" One warden later said it popped like a champagne cork, flying across the water, landing almost at the feet of the waiting family on the far side. The appalled wardens immediately ran over to cover the man before anyone went into shock. The suddenness of the solution surprised everyone, but the family took it in stride. They were so appreciative of the stout efforts from the wardens to recover their son, that all they had was praise for the outcome. Derek was pleased with this reaction, reflecting that sometimes it was necessary to go the extra length—even for a body.

THE YEAR OF 1997 CLOSED with one other major change in the administrative structure. The downsizing in Regional Office in Calgary extended to the field, which directly affected Yoho and Kootenay. The effort to reduce upper management resulted in the amalgamation of Yoho and Kootenay with Lake Louise, effectively splitting Banff National Park administratively. The new region of Kootenay, Yoho and Lake Louise, now known as KYLL (or the "kill" zone) now had only one chief park warden and superintendent. Other positions that were eliminated were the heads of different functions such as fire, backcountry and public safety. Gord Irwin was put in charge of public safety for the amalgamated region, thus greatly extending his responsibility. He still had the resources from those parks, however, to handle the increased rescue, training and administrative load. The shuffle had reduced the number of wardens who had a direct hand in rescue work as they were now handled out of Lake Louise. This was now possible as the technical improvements with helicopters gave them the power and speed to respond efficiently throughout the region.

By 1998 the question of cost recovery in public safety was grinding its way to a final resolution, but the idea that people must pay for their mistakes was a hard one to abandon for those who saw risk sport as an elevated level of social irresponsibility. But if there was still some uncertainty about sending a bill to the family to recoup costs for rescue efforts, it died a final death with the loss of Michel Trudeau, son of former Prime Minister Pierre Trudeau. After skiing with friends in the Kokanee Glacier area of B.C., the group was hit by an avalanche on the trip out. The route back to civilization had taken them around a small frozen lake, requiring they ski beneath the bottom slope of a sizable avalanche path. The avalanche conditions were poor, making the crossing a tricky adventure that ended in tragedy. The avalanche swept Michel Trudeau into the freezing water, leaving no possibility for survival. Three of the friends remained while the rest skied out for help, reporting the accident to the RCMP in Nelson. But as is so often the case, the weather moved in and the hazard increased, making it impossible for a ground party to reach the site. In fact, the RCMP were now quite worried about the survival of the rest of the party. They immediately called the Banff warden office to see if they could help.

Letters of thanks are rarely received by the Warden Service, so the one sent by Sergeant

284

Wayne Buck of the Nelson detachment after the event was happily put in the rescue report in the Banff files. He wrote: "When the avalanche was reported to our office we were unable to respond by air due to the weather conditions at Nelson. Our ground parties were stalled due to the avalanche threat and might not have been able to reach the avalanche site. When your staff were contacted for assistance the response was immediate and their actions resulted in the safe recovery of three victims. Without the assistance of wardens Mark Ledwidge, Scott Ward and helicopter pilot Ken Gray the three who survived the avalanche might well have perished. The dedication displayed went well above the line of duty and has not gone unnoticed. Please convey my sincere appreciation to those involved."

Because the wardens flew in from Banff, they were able to fly north around the storm engulfing the Nelson area, where they found a hole in the clouds that allowed them to reach the lake. But it was "tricky flying." Once there, the dog confirmed there was no body in the avalanche debris. The wardens concurred with the party's assessment that Michel had been swept into the lake with the avalanche debris which had plunged well past the shoreline. The weather and the difficulty of searching the icy water, now freezing over, made further recovery efforts impossible, leaving only the possibility of retrieving the body in the spring.

Mark was not surprised to hear that the Trudeau family was prepared to leave the young man to the lake as his final resting place; they certainly did not think it was worth risking anyone's life for the sake of a more formal funeral. Mark did not think a bill for the services rendered was appropriate after such a gracious decision to avoid a difficult recovery.

The fact that it was even in the cards was astonishing. Dan Vedova felt compelled to send a note to Tom Lee, Assistant Deputy Minister for Parks Canada, saying, "Who in this country will present the Trudeaus with a bill for this search?" Clearly no one wished to sign that invoice. It brought to light the debatable issue of deciding who deserves a bill after a rescue situation. It demands blame be laid with a price tag, sometimes at the door of the innocent. Quite conceivably, a family could be presented with the body of a son or daughter along with a rather large bill when the dead person cannot pay up. The incongruity of the whole cost recovery cause was at last put to rest with the decision to make good the monies from the well-distributed gate fees. It was surprisingly little: about a nickel out of every 10 dollars. When Parks Canada assumed the role of agency in 1998, the solution was solidified and has not yet resurfaced.

It was during this time that management began making moves to settle the public safety positions in Jasper as well. Will Devlin had been acting dually as head of public safety and as a dog handler during the interim. Most dog handlers find keeping up with the dog work more than sufficient, and as Will says, he "put in a lot of long hours." It was time to resolve the staffing issue. But Will had enjoyed the work; he was a good administrator and was well liked by his staff. There had been no problems with the park's ability to perform rescue operations with efficiency and competence, and the park management had no objections when Will put in for the job. He won the position, but concern was raised about his lack of full guide status. More than any other event, this competition illuminated the requirement for accredited certification.

The decision was appealed then re-appealed by Will. In the end, he retained the job, but it was a bitter win. He was not supported in the role externally, and in the end he opted for a job at the equivalent level (Ski Hill Liaison Officer) in Lake Louise.

When the competition came up for the supervisory position, Steve Blake placed first. As a full guide, and an equally good administrator, Steve was an ideal choice. A competition for the position of field rescue leader that Steve had vacated came up shortly thereafter and was successfully filled by Rupert Wedgwood.

Filling the two public safety positions in Jasper helped the wardens gain a welcome sense of stability. The alliance between the Warden Service and the guides association was growing stronger and was probably deepened when wardens and guides alike lost a close friend. It was a simple accident that was made difficult to accept for the sheer randomness of the circumstance. But simple accidents can happen anywhere, and in this case one occurred at the base of Mt. Little, one of the many peaks typified by loose rock in the Valley of Ten Peaks above Moraine Lake. The guide, Karl Nagy, one of Canada's most respected climbers and good friend to many, was hit on the head by a rock missile from high above. Despite the fact he was wearing a hard hat, the large rock had fallen far enough to kill him instantly. With dismay the student he was roped to tried to revive him with CPR, but he was beyond all help.

It was a particularly good friend, Gord Irwin, who flew in on the rescue mission, an experience Tim could well relate to. Gord reflected later: "I never thought I'd have to try and rescue a friend, but there was always that possibility." He added: "This trail was not particularly hazardous … we have all commented on how bizarre this accident was."

To add to the difficulty, they were not given the quick uncomplicated body evacuation they had hoped for, considering the easy terrain. As the weather closed in, they were only able to land at 2,700 metres, where they accessed the site by ground. Mark Ledwidge, a member of the rescue party and also a close friend, began to realize they might not get Karl out as easily as they hoped. As the cloud and snow thickened, the only option was to move the body down to the Neil Colgan Hut, where they spent the night, consoled somewhat by mutual commiseration over the loss of such an unassuming yet gifted companion. Their vigil was relieved early the following morning when the weather cleared enough to fly both the rescue party and the body back to the Lake Louise warden office.

The rescues continued unabated through the summer in all the parks. Two significant searches highlighted the occurrences in Banff in the Cascade/Minnewanka area. The first long search in June came to a successful conclusion when a missing hiker was found by aircraft. The second search in July for a young man did not turn out as well for the victim. The body of the scrambler, who had fallen on Cascade Mountain, took a week to find, re-emphasizing the ruggedness of the terrain around this popular mountain.

Jasper had more success in a very unusual rescue when a young man was fished out of the Sunwapta River after surviving a tumble over the falls. It was one of the few water rescues that ended in success, due to a well-rigged rescue line and the willingness of one water-wise warden to attempt the rescue. The accident happened the way so many did near waterfalls: A young man climbed over the railing to get a closer look, slipped on the rocks and plunged over the falls. The usual number of tourists saw him go over, but were astonished to see him bob to the surface, where he clung to a log jammed against the rock wall under the overhanging cliffs. Calls for a rescue went out the minute the man went over and the response was immediate.

Al McKeenan was a kayaker who knew a lot about fast, turbulent water and volunteered to be lowered down to the hapless man below. He was not thinking of Tim Auger's warning about water rescue, but agreed with Tim's view that water "has a sting in it"—an unpredictable element that could catch the rescuer off guard. Steve Blake directed the setup of the rescue lines to bring Al as close as possible to the victim. Fortunately, the massive overhang forming the canyon below allowed the rescuer to be lowered to within six metres of the man. Al was outfitted with a wet suit and a radio strapped to his chest. When the lowering and raising apparatus was assembled, Al went down, continually communicating directions to the team, apprising them of his location in relation to the pool below and the victim. It was his intention

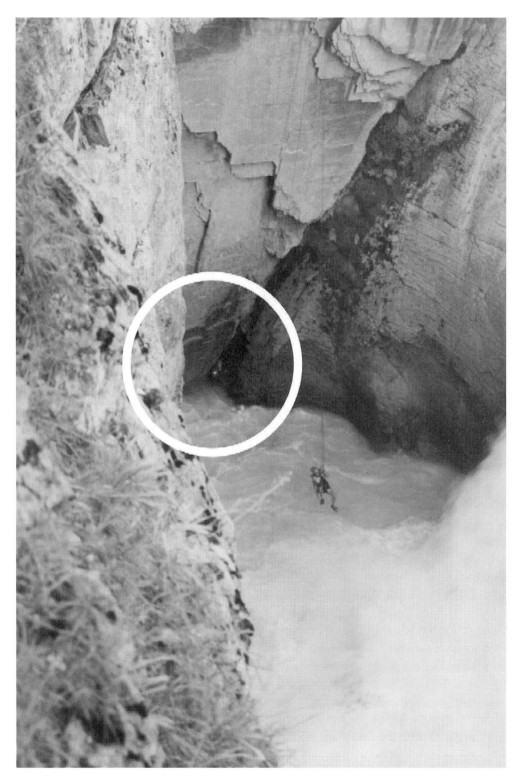

Al McKeenan on Sunwapta Falls rescue. JASPER WARDEN ARCHIVES to scoop the man into a diaper-type rescue seat once he reached him.

The minute he landed in the pool, however, the force of the water filled the rescue seat and began to drag him under. The tremendous power of the current forbade any attempt at swimming, and he soon found he was struggling to keep above the water. It also hampered his attempt to get at the radio. He finally got the mike close enough to his mouth to give urgent instructions to raise him up as quickly as possible. Steve was on top of the situation and soon had Al free of the deadly current. It was apparent that swimming over to the man was not going to work.

But Al realized he was not that far away from the man, who had watched his every move. The next solution was to toss a throw bag to him to establish a hand line that Al could use to pull himself over. The roar of the huge waterfall was deafening and spectacular, keeping the adrenaline running through his system, almost but not quite helping him to forget how cold the water was. The young man clinging to the log had no problem understanding that he was to grab the throw bag and secure it to the log. He caught it on the second toss and immediately wrapped the rope about the exposed wood. With the line in place it was not a problem for Al to haul himself over to the grateful victim.

The next stage went smoothly, but it was a spectacular sight for the tourists that day. Al got the man in the rescue seat and calmly told the boys to raise away. The sudden upward pull launched the man into space where he swung against the backdrop of the cascading falls as he spun upwards to safety. It was Al's turn next, and his departure was even wilder as he almost spun into the down rushing water of the falls. But he went up quickly and avoided a drenching in the heavy spray. It was over within minutes of reaching the man.

People in the rescue business are always amazed at how quickly the rescued person tries to leave the scene before accounting for what happened. The young man was not hurt at all except for being a little chilly, and once on firm ground, he tried to get to his car. Steve managed to slow him down, saying they needed to get a few questions answered. The man had clearly broken the rules by jumping over the barricade. The wardens also wanted to know how he had survived almost certain death. It turned out that he had hit the current exactly right. The main force of the water drove him to the bottom of the pool. When he looked up he could see light above him and he shot up, hitting the one eddy that pulled him to the log. Normally victims get caught in the whirlpool back current that keeps them circulating below the falls where they drown—if the impact doesn't kill them. The comment on the rescue sheet is succinct: "The dude who survived this was very lucky indeed."

THE YEAR 2002 SAW THE BEGINNING of huge changes in the way Parks Canada would handle rescue training and standards and doing business with the public. But before these changes were set in motion, the wardens were involved in two interesting rescues that highlighted their dedication and their personal risk. The first was in Rogers Pass on Mt. Sir Donald. The rescue involved high drama seen by no one except the victim who sent the park a remarkable letter of thanks that illuminated his side of the story.

He began his letter by informing both Don McTighe from Alpine Helicopters and the rescue staff from Glacier National Park that he was well on the way to recovering from "two fractures to the upper left side of the skull, a broken right wrist, a puncture wound to [his] left abdomen, a broken nose and several obvious good cuts to [his] face." The letter related how he and his partner reached the summit at 1:00 p.m. after a snowy ascent from the bivi site below the Uto-Sir Donald Col. Despite deep snow covering the upper 300 metres of the mountain, they descended quickly until they reached the steep part of the ridge. He had just gathered the excess rope and was putting in a nut after clipping through old rappel slings to protect his descent, when he noticed the rock was quite slippery. His next waking sight was of Mt. Uto in the distance as he hung from his harness well down the yawning face.

His buddy quickly rappelled down to him, only to find him incoherent and babbling with little memory of the climb. His friend managed to secure him on a small ledge where he set a good anchor. By now the injured man was becoming more focussed, and he realized his injuries made continuing down out of the question. Shock and hypothermia sent him into violent shivers after his friend left for help. It does not state in the letter that the partner had been pulled off his stance by the fall and had only been saved by the rappel sling.

Jordy Shepherd got the call after returning from a search for an overdue hiker in Mt. Revelstoke National Park. The weather was indeterminate when he called Don McTighe to come from Golden to fly the route, looking for what he was sure would be a body. After hearing the extent of the injuries the man had suffered, he did not think the man could have survived the chilling storms of the previous night. The flight revealed the mountain to be as ugly as it could get in early August, which made Jordy sit back a little stunned when they saw the man waving at them through the snowy mist. He thought suddenly: "Now we have a *real* rescue." The weather was so closed in he doubted if they would be able to get him off with the helicopter as they flew down to reassess the situation. Jordy was already considering climbing in to reach the man, wrestling with all the thoughts that besiege a man about to risk his life for a climber who didn't die.

Eric Dafoe with whom he would normally undertake this level of climb was away, so after consulting with Don, he decided to first give the sling a try. Though the mountain was shrouded in cloud, there was no substantial wind, which made it possible to get in if they had visibility. He was accompanied by Brian Higgins, who really hoped they wouldn't have to climb the route. They took in gear in case that had to be the option.

After Jordy returned to make the first of many passes on the end of the sling, the victim gave a thumbs up, hoping the warden knew he needed help. But he was worried, writing later, "After an hour, I began to worry that my waving had been interpreted as 'I'm okay, don't worry about me.'" Confusion and doubt now plagued the freezing man, who was slowly becoming conscious of how much pain he was in. But he did what he could, putting his pack in order and attempting to cut the rappel rope that held him in case the rescue efforts worked.

Jordy was going nuts with the miasma of fog that clung to the black rocks, revealing from moment to moment the vertical face sliding away to the distant glacier, then engulfing them so completely he could not even see the tail rotor. The slinging was made all that more difficult as he needed to go in with a full pack in case he managed to land but could not be picked up. At one point he was able to get close enough to show the man he had a separate rescue attachment for him that he would just clip into the harness.

As the clouds engulfed them, they would fly off, only to return when the shadowy black forms materialized into the rock face that sheltered the fallen form moving more feebly now. But not only were they plagued with erratic visibility, when they could get a bearing on the man's position, it became apparent that the rock was so steep Don would not be able to get close enough to lower Jordy directly in without hitting the blades. He would have to pendulum the rescuer in if he got the chance. But their persistence paid off when suddenly they got the break they needed. Don got close enough to tip him in, giving him a very small window in which to free the man before swinging into the void below.

Jordy quickly clipped the man on, asking where the anchor was. The happy climber, trying to grin, said he had cut it. But experience or instinct made Jordy look for himself. "Whatever it was I saw, something looked weird—not right, fatal. I had the knife with me and I just slashed it." What he

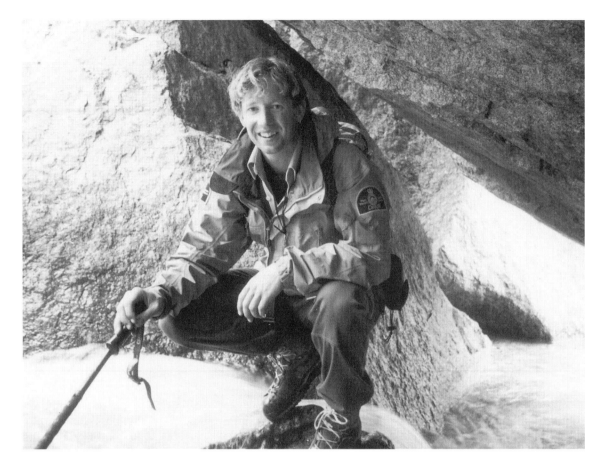

Jordy Shepherd. STEVE BLAKE COLLECTION

slashed was the deceitful rappel rope. The man had indeed cut the climbing rope his partner had tied him in with, but he was still attached to the rappel line. With Don urging them to go he gave the all clear sign, and the two men dove into the fading day in a falling descent that relieved Don greatly.

Neither Jordy nor Don feel they did anything heroic. Both emphasize that the rescue went smoothly despite the underlying tension not to "screw up." Jordy was confident that things would go well as long as he did everything right. Don also feels it went well; he was only flying as he was trained to do. But the man who wrote the letter from the hospital felt differently. "I owe my life to all of you, along with Matt [the climbing partner]

and everyone involved in the rescue. Know that your skills and dedication are very much appreciated."

Don McTighe is proud of this letter. Every once in a while it is nice to know that the work you do is recognized by those who have the most to gain.

A similar dedication was demonstrated by Mark Ledwidge under much different circumstances. It was not the dramatic mountain rescue with a quick recovery, but a long drawn-out search for a missing hiker that only came to a happy conclusion through Mark's persistence. It first came to his attention that a young woman was missing when her mother called from Texas saying she had not returned home for her birthday. She only knew that her daughter's plans were to hike in the Banff area in Canada. With not much more to go on, and wondering why the mother was so reticent about any detailed information concerning the missing woman, Mark started by checking backcountry permits to see if she was registered out. He found no recent registration, but did find a couple of old park use permits that had been returned. When the mother called back a day or so later, he felt it was time to be blunt. He told the mother that if she did not fill him in on the woman's background, they could be of no further help. It slowly emerged that she was diabetic, had a history of schizophrenia, was recently divorced and had been depressed and withdrawn after quitting her job in the family business. With this encouraging information, Mark felt they had better step up the efforts—it was beginning to sound like a medical emergency, possibly a suicide.

Mark started again, now going to the hostel where she had last stayed, hoping to find a clue from someone there. The RCMP were also investigating her disappearance from a criminal aspect, and he was able to check on the use of her credit card. On her first permit she was registered out alone, but on the second trip, she travelled with two other people she had met. She had checked out of the hostel and was not registered at any other accommodation, indicating she may have already left the country. It is difficult not to get jaded in such search scenarios when so many people turn up at home or in the bar, completely unaware that there is a search on—or more discouraging, happy for the dubious attention they are getting. By now everyone else was patting him on the back with cynical encouragement, essentially leaving him alone in pursuit of the girl's fate.

His head down, like a dog with a bone, Mark went back to the visitor centre and checked all the registrations for August to see if he could find anyone who could remember her and possibly give him a last seen location. His enquiries did reveal that two backcountry wardens had seen her on a trip she had returned from, but other than reinforcing the idea that she seemed weird,

they could add little to his knowledge. Despite comments like "Give it a rest!" he returned to the registrations and began calling anyone who had been out in the time period she had been missing. Feeling like a misunderstood Sherlock Holmes, he phoned all those he could track down with no result until he chanced upon one man who did help. The man revealed he had seen the girl on the final day of his hike—10 days after everyone else thought she had left the country.

The man had met her at the campground near the warden cabin, saying he remembered her because she seemed "quite unique." As they were both headed for the highway that day, he offered her a ride to town, but in the end she did not go out with him, and he assumed she had gone out later. Visions of a diabetic lying in her tent, possibly in a coma came to mind. And this was pretty much what he found when he arrived shortly after by helicopter, accompanied by dog handler Mike Henderson. Amazingly, she was still alive, though hallucinatory and very weak. She had lain there for 10 days, crawling occasionally to the creek for water, but was never spotted by any hikers though they must have seen her tent.

Though she had run out of food and insulin, she seemed to be trying to stay alive, but was clearly at the end of her tether. In no time, they had her in the hospital, and before long she was able to return to Texas. Mark felt good about his persistence; it gave him the lift rescuers need and a reason to keep doing a sometimes depressing, often thankless job. It was therefore with deep regret that he later found out she had killed herself that Christmas.

By 2002, THE WARDEN SERVICE, and in particular the public safety staff, had dealt with some serious setbacks. Many hoped that the 21st century would bring stability and a chance to revive the program with the recruitment of younger personnel needed to replace an aging staff. Having Jordy working on his guide exams in Glacier was a great boost, and they looked forward to involving other young people who showed promise in this demanding occupation. One of these was Mike Wynn, a new member of the Warden Service in Jasper, who was working at Sunwapta with Randy Fingland. He had enthusiasm and a winning personality that made him popular with all those he worked with. His outdoor skills were being honed with each trip he took with his mentors in the field, and he loved to ski.

Another warden showing interest in improving his skiing and avalanche skills was Brad Romanuk. He also had worked at the Sunwapta Warden Station, but was working out of the Jasper townsite when he decided to join Randy and Mike on a day trip up to Parker's Ridge to do a snow profile and get in some good training turns. Brad remembers that "It was a day like any other day on a field trip." He joined the Sunwapta crowd early in the morning to head up the hill and was pleased to learn that Mike Eder and others would be skiing in the area also. They all planned to meet at the end of the day to relax and visit before he had to go back to town.

Their intention was to ski to the upper slopes of Parker's Ridge to do a full profile to check the hazard for the avalanche paths called Parker's 1–5. The slopes in question were south of the youth hostel at Hilda Creek, just above Bridal Veil Falls parking lot. The well-broken ski trail took them through safe ground to the left of Parker's 1 and had been flagged by wardens who had worked at the station in previous years. It may have even seemed more casual when Randy brought his small dog Tupper along for the exercise. Eder and his friends were skiing nearer the youth hostel, close to the summer trail that led to the ridge.

As Brad recalls, they stopped to do a quick snow pit halfway up to examine the snow layers, then proceeded to the slopes just above treeline to do a full profile. They found no indication of a serious hazard, recording only a moderate avalanche hazard that might result in a slide on steep slopes. There were no other indications such as natural releases or collapses in the snowpack. With the prospect of finding some good snow near the climbing track, they headed down. Brad remembers they were skiing about 20 metres off the track when they came to an open area transected by a small bench about 20 degrees in steepness. The bench was a natural line between the steeper slopes above and the trees below. Randy Fingland, having the most advanced training, was leading the group that day and cautioned them to spread out while he skied across the slope first.

Brad's memory of the next events remains very clear. He saw Randy ski below a small rock outcrop then turn and wave to indicate he should follow. As he stepped forward, he suddenly noticed the slope fracture about six metres above him. Instantly Mike Wynn, who was standing metres behind and above him called "Avalanche!" From that point on, all of Brad's training kicked into full gear. He immediately released his skis and abandoned his ski poles just as the first wave of snow hit him. He remembers swimming through the snow, treating it like a liquid medium in which he could stay afloat—and thinking "This isn't bad at all." It almost seemed that no harm would come to any of them. But one thing he was very aware of was the speed at which he was carried down. As the motion slowed he was aware of a second and third wave of snow and suddenly he was completely buried. When everything stopped, he opened his eyes and saw light. Abruptly he sat up to discover he had been covered by about a half a metre of snow. He had been sieved through some small trees, but had no injuries other than a few bruises and scrapes.

The second thing that assailed him was the absolute stillness. There was not a sound. No traffic, no birds, no voices or barking from the dog, not even the sound of the wind in the trees. He had a sudden feeling that everything alive had abandoned the world and he was left alone. As soon as he moved, he realized his pack was still on his back, and the reality of what had happened broke over him like a thunderclap. His first action was to dig his radio out of the pack and call Jasper. With a brief message he called in the accident then turned his transceiver on to receive. Looking around, he thought that he had been carried the farthest, and the signals from up the hill seemed to confirm that. But as soon as he tried to head up the hill, he was slowed by the loose unconsolidated snow which made progress agonizingly slow.

His first thought was that the closest signal came from Mike who had been right behind him when the avalanche hit. As he wallowed upward he came to a small cluster of trees where he spotted a ski, then fingers sticking out of the snow. He recognized Randy's ski and hurried over. By now the snow was consolidating, and he could travel more easily, but it made digging that much harder. Following the arm, he struggled to free Randy's head, hoping he was alive. Fortunately he was, but just barely. Finding him unconscious and already blue, Brad gave him one big breath after clearing the air passage of snow. That was enough to elicit a cough and spontaneous breathing.

Without hesitation Brad left him, hoping he would revive, while he looked for Mike. For one brief second he thought, "Maybe, I should turn off Randy's transceiver so I can find Mike easier." As he turned, though, he realized that would be a huge mistake if another avalanche were to come down. Concentrating now on the more distant signal, he moved on until he located a second spot, where he had to turn down the volume to receive the signal. It was diffuse, however, and he decided to probe the general area rather than waste time trying to refine the source. Very quickly he hit Mike and began to dig.

His digging was hampered by dislodged trees mixed in the now solidifying debris. It seemed to take forever to free him, because he was buried deepest, down over a metre and a half. Mike was lying face down, making it very difficult to free his face. Suddenly Brad saw movement in his peripheral vision and was gratified to see Randy now moving more freely and beginning to yell.

He hollered to let him know he was there and was digging for Mike. Throughout the whole episode, he was getting maddening communication over the radio and repeatedly had to break off to give directions.

Randy was hurt, but despite this, he managed to drag himself out of the hardening snow and crawl over. He was very cold, suffering from hypothermia, a leg injury and a rapidly freezing hand. Brad stopped momentarily to give him a glove while trying to maintain CPR. With Randy's assistance, they dug the trapped man out and administered CPR more effectively.

By now the silence that had enveloped him when he first sat up from under the weight of the avalanche, was replaced with the drone of overhead helicopters. Three machines arrived within minutes of each other as the rescue team slogged up toward them. Mike Eder, being closest at hand when the accident occurred, was first on scene. Shortly after, everything was out of Brad's hands. He had done all that he could and now only wanted to fade away quietly from the bedlam.

He and Randy were quickly slung out, with Randy diverting most of the attention with his more prominent injuries. Brad was rather surprised that he almost made it to his truck unnoticed, but at the last moment he was spotted by Chief Park Warden Brian Wallace and put in the ambulance with Randy. In the end, he was grateful for going to the hospital for observation, because the two men were kept in the same room where they could quietly talk out all that had happened. He was also happy to learn that Randy's dog Tupper had been thrown clear of the avalanche and was first to greet the rescue party down by the highway.

Mike Wynn was not officially deceased when he arrived at the Banff hospital. The effort to revive him had kept the heart circulating the blood, but soon after, he suffered massive kidney and liver failure. He was pronounced dead later that night when his heart stopped. The autopsy showed he had had little chance of surviving the accident,

293

as the weight of snow had compressed his lungs immediately, leading to asphyxiation. No one with any experience with avalanche rescue was surprised by the young warden's death, but it was hard to accept. He was the first to leave a young wife and children behind.

The honours given him following his death were unprecedented for the Warden Service. Mike was removed to Calgary before he died, and it was from that city that the Jasper wardens claimed him. A cavalcade of eight warden vehicles came down from the park to pick up the body for the funeral in Jasper. They drove through the city escorted by the city police, with the red and blue lights signalling the procession. They were met at the city limits by the RCMP, who picked up the escort beyond the city. It was the passage through the national parks (Banff and Jasper), though, that impressed Sylvia, Randy and Brad the most. They were in the front of the procession riding together in one truck. At every overpass, side road or pull out, the wardens had turned out, dressed to symbolize the various functions of the job, to honour the cavalcade. At one station, Mike Henderson saluted their passing with his new dog Attila; at another, wardens on horseback with a pack outfit greeted them. The fire brigade was out in full display as were the wardens in public safety uniforms; Wardens on snowmobiles waved as they passed—and so on.

The overpasses also saw other sister agencies out to salute the procession— Kananaskis Country rangers, the Banff ambulance attendants and the

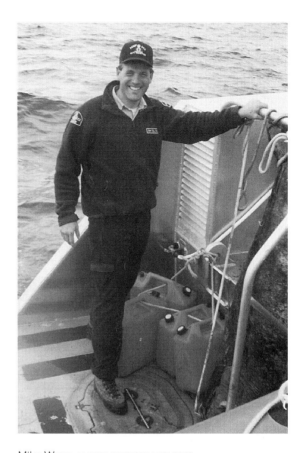

Mike Wynn. JASPER WARDEN ARCHIVES

RCMP. This continued till they reached the Icefield Parkway, where they proceeded up to Jasper. Then at the Big Bend just below the Columbia Icefield where Mike lost his life, another large procession from town greeted them to bring the body back to the funeral home for the service.

11 Risk, Responsibility and Stress

ON A QUIET AFTERNOON toward the end of November, 2002, when the weather was merely overcast but not snowy, Hans Gmoser reflected on what sort of year posed the greatest hazards to running a big heli-ski operation in the mountains. Looking out his window at the bare slopes of Mt. Rundle, he thought back and said, "Well … one just like this." The slopes had not yet received the early critical layers of insulating snow so vital in forming a solid snowpack for good skiing in the winter to come. The interior ranges of the Purcells and Selkirk Mountains normally start collecting these significant layers in October, but by November seventh, they still had only trace amounts on the upper peaks. The temperatures remained mild, leading to precipitation in the form of mixed rain and snow as the days slid toward December. By November 25, rain had percolated through the surface snow layers, forming a melt-freeze lamination of facetted crystals, thus providing the first persistent weakness in the developing snowpack. This was followed by a two-week drought, exposing the exterior layers of snow to cold temperatures, causing them to metamorphose into surface hoar crystals. The Snow Research and Avalanche Warning Section boys would trudge up daily to the snow plots

through the silvery world of the glittering, deadly filaments, admiring their beauty while dreading their significance. For these brittle octagonal structures that grew into elongated columns of sun-reflecting ice diamonds, are surprisingly tenacious and remain within the developing pack as it deepens with the winter snows.

The first serious avalanche calamity of the winter occurred on January 20 when a group of 21 skiers were hit by a large slab avalanche on the Durrand Glacier in the Selkirks. Though a snow profile conducted by the head guide gave him no cause for concern, the slab that had been building up on the buried facet crust layer released when the party skied onto thin snow near the ridge. The result was that 13 people were buried and seven were killed. The snow set up solid as concrete, making some of the excavations quite lengthy, devastating to one guide who survived but was not dug out for over an hour. By a fluke, a slab of snow had lodged above his head, creating a pocket of air that allowed him to live. Not so lucky were the seven people who died in the avalanche.

It was the first avalanche disaster of that magnitude in years, but it would not be the last. By the end of January, the Snow Research and Avalanche Warning Section team looking after the highway at Rogers Pass registered a significant avalanche cycle leading to an intense period of control work, during which 240 slides were recorded in the traffic corridor. Though this was not unusual, it was indicative of the problems established early in the winter. But as the storm passed and avalanche activity subsided, the avalanche danger rating was lowered to moderate below treeline.

Despite the lower rating given for areas below treeline, the significant danger in the alpine kept the heli-ski operators busy seeking hidden corners of safe terrain to ski. Lack of fresh snow and the prevailing danger taxed their expertise to the limit as run after run was skied out. The guides' diligence paid off, however, as only one of the 29 deaths caused by avalanches in the winter of 2003 occurred in the heli-ski industry. With the severity of the conditions that year, this was a remarkable achievement, indicating how far the industry had come in dealing with the perils of the trade.

Grant Statham, an ACMG guide working part-time for the Canadian Avalanche Association (CAA) as well as various heli-ski companies, recalls the winter with wonder. "I think that year could be a book in itself. So many stories …" Lloyd Gallagher, who had retired from Kananaskis Country but had kept his hand in guiding for CMH recalled that winter with a shudder. "There were too many unknowns … we had guides that were working with us for 30 years, but this year they couldn't get a reading on the snowpack. It was a bad year to do anything in terrain you hadn't skied before … "

But even guides have no absolute corner on determining for certain when an avalanche will occur, and they, like most people, are susceptible to the "heuristic traps" of everyday thinking. A recent study by Ian McCammon on the influence of this shortcut thinking in relation to avalanche accidents was presented to the International Snow Science Workshop held in Penticton, B.C. in October of 2002. Heuristics, or, "the simple rules of thumb people use to navigate the routine,

complexities of modern life," often replace the more time-consuming process of evaluating data, weighing alternatives and making a cogent decision based on observations and facts. The heuristic trap is "set when we base our decisions on familiar but inappropriate cues which lead to catastrophic results." Such cues for avalanche terrain include broken trails, familiarity with the country and the presence of others. McCammon feels there is too high a correlation between heuristic thinking and accidents to ignore, saying, "It seems highly likely that heuristic traps not only contribute to avalanche accidents, but that learning about them is crucial in preventing future accidents." He found it "disturbing that the victims in this study that were most influenced by heuristic traps were those with the most avalanche training."

These misleading cues may have influenced the school group from Calgary to venture into the Connaught valley two weeks after the tragedy at the Durrand Glacier. The trip was part of an outdoor curriculum the students of the Strathcona-Tweedsmuir School had engaged in for 17 years, and they knew the valley well from previous excursions. There was a well-broken trail up the valley, indicating that several other parties had gone on before, and indeed on that day, two experienced guides skied past the school group. Though Grant Statham was cautious that winter, he felt he would have gone as well. Clair Israelson, backing this sentiment, stated in an interview, "I would have gone up there too and felt entirely confident in that decision based on my training and experience from tromping around the mountains almost every day in wintertime for the past 30 years." But Clair added, "And I would have been wrong." The problem of familiarization coupled with the presence of other people is one of perception. Grant Statham considered that his reading of the vast expanse of open avalanche slopes in the upper valley, with a broken track and other skiers ahead, would have been much altered under different conditions. He reflects: "If I had seen that valley for the first time from the top of Balu Pass on a

10-day ski trip, I would have thought twice about crossing it." Jordy Shepherd, well on the way to being a full guide, concurs. The white expanse of an unfamiliar valley stretching out through obvious avalanche terrain would not be so inviting. This corresponds with McCammon's findings: "In unfamiliar terrain, people with advanced avalanche knowledge appeared to use their risk-reduction skills to their advantage. But in familiar terrain, these same groups exposed themselves to the same level of hazards as other groups with less or no training."

The school group, who had spent the previous day learning about snow profiles on the slopes above Rogers Pass, had already found variable results. They had also checked at the Rogers Pass Discovery Centre on Friday to discuss route options, collect weather and snowpack information and consider options for Saturday, the 1st of February. The fact that seven people had died not far from the Rogers Pass area only 10 days ago was a concern for one parent, who must have been happy that the leaders had advised them to give their children money to ski at the Kicking Horse Ski Area in Golden if conditions were not favourable for the planned tour. But the information they received did not indicate an extreme avalanche hazard. The Avalanche Danger Rating was posted as:

Below Treeline—Moderate
Treeline—Considerable
Alpine Areas—Considerable

With travel caution only advised for steeper terrain in areas above treeline, the leaders of the school group felt they would be safe in the valley despite having to cross avalanche runout paths. The lengthy discussion in the avalanche bulletin did warn of a "potential for a triggered event to step down to one of the deeper instabilities," but predominantly, there was a trend to more stability in the snowpack. Neither did Abby Watkins and Richard Marshall, two experienced guides from Golden B.C. who were also skiing in the valley that day find any reason for concern. Rich later reported: "There was nothing that day to tell us we shouldn't go to that particular area."

They left around 9:30 a.m. and travelled single file through the mature forest before reaching the open avalanche runout zones. The guides passed the group before leaving the trees and headed for the open slopes to a clump of trees, where they stopped for a rest. As they were leaving the trees on the upper trail, the pair saw a powder cloud of snow form high up on the slope of Mt. Cheops. Realizing it was an avalanche, they looked for the school group who were not far back. Spotting them directly below the thundering wall of snow racing down the mountainside, they yelled "Avalanche!" three times. Both guides were convinced the slide would engulf them too, but at the last minute a slight rise in the terrain deflected the mass of flowing snow down the valley. Their yells caused the lead skiers to look up, but they had no time to respond. When the dust cloud cleared, Abby and Rich saw no one standing. Everyone in the group below was either fully or partially buried.

Suddenly, the years of avalanche rescue training replaced all other thoughts as they skied down to the devastation. One of the most difficult tasks facing guides trained to recover avalanche victims is determining who can be saved and who can't. Only those left near the surface can be dug out quickly enough to be saved. Knowing this, and able to determine the relative proximity of the individual to the surface from the strength of the avalanche beacon signal, Abby and Rich had to make choices. It was a triage situation where the minimum was done to dig out the upper victims before they went to the next. Abby later recalled: "There was no time to attempt resuscitation. There's another 5 beacons to find. If they don't respond without CPR, then that's it. You have to move on, because you might find somebody who will resuscitate on their own." It required discipline to skip over fainter signals but it saved five people who would otherwise have died.

Unbelievably, one of the first victims they found was the lead instructor near the upper end of the deposit. His hand was protruding from the snow, making him an easy target and Rich quickly had him out. "He had a look of great relief on his face," Rich later remembered, but more important, he had a satellite phone. His first response was to phone the warden office and report the accident. Abby, meanwhile had uncovered the first of the students, whose leg was protruding from the rapidly congealing snow. But now they had help when two other skiers who had also seen the slide arrived on scene. The first thing Anders Blakstveldt saw was two teenage girls frantically digging with a shovel for those still buried—but the shovels barely penetrated the almost ice-dense snow. They were momentarily confused when he asked how many more were buried, as his transceiver was picking up signals everywhere. Picking one, he began to dig.

When warden Simon Hunt, who had seen far too much death that winter, picked up the phone at Rogers Pass at 11:45 that morning, he did not know that the call would instigate one of the biggest avalanche rescues since the Granduc mine. But before he could clarify how many people were missing, the teacher said he had to return to the rescue efforts and turned off the phone. Simon immediately alerted warden Tim Laboucane who took over as Incident Commander. With the help of dispatcher Carolyn Pollock, they burned up the phone lines notifying everyone on the call-out sheet about the accident.

The first warden Laboucane reached was Eric Dafoe, who was at the carport heading downtown and almost did not take the call. The winter had been stressful and he cherished his days off, but some inner thought, or possibly the tone of his wife's voice prompted him to return. The words "Hey, guess what, you're going to work," settled on him like a stone as the details emerged and the implications materialized. Even as he was out the door to pick up teammate Jordy Shepherd, he knew the catastrophe would have long-reaching consequences. By 12:35 they were en route with Kokanee Helicopters and soon spotted the appalling wreckage below with rescuers already on-site. If the school group had run out of luck with the avalanche, other things had clicked into place. The accident happened on a Saturday around noon, just when all the heli-ski companies were changing ski groups for the coming week, and the guides plus the helicopters were instantly available. When Eric left Jordy to take over field command, Bruce McMahon (avalanche forecaster for Snow Research and Avalanche Warning Section) had established lookouts for further avalanche activity and was continuing with the rescue efforts. They were very concerned over the building threat of a second avalanche, but all they could do immediately was post spotters and locate escape routes.

Both Jordy and Bruce were impressed with the work accomplished by Abby and Rich. By the time they got there, the two guides had already worked down the entire length of the deposit, locating surface clues, excavating persons near the surface and pinpointing deeper burials for others to work on. But the life saving was over. Now began the tedium of digging out the unfortunate who were buried too deep to save, the shallowest being nearly a metre down. Other people began to arrive in droves, making the logistics of co-ordinating search efforts a nightmare for Eric, who was in charge of the rescue operation. With over 50 people and eight helicopters moving through the narrow valley, communication became the greatest challenge. The guides who had arrived all had their own radios, the batteries on the park radios were not always reliable, the helicopter pilots had to be monitored to be sure there was no collision in the fading light, the media clamoured for details and frantic parents demanded to know the fate of their children. At one point, when there was serious concern about the impending avalanche danger, Eric could not contact anyone in the field. This was especially aggravating to John Kelly, who was monitoring the situation but could not reach anyone for over 20 minutes. The wind that had caused the buildup of snow high on the mountain leading to the initial release continued to blow, alarming the observers who needed to signal the workers at the least sign of avalanche activity.

As the distracting chorus of beeps from transceivers thinned to nothing, one body could not be accounted for. It was later discovered, but not communicated immediately to the searchers, that the young woman had already been flown out when the activity was at its most hectic. It was over an hour before this oversight was corrected. It turned out to be a minor glitch in a remarkably well-run rescue operation for which the wardens had no precedent. Although the field efforts concluded around 3:00 p.m., dealing with the consequences of the deaths of seven students had only just begun. Grief counsellors made their way to the pass while Eric and Jordy prepared for the media conferences in Revelstoke. As Canada reeled from the news, the only thing that competed with the horror of the event was the equally tragic loss of seven people on board the space shuttle *Columbia* during the same time frame.

ALTHOUGH THE TEACHERS who led the children into the Connaught drainage that fateful February day might not say they took a calculated risk in going there, that was what they did. But calculated risks are a part of life; one every individual undertakes every day just getting out of bed in the morning and driving to work. Risk, as defined in the Avalanche Risk Review written for Parks Canada following the Balu Pass accident is considered to be "the chance for loss (or gain)." Glenda Hanna, author of *Outdoor Pursuits Programming: Legal Liability and Risk Management*, refines this distinction by differentiating between pure and speculative risk, where "pure risk describes situations which involve either a chance of loss or no loss, but not an opportunity to gain. Speculative risk, on the other hand, involves a calculated gamble where one also might lose, but one might gain." Outdoor programmers "accept and even seek a certain level of risk in order to achieve individual and/or program challenge objectives."

Though many schools and institutions recognize this and build it into their outdoor programs, the degree to which risk is understood and accepted is often more complex than many people realize. Risk tolerance was discussed in the Strathcona-Tweedsmuir School Outdoor Education Program Review compiled by Bhudak Consultants Ltd. for the board to consider after the fatal accident. It was recognized that it is easy to philosophize about the benefits of providing a challenging program that has potential risk; it is also well documented that students thrive on adventurous activities where the potential risks in the program are acknowledged. But the consultants cautioned that the "benefit-focussed approach" might not have given enough consideration to the "potential cost" of the risk resulting in an accident. The potential cost can and often does, lead to catastrophic risk (loss of life)—often unanticipated when danger is not recognized.

But what about those people who do not think they are taking a risk, yet pay the ultimate price? Many tourists inadvertently walk into traps that don't appear to be hazardous despite many warning signs and fences. The most common places for the average citizen to meet their final fate are rivers, waterfalls and canyons—or, in Jasper, on the icefields. A reasonable person will acknowledge that if they cross a barrier protecting them from the edge of a cliff or falling water, they may be putting themselves into some form of jeopardy, but few recognize the hidden danger of a snow-covered crevasse on a flat surface.

Unfortunately, it is often children who suffer if adults fail to perceive this risk. One such case involved a family from Calgary whose young child fell into a narrow crevasse on the toe of the Athabasca Glacier in the summer of 1990. There were signs indicating that crevasses were present and that care must be taken, but few understood that falling into a crevasse can lead to death.

The opportunity to walk on the ice was taken by the family toward the end of July of that year, but without the aid of a guide or appropriate equipment. Because it was a warm day the family was dressed in light clothing. As the young ten-year-old boy was skipping happily across a narrow opening in the ice, his footing failed and he slipped suddenly into the crevasse. The constriction that halted his fall wedged him in solidly, beginning the process of melt-freeze that would hold him even more firmly with the passing minutes. The thin T-shirt and shorts gave little protection from the cold.

The father was frantic once he realized his son had fallen into the crevasse but had enough presence of mind to seek help. The first person to respond was Rod McGowan, a guide who worked for the Icefield tour group. Earlier in the day Rod had already pulled out one young man who had sunk up to his shoulders in a crevasse and when the father waved to him for help, he hoped it would be a similar situation. Rod went to the site of the accident thinking a simple rope raise would be sufficient, but what he saw stopped him short. His immediate thought on seeing the slim child wedged head down in the narrow slot was "He's dead." He immediately radioed Parks, then sent the mother and daughter down to the toe to direct the incoming help. One of the bystanders happened to be a doctor who had experience with

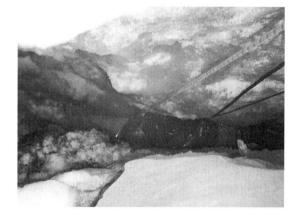

Rescue on Columbia Icefield. JASPER WARDEN ARCHIVES

exposure victims, which made Rod feel much better. To save time he then made a loop in the rope and was able to secure it to the child's ankle.

Because the boy was wedged so firmly in the ice, it caused him pain when they tried to pull him out. The screaming was too much for the father, and he refused to allow them to continue, asking instead to go down to see what he could do. But this delay had serious consequences. Rod was very reluctant to send the father down, but the man insisted. There was little need for concern, however, as the large man could barely go below the lip of the crevasse before he called to be brought back up.

When Terry Damm received the call, he knew he would need backup and contacted the Jasper warden office to see who was around. The ever alert Murray Hindle stationed at Athabasca Falls, overheard the conversation and immediately responded. He yelled at Bill Hunt to grab his gear and prepare to go into the crevasse once they got there. When the Athabasca team arrived, Terry was already heading up with a crushingly heavy pack that made him think he was moving through sludge. When he got to the accident site, the first thing he saw was the father clinging to the rope that led to his son, with tears streaming down his face.

Once the second team reached the crevasse they lowered Bill into the narrow slot, but when he reached the child, there was no response. With only about a 20-centimetre clearance in which to work, Bill tried to have the rescuers pull him up while he tugged on the boy but he could not budge him. Eventually, after resecuring the original rope, they decided to pull on it again with Bill assisting as much as possible. This time they managed to dislodge the child and, with a steady raise, brought him to the surface. The doctor who had remained on scene started CPR, which was maintained throughout stretcher transport to the highway. Despite the efforts, the child had been too long in the crevasse and did not survive.

The park assessment that "lack of respect or understanding for warnings and dangers of glaciers" clearly lays some of the responsibility with the parents; however they did not see it that way. Within a year everyone who participated in the rescue, as well as the major organizations of Parks Canada and CMH (for whom McGowan worked at other times of the year) were named in a lawsuit. The lawsuit was not upheld, but it did require Parks to justify the rescue response, essentially putting the whole public safety program under the scrutiny of the courts. It was deemed that one person on standby at Sunwapta Warden Station was not sufficient for a major response to the frequent callouts for crevasse rescue at the Columbia Icefield. It was also felt that the signage was not adequate to convey the message of the dangers of exploring the toe of the glacier without protection. In response, a larger sign was put up and another person was assigned to work at the station. Since that time, much more work has been put into directing people away from problem areas, thus significantly reducing the number of incidents that plague the wardens.

THE MAJOR TRAP FOR THE AVERAGE non-risk-taking tourist is water. A simple, all too common, incident in one of Canada's eastern parks motivated one young park warden to investigate the concept of Hazard Assessment in hope of preventing tragic accidents. Jenny Sparks, a seasonal park warden in Pukasaw National Park, found herself dealing with the death of a child (who had drowned in Lake Superior) of a close family friend—a devastating experience that took her out of search and rescue, but not without a promise do all she could to prevent similar accidents. Her research led her to think that what was lacking was a site specific hazard warning to the unwary. This brought her to the problem of how to successfully inform the public of local hazards. Her efforts caught the attention of management, and soon she was carving out the principles of Visitor Risk Management for various parks.

In 1990, she was offered a term job in Ottawa to evaluate how national parks across Canada were dealing with a risk assessment for hazards within their boundaries. Eventually a pilot program was conducted in Banff using the large database assembled from the public safety accident files. The recommended management actions taken to minimize risk were to be incorporated in the Public Safety Management Plan for each park.

Parks Canada began to take steps to communicate hazard awareness to the public, but later accidents proved there was still much to do in this field. In 2001, just shy of the 11th anniversary of the child's death on the toe of the Athabasca Glacier, another child suffered the same fate. The *Calgary Herald* write-up stated: "Frantic efforts by rescuers failed to save the life of a nine-year-old boy stuck in a glacial crevasse in the Columbia Icefield for nearly four hours … He died of hypothermia." In this case, the boy stepped on a rotten snow bridge covering a narrow 15-centimetre slot that broke, sending him five metres down the narrow crevasse. The wardens had to chip him out of the encasing ice, but even with the heated glycol now available to enhance the extrication, it still took two hours with four men working to bring him to the surface. It was a cold, frustrating job that was difficult for all concerned. Steve Blake, who was field rescue leader stated: "It involved people hanging upside down and sideways in the crevasse digging him out by hand through ice and snow … we're talking a space of six or eight inches wide, so your chest is pressed against both walls and you have one hand to work with to try and manipulate tools to dig." Each time a person had to be brought up and another rescuer lowered down, more time slid by. With growing concern, Steve saw the small boy's life slip away, but could do little more than send people down and wonder if the signs posted at the glacier toe were of much use. That a language barrier was probably the main reason the family had not recognized the danger did little to console him.

The effort to prevent accidents before they happen, and having a prompt rescue effort when they do, has always been an important component of the public safety program. To management it is also important from the position of possible liability. People often want to blame anyone but themselves for accidents they or their families are involved in, and an anonymous government agency is easy to blame. This is not to say that the national parks do not have a responsibility to do all that is reasonable to ensure the public's safety, but the degree of that responsibility is constantly in question. Because lawsuits seem to be a rising occurrence, parks continue to evolve more sophisticated and workable means of accident prevention.

This is a challenge, as the level of responsibility expected by parks of the public and the public's expectation of safety are not always clear. Not even the legal responsibility of parks is tightly defined. The 1983 paper on "Issue Analysis in Mountain Search and Rescue" refers to this, stating: "Precise definition of Parks Canada's legal responsibilities to provide mountain search-and-rescue services is hampered by a lack of directly related Canadian case law and the difficulty of rendering a comprehensive legal opinion which anticipates all possible factual situations."

Despite lack of legal precedence, however, when a national park invites people to come and visit, there is an automatic expectation the park will exercise due diligence for that person's safety. That degree of due diligence becomes muddied, however, if an individual fails to behave responsibly to ensure their own safety. Because it is impossible to eliminate the dangers inherent in the wilderness, what becomes important is the degree to which the park warns the public of danger it can do nothing about. This is so obvious that Judge Whitehall—the Crown's attorney—went almost as far as to say the Crown had no legal responsibility from conditions found in a wilderness setting—the park has complied with due diligence if it has adequately warned the public of the hazards encountered in the natural environment. This relates to the legal concept of "assumption of risk" which an individual accepts if their activity continues after being fully warned of the hazards of that activity. If an accident occurs under these conditions, the individual (or group) can be held responsible for contributory negligence.

This concept was first tested for a public safety event when Parks Canada was sued by the leaders of the boys group from Philadelphia in 1955. They contested that there was no adequate warning given for the conditions on Mt. Temple which led to the death of seven young men. The fact that they never sought the information that was freely available quashed the suit, lending credence to the belief that the leaders fell below a standard of self-protection that should have been given the boys.

It was later tested again after a young girl fell to her death on Mt. Victoria in 1980. In this instance the girl, who was not a climber at all, was convinced by a friend to attempt the summit of this high alpine peak, despite poor conditions. The friend professed to be an experienced climber himself, but subsequent interviews did not entirely support this claim. The third person on the ill-fated trip was another young man who had no climbing experience at all; his previous travels were limited to some high alpine hiking only. Because the registration system was still in place, they did speak to the resident Lake O'Hara warden Al Knowles before they left for the climb, but failed to heed his warning. Al had caught the leader signing out at the self-registration box and advised him of the unstable conditions brought on by a week of wet cool weather which had left the mountains plastered in fresh snow. Al noted with some concern that later that same day a party of seven Alpine Club of Canada climbers returned from Abbots Pass because of the hazardous conditions. The leader of this party also encountered the young group of three and advised them not to attempt Mt. Victoria, telling them the conditions were far too dangerous.

Despite all warnings, the party went anyway, proceeding as far as the Sickle where they encountered very soft snow and finally turned around. But by now it was getting late, and the snow they had crossed earlier was also soft. After reaching the end of the summit ridge where the route begins to descend steeply to the hut, the leader decided the team should unrope, perhaps because there was no opportunity to belay properly in the sloppy snow above the cliffs. But tricky down climbing was too much for the untrained girl, and she fell to her death, tumbling over the long broken cliffs that ring the Death Trap hundreds of feet below.

The frightened boys reacted very differently to the horrific event. The hiker froze and refused to go any farther. The leader ran off, leaving him on his own, and descended in a rush to the hut where he met two men staying there. One of them went down to Lake O'Hara for help while the other two descended to the girl. The weather, which continued to deteriorate, hampered rescue efforts. Clair Israelson was able to get in by helicopter to remove the body and the two climbers but then realized a real rescue was in the making when he learned that the third man was still high up on the ridge. But the man who was left behind had summoned the courage to make his way to the hut, to the relief of the team, who were anticipating a dangerous climb in poor weather to bring him down.

News of the girl's death was hard for the parents, who were quickly convinced that the young leader was not at fault. Consequently the girl's family sought an inquest, claiming that by allowing the boy to sign out for the climb, the park had condoned the trip. An article in the *Calgary Herald* reports the boy's father "took issue with reports that indicated the climbers had been warned against the climb. 'They were given a Parks permit to climb the mountain and also given permission to use the hut.'" The inquest that followed to determine if a lawsuit was warranted, indicated beyond question that self-registration is not a permission slip, nor is registering to stay at a hut an indication that conditions were safe.

One of the greatest areas of contention for lawsuits is the invisible line between "front-country facilities" and the backcountry. In considering the likelihood of a successful lawsuit against the Crown, it has been recognized that more developed areas have a greater potential for liability cases because of a greater expectation of safety. The 1983 Issue Analysis paper stated that: "The more the Crown does to make a particular area safe and attractive for human activities, the more likely the Crown will be legally responsible if the area turns out to be unsafe." This fine line of responsibility is difficult to draw. And there is little case law to refine the distinction.

One case came before the courts to test this issue. During the winter early in the 1980s a middle-aged couple became lost while cross-country skiing on the Pipestone Loop trails near Lake Louise. The loops, located just off the north side of the Trans-Canada Highway, are complex, interconnected trails that do not extend more than three kilometres off the main corridor and are designated as front-country territory. With this in mind, the pair were equipped accordingly, with food, water, maps and matches and some spare clothing. On registering out, they spoke to a park attendant at the information desk who pointed out a secondary trail linking two main trails which would shorten the trip if they wanted to return earlier.

The couple headed off for what should have been a short ski day. Unfortunately they took the wrong trail. This led to a succession of wrong choices until they were unable to retrace their steps at all and became wet, exhausted and completely lost. Finally the woman could no longer go on. They met no one and apparently did not clue in to the traffic noise from the highway not far from where they stopped. The husband left his wife and finally did make it to the highway after dark, and was able to initiate a search effort. However, by the time the rescuers reached his wife she had died of hypothermia. The husband suffered severe frostbite and eventually lost a few toes. The emotional distress, however, was the main motivator for filing a lawsuit.

The husband claimed that the woman at the trail office had misled them. The fact that the park was remapping and signing the trails seemed to indicate some fault prior to the accident. The case was thrown out on the basis of the Crown Liability Act and the Occupiers Liability Act. The plaintiff could not prove the employee had any knowledge of a dangerous situation prior to the incident. The fact that the signs were to be improved was not found valid by the judge, who stated that improving a condition—even after an accident—was not an admission of guilt "merely a matter of common sense." More interesting, however, was the decision that the park trails operated under a different standard of care than that required by landowners (Occupiers Liability Act). Under the National Parks Act, the park has a responsibility to "maintain the parks in a manner which leaves them unimpaired for the enjoyment of future generations." This implies a lower standard of care where signage is actually an unexpected plus not required by parks to provide. The judge ultimately stated that it was not "reasonably foreseeable that a skier on these short, novice level ski trails would become so lost as to lead to a fatal result." In short, even front-country trails can assume the dimension of wilderness that normally applies to land beyond an eight-kilometre limit of a highway.

But although the number of liability actions against parks has been low (which is particularly indicative of the success of the rescue work over the years), management remains concerned about expensive lawsuits. Indeed, if the accident is significant, it can result in changes in policy and directives even if lawsuits are not involved.

In 1987, when Sylvia Forest was still working for the Cadet Camp in Banff, her trips with the young students became severely curtailed after a young girl broke her ankle in Glacier National Park. The leader of the group set her ankle with a splint, then called the Warden Service for an evacuation. Eric Dafoe responded and arrived to sling the victim out, but some time had elapsed between the accident and the arrival of the helicopter. When he reached the highway, he checked her ankle for circulation and realized she had no feeling in her foot. The girl was taken to the hospital, but the lack of circulation had already caused damage and she lost her foot. The repercussion was almost immediate. Suddenly all the extended mountaineering adventures were eliminated, much to the disappointment of both staff and students.

The heli-ski industry has always had to battle with the consequence of risk taking, responsibility and accidents. When Hans Gmoser first developed this exciting approach to skiing, he did not realize how complex snow could be. In the early years he worked closely with the snow gurus of the industry such as Ed LaChapelle and Peter Schaerer to get a handle on the avalanche problems he faced. Despite all the snow pits and stabilization procedures, Gmoser says, they still did not know all the "multiple factors one has to consider to get any kind of appreciation for what they are dealing with." This led to serious consequences when large numbers of people started to get killed in avalanches.

After such events as the St. Valentine's Day avalanche (seven dead), Thunder River avalanche (seven dead) and the Bay Street (nine dead), the government in British Columbia began to get nervous. The operators knew they had to do something to prevent these huge avalanche disasters before the government stepped in. Ed LaChapelle, a leading avalanche expert in the United States, pointed out that an exchange of information between each group would deepen their insights into developing problems.

CMH now had a string of lodges between the Bugaboos and the town of McBride that were connected by radio, so in 1981 they began to exchange information on conditions each evening. Hans stated: "I think that was really the basis for the Info-Ex that the Canadian Avalanche Association then started." It came about after a fatality in one ski area that might have been prevented if knowledge of similar avalanche conditions experienced at a neighbouring area had been available. The idea of sending in daily avalanche data from each operation, which could be accessed by all, meant that greater safety measures could be employed. The information that was available only to CMH staff was soon passed to the CAA in Revelstoke, who then made it available to other operations, thus creating the Info-Ex program.

PARKS CANADA HAS ALSO EXPERIENCED radical changes in policy as a result of mountaineering deaths. In the late seventies, both Mark Ledwidge and Gord Irwin worked as park interpreters and were encouraged to climb as much as possible during work to gain understanding of the landscape. Mark was out climbing with two other co-workers when one man slipped while descending a steep snow slope. The resulting fall led to his death. Up to that point, the interpretive service was able to purchase mountaineering equipment and go climbing, but the accident caused this activity to be reviewed. It was questioned why they were out climbing at all when they had no connection to the public safety program. It was pointed out that none of the personnel were getting training for this type of work and could not guarantee a standard of safety similar to that of the wardens. Within weeks, all the equipment purchased by the Interpreter Service reverted to the Warden Service and climbing activity was cancelled for the interpreters during working hours. Both Gord and Mark, who wished to pursue a career that entailed climbing, soon joined the Warden Service.

Changes came after Mike Wynn's death as well. Because Mike was killed while working, Labour Canada was obligated to investigate his death to determine if negligence had been involved. Had the leader of the trip been found to be at fault, charges could have been laid on the immediate supervisor and those above him. The investigation was thorough and lengthy, leaving everyone on edge and very aware of how potentially vulnerable they were if training standards were not met. As a result, wardens are now not allowed to travel

in backcountry avalanche terrain without having a Level I CAA avalanche course. This, above all, is indicative of the changes in operations from 30 years ago when wardens lived in the backcountry all year round with no formal avalanche training at all.

There have also been adjustments in training standards to meet the liability concerns of park managers. Those wardens who do not receive the requisite number of training courses in public safety are not able to attend technical rescues. This is probably more a result of the stipulations of Labour Canada, which requires all employees be trained to the standard of the work they are asked to undertake. Prior to the year 2000, only the park could be named in a lawsuit. Managers were not held personally responsible for their employees. After 2000, a change in the liability laws meant that if a manager sent an employee into the field without adequate training and it resulted in an injury or death, the manager could be held personally liable.

Other changes came about after the Balu Pass avalanche accident. Park managers were proactive in seeking solutions to the problem of communicating avalanche hazard to the public. They hired full guide Grant Statham to put into effect the recommendations that came out of the Avalanche Risk Review commissioned by Parks Canada and to explore better ways to communicate avalanche hazard. This was a two-year project that ended in 2005. The result was a sweeping change in classification of avalanche terrain, with serious restrictions on travel for custodial groups and clubs in national parks if members younger than 18 are present. Those valleys deemed high in avalanche hazard potential are not open to these groups, period. Other valleys with questionable terrain, require the group be accompanied by a full guide. Only those valleys with no avalanche hazard whatsoever can be travelled by these groups unescorted by a full guide.

THOUGH MUCH OF THE PUBLIC SAFETY work is routine, the chances of being engaged in a high stress incident are quite likely, even if an individual only works in the field for a year or so. The successful public safety worker must learn to deal with stress from many sources, something not readily apparent to those who have not experienced working in this outwardly glamorous field. One not so obvious stress comes from performing work beyond one's ability. Though this is not as prevalent today, because only those people who really want to climb get into the field, it was an issue for the early pioneering wardens. Many of them had no wish to climb mountains, and although most adapted, quite a few never got over the terrors of some of those early schools and were more than glad to transfer to Prairie region.

Currently those working in public safety are gravitating toward the standards set by the ACMG, but becoming a guide can be stressful. Few pass all the exams without failing one, and often it takes a couple of efforts to get that last outstanding course—all of which takes time, commitment and money. Wardens often had the advantage of being sponsored by the government and the opportunity to learn from guides in the Warden Service. Both Jordy Shepherd and Percy Woods for instance, acknowledge the tremendous boost they got from working with their experienced peers. But this does not eliminate the stress of going through the exams, as Sylvia Forest clearly recalls. She did not always have full sponsorship or sufficient time to train for the courses, and in the end she took a leave of absence. She still wakes up with a feeling of great relief that the ordeal is over and she can get on with a life that was put on hold till she attained her goal.

Then there are the rescues themselves. One of the consequences of the tremendously increased capacity of the helicopter is the ability to bring the rescuer very quickly to the accident. When Burke Duncan from Kananaskis Country was called from a barbeque in his back yard to an accident on Mt. Rundle, he realized that one of the traits a person with this job really needed was adaptability. He had to go from a very secure environment to one of exposure, danger and trauma in the space of a few minutes. When Jim Murphy thought about this, his reaction was: "Yah, but then you have to go back to the barbeque!" The challenge for him was to come down from an adrenaline rush that no one around him could relate to. It was usually pointless to even talk about the experience he had just gone through with those who had stayed at the party.

Often the rescues are not rescues at all but recoveries of bodies or body parts. All rescue personnel, be they professional or volunteer, remember the first time they had to deal with a person who died in the accident. Dave Smith immediately recalls spending the night with a young woman who had died at the base of Mt. Rundle. Unpleasant as that was, it was not as hard to deal with as the gruesome results of a long fall over broken terrain. Peter Fuhrmann did not hesitate to send inexperienced wardens to such accidents, reasoning the sooner they got used to it the better. There was no point in spending a lot of time training someone who could not handle death or dismemberment. One of his first recruits to this blood and guts training was Rick Kunelius, who had to have a long talk with himself on one rescue about the value of becoming a butcher at Safeway before becoming a warden.

Coming to grips with the traumatic side of rescue is not always easy but if ignored it can lead to cumulative stress. This was not actually recognized in the early days of rescue work, possibly because it had not yet been recognized during the Second World War. The war veterans dealt with death and maiming in much the same way they had dealt with it in Europe—they accepted the outcome, kept it to themselves and carried on. However, there were rescue critiques following each incident that tended to be anaesthetized by a certain amount of alcohol. Talking about how to improve the rescue work and illuminating what was done well over a few beers was certainly effective in reducing the stress, and many wardens preferred this to more formalized debriefing sessions. One of the overwhelming reasons for this being an effective way of dealing with bad accidents is the opportunity to share the experience with co-workers who were there and who understood. As Darro Stinson observed, no one went home right after a serious incident to sit and stew alone. He made sure everyone went back to the rescue room or to the bar to "unwind," if not to talk, then to listen and enjoy the companionship of their peers.

Reg Bunyan came to realize the value of this companionship, or lack of it, when he returned from the Balu Pass tragedy. It is particularly hard for wardens or anyone else, for that matter, to deal with the death of children or young adults. Reg was one of the wardens called out from Lake Louise to help with the recoveries, but he was also slated for a law enforcement school the day after. No one seemed to think he should not go, but when he looks back on how it affected him, he realized it might have been a mistake. He was suddenly surrounded by people he did not know and who had no ability to relate to the overwhelming experience he had just come from. Deprived of friends and family, he had no opportunity to divest himself of the sadness he felt and found himself unexpectedly depressed over the incident. He had been on many serious rescues, none of which bothered him overtly, and was surprised by how deeply the Balu Pass accident affected him.

One of the first people to recognize the need for critical stress debriefing was Lloyd Gallagher, while he was the alpine specialist for Kananaskis Country. Dave Smith pointed out that Lloyd was particularly sensitive to his employees when they had gone through a rough rescue and always made sure they were doing okay. After Dave spent the night with the body of the young woman, Lloyd made sure he talked about it and then followed up, asking daily how he was doing. It may have almost been annoying, but to this day Dave is very appreciative of his effort.

Parks Canada has had varying degrees of success with critical stress debriefing. Because war-

dens dealt with rescue trauma largely in-house, the importance of having professional help was not immediately recognized. The first major occasion to seek professional help was after the death of Pat Sheehan. But the park managers did not spend a great deal of time finding an appropriate counsellor. The session did little for Gerry Israelson, who found that the presence of many government workers who had little to do with either Pat or the rescue, stilted his desire to say anything meaningful. Dale Portman, who knew Pat well, was much more emphatic about the failure of this proceeding, saying he found the whole thing stiff, formal and ultimately hollow.

Perhaps it was the criticism of this debriefing or a change in managers that led to a big improvement in counselling after Mike Wynn's death in 2002. Parks recognized that the counsellor should have a good understanding of what wardens do and be able to relate to them at a field level. They also recognized that the large group debriefing was not appropriate in all cases, and took a three-tier approach. Wardens could receive one-on-one counselling or attend more formal sessions depending on need. More important, the families of the victims were also included in the counselling. One of the critical elements of dealing successfully with grief and loss is recognizing the role wives and families play in the recovery process. Managers also recognized that the trauma of such an event often has long-term effects, and made counselling available for as long as it was needed.

But Mike's death and the dealings with the families and co-workers left Steve Blake with a feeling that more could be done, particularly in the future, when less experienced managers might be involved. This initiated the development of an Incident Stress Plan that allowed managers to follow correct procedures immediately from the ground up. It was essentially a checklist of what and what not to do and when. It contained simple things like ensuring that death benefit cheques sent by mail are identified. It also emphasizes that managers are not always the best judge of what is good for the employee.

Another stressful part of the job is dealing with the families of victims, though in some cases it can also be rewarding—almost consoling. Family members can be particularly difficult to deal with if they are present while rescuers are trying to save the victim. Family members may also exhort rescuers to continue in an effort to recover a body when it is too dangerous to do so. On one occasion when a young son of the Vanderbilt family went missing on Mt. Robson, his pals from the Harvard Mountaineering Club thought their own efforts might produce results when the wardens failed to find him. Nicolas Vanderbilt was a writer, apparently working on a screenplay about climbing and had set off with a friend to climb Mt. Robson to gain insight for his proposed play. Family and friends rated them as skilled climbers with only limited experience in the Rockies, though this was Vanderbilt's second attempt on the mountain. They were last seen by another party high up on the Wishbone Route on Wednesday, August 22, 1984.

After they failed to return on Monday the 27th, the Robson rangers and RCMP initiated a search. But by Friday, after having found nothing, they called Jasper for assistance. Gerry Israelson responded but in the interim the weather had deteriorated, making search efforts by helicopter quite limited. The following day Willi Pfisterer arrived and so had the family and three members of the Harvard Mountaineering Club. When the three announced they would like to mount their own search effort, Willi was more than happy to let them try. The Vanderbilt family hired a helicopter and off they went. A much chastened crew returned a few hours later having seen the scope of the mountain; they had realized the magnitude and difficulty of the terrain their friend had disappeared in. They happily handed the task back to the wardens, but by now it was obvious that the pair had died. Gerry wrote: "It is my opinion that the mountain was searched very well. It is also my feeling that if the missing climbers were alive they would have been located by us." Willi then flew the mountain one last time with Mrs. Jean Vanderbilt who went home satisfied that everything possible had been done.

Although the Vanderbilt family went home satisfied, other situations were not so easily resolved. Todd McCready recalls many situations where wives were at the rescue base wondering why no one was doing anything. All members of the team, who are equally frustrated at poor conditions, feel this pressure, but it is useless to risk more lives by sending people out under dangerous conditions—particularly if the individual is dead. Unfortunately, that is often difficult to determine if the body is not recovered. Despite the slim chance of surviving a long fall, it cannot be ruled out and wardens often continue to look despite the dangers.

But being aware of the need to understand why a family member has died is one of the strengths of the Warden Service. Wardens go to great lengths to explain to grieving family members exactly what happened and will often fly them to the site if it is reasonable to do so. Treating a body with care is also part of overall care given to victims and their families—but sometimes it takes a bit to fully realize how carefully that must be done.

As a new recruit, Al MacDonald had learned the hard way how sensitive people can be. He had been called in to assist an elderly gentleman who had suffered a heart attack at the Columbia Icefield, but by the time he got there the man had passed away. The ambulance had arrived, but the gentleman was still lying where he had fallen, surrounded by the distraught family. Thinking it best to ease their suffering, he covered the man with a blanket, head and all. This brought about a tremendous outcry from the new widow, who was convinced her husband could still be revived. From that time on, he always made sure that the individual was put in the ambulance with all the display possible of maintaining CPR until they got the body to the hospital.

As difficult as dealing with victims and their families may be, it is quite another to face the very real risks encountered either while training or on rescues. Ninety percent of the time rescues and climbs go smoothly. But prolonged exposure to danger will catch up, and most public safety wardens have tales of close calls that kept everyone on their toes.

One potential disaster was doing a crevasse rescue on the Athabasca Glacier beneath the looming icefall that hung off the top of The Snow Dome. The very idea of staying in this bowling alley of calving ice boulders to pull someone out of a crevasse gave Evan Manners a constant nightmare. When he was finally called to help on a rescue at this location, he realized he was one of the more experienced persons there. On the flight in, he kept asking himself why he had just volunteered to go on his nightmare rescue. Other wardens who did not have the same family commitments as he did could have gone.

The rescue turned out to be for a young man who thought he knew a lot about glacier travel, but not enough to rope up. With little sympathy and not wanting to stay in the exposed terrain any longer than absolutely necessary, the team pulled the fellow up, broken bones and all, and flew him out secured in the Jenny Bag. The whole operation was slick, and the whole team got out in good time, but after it was over, Evan realized that as long as he was available for rescues, he would always be in this position. It was ultimately one of the reasons he took the opportunity to work for the Canadian Avalanche Association the following year.

Though most public safety wardens have close calls, Gerry Israelson must surely top the list with a near-fatal experience while on a routine evacuation on Mt. Edith Cavell. It was a nice day when they flew up to the mountain to pick up some members of the British Army who had become stranded when they tried to get off the mountain. Their descent brought them to the top of a large cliff band, where they spent the night on a broad scree ledge calling for a rescue.

The next day Gerry flew up with Murray Hindle, while Willi ran base operations from the Edith Cavell Tea House parking lot. None of the men were hurt or incapacitated in any way, and it appeared to be a routine mission. Gerry got the first pair ready to sling off in the rescue harness, with their climbing packs clipped to the side. What he did not notice was an ice axe secured horizontally across the top of one of the climber's packs. As he stepped back to give Todd the signal to lift off, the action caused the pair to rotate and the protruding pick of the ice axe suddenly became entangled in Gerry's clothing. Sudden he was airborne as the helicopter headed for base. Todd had no idea he had snagged Gerry, and all the hapless rescuer could do was squirm.

Murray saw everything with fascinated horror and reacted quickly by running forward to grasp Gerry by the legs. But by then Gerry was well off the ground and headed for the cliff edge. Willi, who was watching the operation from below could hardly believe his eyes. Not knowing the outcome, he suddenly saw Gerry fall—then nothing. The ice axe released its deadly hold on Gerry's clothing just before they slung off the cliff, and he landed on the scree almost a boot's length from the edge of the 300-metre drop. That night, after a few "pops" to wind up the scary operation, Gerry crawled into bed saying to his sleepy wife, "Well, I almost made you a widow today!"

The public safety job can be hard on families, particularly if they do not buy into the climbing mentality. The wives of wardens or rangers watched their husbands go to work every day, not knowing what dangers would crop up—or they would answer the phone in the middle of the night when a rescue call came in. It seemed to Wanda Ward, Scott's wife, that she was the one who always got the night calls; Scott was usually sound asleep, recovering from his last search. Leslie Israelson remembers the family going into rescue mode: get the food ready and kiss Gerry as he was going out the door. The whole family got caught up in the tension of the moment as dad went on another rescue, often under terrible conditions. One striking thing about the rescue report when the boys were stranded on top of Mt. Robson, was the number of calls made to families saying the guys were still fine. All dutifully recorded with date and time.

Dale Portman, who spent nearly three decades dealing with motor vehicle accidents, mountain rescues, avalanche accidents, murders and suicides, summed it up this way. "You accumulate a lot of baggage over the years and eventually the closet gets full. I went on a call with the dog, tracking a suicidal person who was packing a shotgun. I just didn't want to deal with another grisly body or wonder who the gun was going to be pointed at. I really had to force myself to go. I went, but I knew it was time to go. I hung up my tracking harness shortly after that and took a year off to get away from it all."

Mark Ledwidge is emphatic about the personal sacrifices that have to be made—that sometimes seem to elude management—just to get through the full guide's course. Not many managers are aware of the personal toll on rescue personnel and their families from attending rescues or even trying to pass guide exams. Relationships and families are lost when the cost gets too high, which indicates to him the huge motivation necessary to pursue this work. He reflects on the comparatively clean record Parks Canada has in rescue work. To date, no one has been killed or injured during a rescue. This is something to be proud of, but it makes Mark nervous. He credits the safety record to the tremendous skill of the pilots they have been so fortunate to work with, but is careful to point out that most of the work is still done with helicopters and helicopters have accidents all the time. Helicopters are inherently dangerous, but much more so when pushing the limits of rescue work. Pilots are asked to perform under conditions of high winds and bad visibility and often at elevated altitudes in high-angle situations.

One of his most dramatic experiences combined several of these elements on a rescue for two injured climbers on the north face of Mt. Stephen in Yoho National Park. The climbers were doing a new "aid route" on the face when they ran into trouble, resulting in a badly injured leg. The pilot flying in this case was Kathy Moore. The face was exceedingly steep near the top, making the rescue quite exciting. With tricky face winds and minimal rotor clearance, Kathy placed Mark close to the injured man. Mark got the man in the rescue bag quite quickly, and everyone was off the mountain in short order. He gives the credit for the success of the operation to Kathy who had the tough job of getting him in there, but adds that they were flying at the edge of the helicopter's capacity. He pensively remarked: "Lots could happen in a matter of seconds."

The fact is, in some instances a lot does happen, and it results in the loss of good friends and co-workers—not often, but in the close-knit climbing community of the Canadian Rockies, the chances of knowing at least one casualty in a lifetime of public safety work, is high.

The questions of risk taking, freedom of action, consequence and responsibility are not intended to be answered here, nor is it likely they could be. Clearly there is a need to elevate the level of communication between the public and parks over these issues, but how to do so effectively can be complicated. What is said is not often what is understood and the boundaries between what is acceptable and what is desired will likely be contested for years to come.

12 Then and Now

By the end of 2004 the biggest challenge facing both the Warden Service and the Kananaskis Country rangers was the growing age of the individuals running the programs and the lack of new recruits coming on strength. But they had metamorphosed successfully from cowboys to climbing guides during the first 50 years of offering a professional rescue organization.

Tim Auger, who had overseen 30 years of that evolution, retired at the end of 2003, just two years short of that anniversary. His cheerful presence was missed by all, but it also left a hole that took a while to fill. Cultivating the in-house staff to do the job was the primary method parks relied on in the past. But demanding guiding standards have made this a costly and time-consuming solution, and other options are now being considered.

One option is hiring fully trained guides to augment the program. The idea that it is cheaper and easier to turn a guide into a warden than vice versa has some merit. Another option is to contract the work out to the Association of Canadian Mountain Guides. Clair Israelson points out, however, that this would completely alter the culture so carefully nourished by the Warden Service over the years. Guides hired from outside would bring their own culture and way of doing busi-

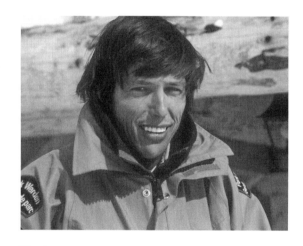

Tim Auger. BOB SANDFORD COLLECTION

ness which may not mesh well with the current Warden Service staff. Another concerns is that guides may be good climbers, but that does not mean they will function well in a rescue situation that requires teamwork.

Gord Irwin, who took over from Tim Auger to run public safety for Banff, Lake Louise, Kootenay and Yoho, does not think hiring more guides is the solution. He would prefer to fill positions such as Tim's with young seasonal staff who can be brought into the public safety program. He feels wardens can be trained to rescue leader status without being full guides.

The training requirements, however, are hard to meet. Every function in the Warden Service is faced with the same training dilemma, and managers of the individual functions are reluctant to let people go to all the training sessions required of them. Gerry Israelson pointed out that the problem is one of losing the middle section of the response personnel pyramid. He always felt the wardens called upon to respond to public safety issues should be structured like a pyramid with the lead guides on top, backed by the well-trained support wardens who could operate confidently under most field conditions. They, in turn had the backup of the third layer of wardens or support personnel who looked after gear, supplies and communications. All levels are critical in most rescue operations, but particularly for searches or complicated rescue scenarios. It has been maintaining the support ranks that has been a problem for the public safety program over the years.

Keeping a viable professional rescue organization operating in both national parks and Kananaskis Country has also been plagued by a lack of younger personnel coming on staff. The ability to maintain younger staff has been truncated by hiring freezes. The loss of people like Pat Sheehan, Simon Parboosingh and Mike Wynn is being acutely felt today. The thinning of trained people means that the loss of even one individual is significant in the organization.

By 2005, staffing change in each park has tried to accommodate working with limited personnel. Glacier National Park is fortunate in having Sylvia Forest, who has her full guide status, in the public safety position. Glacier is doubly blessed as Jordy Shepherd, who moved briefly to Jasper, has also completed his full guide status and is back working in that park.

For a brief period, it looked like Waterton was in good hands when Lisa Paulson took the public safety position there. However she has since moved to backfill the vacant public safety position in Lake Louise. Though she does not have her full guide status, she is partway there and will possibly finish in the next couple of years. The public safety position in Waterton is now filled by Edwin Knox in the acting supervisory position until the job is filled permanently. Though Edwin has no training as a guide, he has considerable experience and can call on old hands for most non-technical rescues.

Banff now has four full guides in the public safety position. Though it is sufficient to ensure that one person is always covering, the area they respond to is significant. They must provide rescue assistance to all of Banff, Yoho and Kootenay national parks. Though the two smaller parks, in particular Kootenay, have few major incidents, events such as major avalanches involving many people can happen at any time. Banff, however, will have to respond to any technical rescues in Waterton as well, being the closest source for people trained to that level outside of the Kananaskis Country rangers. In addition, the park has been asked to respond to many B.C. parks with the potential for serious accidents such as the Bugaboo and Assiniboine provincial parks.

Jasper National Park is currently staffed with two full guides, but only one of them is in the public safety position. Steve Blake has moved on temporarily to cover the CPW position running the Warden Service, while Rupert Wedgwood backfills the public safety position for him. The wardens had had temporary coverage for Rupert's job as field leader, but nothing is permanent. Jordy Shepherd worked in that capacity for three months and has now been replaced by Brian Webster from Canmore. However, the position is only offered for three months, making it difficult to fill.

Jasper does have a very good rescue leader at Sunwapta, who has been in and out of the public safety training program for many years. Garth Lemke is a young warden who started out in Jasper before Gerry Israelson left and was selected to fill the public safety training position at that time. He was hired on only as a term warden, however, and needed to upgrade his status to remain in the position. This he did, and in the interim he worked as a park ranger in Bugaboo Provincial Park. His earlier training in Jasper stood him in good stead, and he functioned there as a rescue leader. It also gave him plenty of opportunity to upgrade his climbing skills. When the opportunity to move back to Jasper at Sunwapta in a public safety position came up, he jumped at the offer. Since then he has become the right-hand man for Rupert and is on call when either of the two full guides are away. His only restriction is that Banff must be called to take a lead hand if the rescue mission requires someone with full guide status to respond.

The current status in Kananaskis Country, the other professional mountain rescue service in Canada, has not changed much since Lloyd Gallagher's retirement. George Field and Burke Duncan still run the program and train the rangers under them. They also face a shortage of younger rangers with an aptitude for public safety. Along with diminished budget, the challenge as they grow older is similar to that faced by the national parks. George, however, is quite creative and has no problem recruiting help from many resources in the area. Banff is right next door, and there are also the Canmore guides who have helped on numerous occasions. He also enlists the aid of the RCMP and ambulance paramedics. Certainly Mike Henderson, the dog handler in Banff, has gone out on several occasions. But George is concerned about how things will be handled in the future. Again, there seems to be no proactive effort from management to deal with long-term replacement.

George is not the only person to enlist the aid of outside agencies. Eric Dafoe at Glacier National Park received considerable support from heli-guides for the Balu Pass search. Glacier is uniquely surrounded by many heli-ski companies and has a memorandum of understanding with most of them. There is a reciprocal agreement

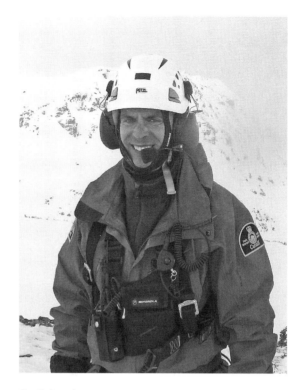

Garth Lemke. JASPER WARDEN ARCHIVES

that the park will respond to any accidents they have and vice versa. The park also has a standing agreement to give and receive aid from Kicking Horse Ski Resort, which has trained professional patrol people as well as two dog handlers. These CARDA dogs are actually the closest at hand for immediate response.

Provincial Emergency Program volunteer groups are also available and several local groups are looking at expanding their response capability. With the evolution of the dual release sling capability, the Revelstoke, Golden and Nelson regional groups hope to start using this resource as well. They also are becoming more active in avalanche search and rescue. One thing that concerns Dave Smith with B.C. Highways, however, is the departure from having searches overseen by persons with CAA level II training. Many times this was a guide from a nearby heli-ski company who responded to a call from the RCMP.

Another area of consideration for future rescue coverage is the accessibility of remote country to a growing population. Alberta, in particular, seems to be experiencing a mini-population explosion, and the economic prospects for that province indicate that it will only increase. The countryside is being explored by many resource extractors, as a result they are opening up wilderness areas at an alarming rate. British Columbia is also experiencing an opening up of the province with mining, logging and a significant increase in backcountry ski and hiking operations. Places like Revelstoke are becoming the snowmobile capitals of Western Canada, which makes many wardens in Glacier nervous. The capacity of these machines to access avalanche terrain is huge and the popularity of their use is growing exponentially. The potential for accidents may someday exceed the capacity of rescue personnel to respond.

After 50 years of evolution, the professional rescue organization of public safety within Parks Canada can claim a respectable safety record. Both Tim Auger and Mark Ledwidge like to keep things in perspective, however. They do not claim to be an elite world-class rescue service. They are quite humble when they consider what their counterparts in heavily populated countries of Europe deal with daily. In fact, as a professional federal rescue organization, the Warden Service plays a very small role nation wide. They are a tiny cog in the National Search and Rescue Program as compared to the Canadian Military or Canadian Coast Guard that deal with rescues right across the country. But despite keeping a reasonable perspective on their achievements, both men are quick to point out that rescue helicopter pilots in Canada are among the best in the world, and they give much of the credit for a significant safety record to those men and women.

Often Europe and the United States are looked upon as yardsticks for what can be expected in Canada. Should the population grow to even a small portion of what those countries deal with, the need for rescue organizations will not fade. And there will be people to respond, be they wardens, rangers, PEP, RCMP, CARDA, other volunteer agencies or ACMG guides. The wheel still turns, creating more history and more stories.

List of Abbreviations

ACC	Alpine Club of Canada
ACMG	Association of Canadian Mountain Guides
BCIT	British Columbia Institute of Technology
CAA	Canadian Avalanche Association
CARDA	Canadian Avalanche Rescue Dog Association
CFB	Canadian Forces Base
CMC	Calgary Mountain Club
CMH	Canadian Mountain Holidays
CMRG	Calgary Mountain Rescue Group
CNR	Canadian National Railway
CPR	Canadian Pacific Railway
CPS	Canadian Park Service
CPW	Chief Park Warden
CSPS	Canadian Ski Patrol System
DOT	Department of Transport
DPW	Department of Public Works
EKMR	East Kootenay Mountain Rescue
EMT	Emergency Medical Technician
HFRS	Helicopter Flight Rescue System
IKAR	International Commission of Alpine Rescue
NRC	National Research Council
PEP	Provincial Emergency Program
SRAWS	Snow Research and Avalanche Warning Section
TCH	Trans-Canada Highway
VHF	Very high frequency; a radio

Glossary

aid climbing   Climbing a vertical rock wall using artificial assistance such as pitons or bolts.

aid route   A climbing route that requires artificial assistance such as pitons or bolts.

anchor   A solid attachment placed by the climber on the mountain.

arête   A narrow ridge of bare rock situated between two or more deep smooth-sided semicircular areas (cirques); found in mountainous areas that have been glaciated.

avalanche cord   A long cord dragged by skiers while in avalanche terrain in hope that some portion of it will be left lying on the surface if they are buried by an avalanche.

avalanche probe   Metal rods that can be fastened or screwed together and pushed into the snow to locate avalanche victims.

avalauncher   A tool which uses compressed gas to launch an explosive projectile up onto an avalanche slope.

avalanche transceiver   *See* rescue beacon.

backcountry warden   A warden who is assigned to patrol the wilder, more out-of-the-way regions of a national park.

base rescue leader   The rescuer who is in charge of a rescue at the base rescue site. This can be located in an office or in a temporary field location or command centre.

belay   To fasten or control the rope to which climbers are attached.

bergschrund   A large crevasse formed at the head or upper end of a glacier.

bivouac   A temporary camping spot above treeline used by climbers to get an early start.

bolt kit   A kit containing a hammer, drill and bolts, which is used to drive an anchor into rock.

cargo hook   A hook located on the underside of a helicopter that loads can be fastened to.

chalk   A small metal object resembling a bolt or a nut that has a sling attached and can be placed in a rock crack. Often used in place of a piton.

chalk stone   A small natural stone that is used in place of artificial chalk in a rock crack.

chimney   A crack in the rock face wide enough that a climber can use it as a route up.

crevasse   A deep crack or fissure in the ice of a glacier.

col   A low point in a ridge of mountains, often forming a pass between two peaks.

corn snow skiing   Skiing on frozen snow that is just beginning to melt on the surface in the spring.

cornice   An overhanging mass of snow or ice formed by wind action.

couloir   A deep mountainside gorge or gully often full of summer snow and sometimes used as a route up a mountain.

crampon   Metal spikes attached to the sole of a climbing boot for climbing and walking on glacier ice.

deadman   A metal plate or other object that is buried in the snow to provide a solid anchor.

defile   A low gully on a mountainside.

depth hoar   Large cup-shaped crystal structures that usually form in the bottom layers of a snow pack as a result of cold weather, generally resulting in an unstable snowpack.

detonation cord   An explosive cord that can be used in place of dynamite.

field rescue leader   The rescuer who is in charge of rescue operations at the actual rescue site.

first party   The first group of rescuers sent to an accident site accompanied by the field rescue leader.

flying using vertical reference   A method by which the helicopter pilot uses a fixed reference point to determine his vertical distance above a point on the ground or mountainside.

frontcountry warden   Wardens assigned to high visitor use areas in a national park (typically townsites, highways or motor accessible campgrounds).

Gazex station   A station erected in avalanche trigger zones that employs expanded gas to trigger an avalanche.

glass   To glass is to look for objects through binoculars or a spotting scope.

high-angle rescue   A rescue that takes place on very steep rock or ice; generally over 45 degrees.

howitzer   An military artillery piece used in Rogers Pass that recoils when fired.

jumaring   A method of ascending a rope with movable metal clamps or prussic slings that are attached to the rope and that provide slings to stand in. The climber moves up the rope as he steps and moves the jumar upward.

karst   Limestone rock landscape, characterized by caves, fissures, and underground streams.

ladder pitch   A steep rock section in a cave that usually has a fixed ladder to aid in the ascent and descent of that section of the cave.

last seen point   The location where a victim was last seen in an avalanche.

lead   A short climbing section (usually a rope length long) that the first climber on the rope (the leader) ascends.

leader fall   A fall taken by the first climber (the leader) which is not held until the fall is arrested by the first piece of protection.

Magic Pantry   A commercial product wrapped in aluminium foil that is boiled to provide a meal. Often used by backpackers and climbers.

mine stretcher   An old fashioned stretcher originally used in mine rescue situations.

moraine   An accumulation of boulders, stones or other debris carried and deposited by a glacier.

mountaineer   One who climbs mountains for sport.

park ranger   That member of a provincial park staff who enforces provincial park statutes. Rangers have several responsibilities including mountain rescue. In Canada they are usually provincial park employees while in the U.S. they are usually federal park employees.

park warden   An employee of a national park who is responsible for enforcing the National Parks Act and the park's regulations. The responsibilities are many and include mountain rescue work. In Canada wardens are usually federal park employees while in the U.S. they are usually state park employees.

pass   A low point between two mountains, which can usually be navigated on foot.

Pieps   A commercial brand of avalanche beacon.

piton   A metal spike, which can be driven into ice or a rock crevice, and which has an eye at the end so that a rope can be passed through it and then be secured.

Primacord   Commercial name for detonation cord.

protection   The use of a piton, bolt, chalk, stone or other device that can be anchored to the mountain and through which a climbing rope is passed to protect a climber from falling too far.

317

prussic knot   A special knot used to tie a prussic sling to a climbing rope. It can be easily slid along a rope's length but when weight is put on it, it binds to the rope and does not slip.

prussic sling   A thin cord similar to a climbing rope but much smaller in diameter that can be used on a climbing rope for ascending purposes (much like a jumar) or as an anchor.

rappel   The act or method of descending from a mountain or cliff by means of a rope using either the body or an artificial aid as a friction device.

recoilless rifle   An artillery piece used in avalanche control that requires some sort of tower or structure that will accommodate a back blast from the gun, rendering it recoilless.

rescue beacon   An electronic homing device that is used in searching for avalanche victims.

scree   A slope covered in smaller rock debris that usually moves when stepped on.

serac   A ridge, pinnacle or block of ice in the crevasses or slopes of a glacier.

Skadi   A commercial brand of avalanche beacon.

ski cutting   The act of skiing horizontally across a snow slope to release the tension in a snow pack, allowing the snow to avalanche, thus stabilizing the slope.

skid   A tubular assembly on the undercarriage of a helicopter that provides stability and rests on the ground or landing pad when the helicopter is not in the air.

skins   Strips fastened to the bottom of skis providing traction when climbing up a hill.

sling rope   A four-strand rope of varying length that can be attached to the underside of a helicopter for a rescuer to hang from in flight.

snow pack   The successive layers of snow formed during the winter with each new snowfall.

snow pit   A deep pit dug down into the snow pack which reveals the successive layers of snow formed during the winter.

snow profile   A diagram of the snow pack produced by examining the different characteristics of each significant layer of snow which is then plotted and measured.

surface hoar   Cookie or wafer thin crystals that form on the surface of snow after lengthy durations of extremely cold and windless periods.

sweeper   A branch or tree that extends low out over the surface of a river that can sweep people from water craft or prevent the passage of the water craft down the river.

talus   A slope covered in larger rock that tends to support a person's weight.

tarn   A small body of water found in alpine or sub-alpine landscapes.

technical climb   A climb on a mountain or rock face that requires a rope and some form of protective aid to be climbed safely, and which requires greater mountaineering skill.

The Pass   A local term for Rogers Pass in Glacier National Park.

traverse   To travel horizontally across a slope.

verglas   Very thin ice that coats rock after a storm and which is prone to being very slippery.

wand   A three-foot piece of thin green bamboo (often found in garden centres) placed in snow or on glaciers at regular intervals to mark the route taken by a climbing (skiing or hiking) party. Its top is usually flagged with flagging tape for visibility in a storm.

Bibliography

Books, Articles and Pamphlets

American Alpine Club. *Accidents in North American Mountaineering*—1969 (1970): n. pag.

Atwater, Montgomery. *The Avalanche Hunters.* Philadelphia: Macrae Smith Company, 1968.

Banff National Park. "Rescue Report: Mt. Blane." Banff National Park, 1961.

Beers, Don. *World of Lake Louise—A Guide for Hikers.* Calgary: Highline Publishing, 1991.

Blades, Kevin. "Avalanche Teaches Quality Lessons Despite Losses." *Viewpoint Magazine* (1990): n. pag.

Blake, Steve. "Incident Stress Plan." Jasper: Parks Canada, 2002.

Bonatti, Walter. *On the Heights.* London: Rupert Hart-Davis, 1964.

——. *The Great Days.* Trans. Geoffrey Sutton. London: Victor Gollancz Ltd., 1976.

Strathcona-Tweedsmuir School Outdoor Education Program. Kamloops: Bhudak Consulting Ltd., 2003.

Burns, R.J., and Mike Schintz. *Guardians of the Wild.* Calgary: University of Calgary Press, 2000.

Canadian Park Service. "Dos and Don'ts of Winter Travel." Ottawa: CPS, n. dat.

Dornian, Dave, Ben Gadd, and Chic Scott. *The Yam: 50 years of Climbing on Yamnuska.* Calgary: Rocky Mountain Books, 2003.

Engel, Claire. *A History of Mountaineering in the Alps.* London: George Allen & Unwin Ltd., 1971.

Everts, Christine. "The Canadian Avalanche Association's Oral History Project." Revelstoke: Canadian Avalanche Association, 2003.

Fraser, Colin. *The Avalanche Enigma.* London: John Murray, 1966.

Gailus, Jeff. "Weapons in the War Against Snow." *Mountain Heritage Magazine* 3.4 (2000/2001): n. pag.

Goldestzer, Torsten, and Bruce Jarnieson. *Avalanche Accidents in Canada. Volume 4 1984–1996.* Revelstoke: The Canadian Avalanche Association, 1996.

Hanna, Glenda. *Outdoor Pursuits Programming: Legal Liability and Risk Management.* Edmonton: University of Alberta Press, 1991.

Harrer, Heinrich. *The White Spider: The Classic Ascent of the Eiger.* New York: J.P. Tarcher/Putnam, 1998.

Hein, Phil, William Leiss, and Denis O'Gorman. *Parks Canada's Backcountry Avalanche Risk Review.* Calgary: Parks Canada, 2003.

Jasper National Park. "Rescue Report: Mt. Brule." Jasper National Park, 1967.

Kershaw, Robert. "Noel Gardner and the Birth of Avalanche Science." *Mountain Heritage Magazine* 3.4 (2000/2001): n. pag.

Lundberg, Murray. *Death Came Silently: The Granduc Mine Disaster.* Explore North. 24 Aug. 2004 <http://www.explorenorth.com/library/yafeatures/bl-granduc1.htm.>

MacCarthy, Albert. "The First Ascent of Mount Eon and Its Fatality." *Canadian Alpine Club Journal* 12 (1921–21): n. pag.

MacInnes, Hamish. *High Drama: Mountain Rescue Stories from Four Continents.* Toronto: Hodder & Stoughton Ltd., 1980.

May, W.G. *Mountain Search and Rescue Techniques.* Boulder: Rocky Mountain Rescue Group Inc., 1972.

Mayberry, Kim. *Romance in the Rockies: The Life and Adventures of Catharine and Peter Whyte.* Canmore: Altitude Publishing Canada, 2003.

McCammon, Ian. "Evidence of Heuristic Traps in Recreational Avalanche Accidents." International Snow Science Workshop. Penticton, 2002.

McClung, David, and Peter Schaerer. *The Avalanche Handbook.* Seattle: The Mountaineers, 1993.

Merrill, Alex. "Granduc: The Silent, Deadly Slide." *Mountain Heritage Magazine* n.d. n. pag.

National Parks Service. "Operational Policy Directive: Public Safety—Organization and Objectives." Ottawa: National Parks Service, 1969.

Parks Canada. "Issue Analysis in Mountain Search & Rescue." Ottawa: Parks Canada, 1983.

Perren, Peter. "The View from Inside an Avalanche." *Mountain Heritage Magazine* 3.4 (2000/2001): n. pag.

Portman, Dale. *Rescue Dogs: Crime and Rescue Canines in the Canadian Rockies.* Canmore: Altitude Publishing Canada, 2003.

Portman, Dale, and Scott Ward. "Dog Training Standards for Canadian Parks Service Search and Rescue Dogs." Banff: CPS, 1991.

Ross, Peter. "The Season of the Hundred Year Avalanches—Interview with Peter Fuhrmann." *Mountain Heritage Magazine* 3.4 (2000/2001): n. pag.

Roth, Arthur. *Eiger: Wall of Death.* Toronto: George J. McLeod Ltd., 1982.

Royal Canadian Mounted Police. "History of the Police Dog Service." Ottawa: Royal Canadian Mounted Police, n.d.

Sandford, Robert. *The Canadian Alps: The History of Mountaineering in Canada* 1827–1906. Banff: Altitude Publishing, 1990.

——. *The Highest Calling—Canada's Elite National Park Mountain Rescue Program.* Canmore: The Alpine Club of Canada, 2002.

Schaerer, P.A., and C.J. Stethem. *Avalanche Accidents in Canada I. A Selection of Case Histories of Accidents* 1955 to 1976. Ottawa: National Research Council of Canada, 1979.

——. *Avalanche Accidents in Canada II. A Selection of Case Histories of Accidents* 1943 to 1978. Ottawa: National Research Council of Canada, 1980.

——. *Avalanche Accidents in Canada III. A Selection of Case Histories of Accidents* 1978 to 1984. Ottawa: National Research Council of Canada, 1987.

——. *Avalanche Studies Rogers Pass* 1956-1961. North Vancouver: Self Published, 1995.

Scott, Chic. *Powder Pioneers: Ski Stories from the Canadian Rockies and Columbia Mountains.* Calgary: Rocky Mountain Books, 2005.

——. *Pushing the Limits: The Story of Canadian Mountaineering.* Calgary: Rocky Mountain Books, 2000.

——. *The History of the Calgary Mountain Club.* Calgary: Self Published, 1987.

——. "Tragedy on Mount Temple." *Mountain Heritage Magazine* 3.4 (2000/2001): n. pag.

Simmons, Jack, ed. *Murray's Handbook for Travellers in Switzerland* 1838. New York: Humanities Press, 1970.

Stethem, Chris. "Getting Started with Avalanches." *Mountain Heritage Magazine* 3.4 (2000/2001): n. pag.

Tetarenko, Lorne and Kim. *Ken Jones—Mountain Man.* Calgary: Rocky Mountain Books, 1996.

Ullman, James Ramsey. *The Age of Mountaineering.* London: Collins, 1956.

Waterton Park. "Rescue Report: Mt. Cleveland." Joint Canada/U.S. report. Waterton Park, 1969.

Whelan, John. "Frozen Hell on Earth." *Mountain Heritage Magazine* 3.4 (2000/2001): n. pag.

White, Brad. "Development of Avalanche Safety and Control Programs in the Canadian Rocky Mountain National Parks. An Historical Perspective." International Snow Science Workshop. Penticton, 2002.

Wills, Alfred. *Wanderings Among the High Alps.* London: R. Bentley, 1856.

Interviews and Personal Communication

Anderson, Andy — chief park warden

Auger, Tim — park warden/public safety specialist/ alpine specialist/mountain guide

Balding, George — park warden/park superintendent

Barter, Terry — RCMP dog handler

Beers, Don — author

Bjorn, A.J. (B.J.) — park warden

Blake, Steve — park warden/public safety specialist/ mountain guide

Blanchard, Barry — mountain guide

Brown, Anna — park warden

Bunyan, Reg — park warden/public safety specialist

Burns, Gord — RCMP dog handler/civilian S&R dog trainer

Burstrom, Alfie — park warden/dog handler

Callahan, Matt — helicopter pilot

Calvert, Katherine — park warden

Cooper, Lance — park warden/helicopter pilot

Crocker, Gordon — mountaineer

Dafoe, Eric — park warden/public safety specialist/ avalanche technician

Damm, Terry — park warden

Davidson, Tom — park warden

Davies, Jim — helicopter pilot

Devlin, Will — park warden/dog handler/public safety specialist

Duncan, Burke — park ranger/public safety specialist

Eder, Mike — park warden

Enderwick, Peter — park warden/lawyer

Field, George — park ranger/public safety specialist/ alpine specialist

Fingland, Randy — park warden

Forest, Sylvia — park warden/public safety specialist/ mountain guide

Forman, Gary — helicopter pilot

Fortin, Gaby — chief park warden/park superintendent/director general

Fuhrer, Hans — park warden/public safety specialist

Fuhrmann, Peter — mountain guide/alpine specialist

Gallagher, Lloyd (Kiwi) — mountain guide/alpine specialist

Gmoser, Hans — mountain guide/heli-ski operator

Halstenson, Joe — park warden

Haney, Bob — chief park warden

Hansen, Bob — park warden

Henderson, Mike — park warden/dog handler

Hendry, Russ — S&R coordinator

Hermanrude, Ollie — chief park warden

Hindle, Murray — park warden/law enforcement specialist

Holroyd, Jack — park warden/park superintendent

Horne, Greg — park warden

Irwin, Gord — park warden/public safety specialist/ alpine specialist/mountain guide

Irwin, Sharon — park ranger/park warden

Israelson, Clair — park warden/public safety specialist/alpine specialist/mountain guide/ director CAA

Israelson, Gerry — park warden/public safety specialist/mountain guide

Jacobson, Perry — chief park warden

Jones, Ken — pioneer/mountain guide

Klettl, Tony — park warden/public safety specialist

Kosechenko, Brent — park warden/public safety specialist

Knox, Edwin — park warden/public safety specialist

Kun, Steve — park superintendent

Kunelius, Rick — park warden

Laboucane, Tim — park warden

Larson, Arnor — photographer/rope rescue specialist

Lawrenson, Art — park warden

Ledwidge, Mark — park warden/public safety specialist/mountain guide

Leeson, Bruce, Dr. — environmental coordinator

Lemke, Garth — park warden/public safety specialist

Locke, Charlie — mountain guide/ski area operator

MacDonald, Al — park warden

Manners, Evan — park warden/avalanche specialist

Marino, Dale — RCMP dog handler

Martin, Duane — park warden/law enforcement coordinator

Mathews, Ron — RCMP dog handler

McCready, Todd — helicopter pilot

McGowan, Rod — mountain guide

McKeenan, Al — park warden

McKnight, Mike — assistant chief park warden

McTighe, Don — helicopter pilot

Michaud, Lyn — mountaineer/search and rescue specialist

Mickle, Don — park warden

Millar, Marv — chief park warden

Moore, Al — RCMP officer

Morton, Jay — park warden

Murphy, Jim — park warden/chief park ranger

Niddrie, John — park warden

Paulson, Lisa — park warden/public safety specialist

Pawson, Ken — mountaineer/search and rescue specialist

Pendlebury, Rod — CARDA dog handler

Perren, Peter — park warden/lawyer

Peyto, Gord — park warden/dog handler

Pfisterer, Willi — mountain guide/alpine specialist

Portman, Dale — park warden/dog handler/author

Pugh, Jay — CARDA dog handler/instructor

Ralf, Rick — park warden

Romanuk, Brad — park warden

Rutherford, Gordon — park warden

Schaerer, Peter — engineer/avalanche consultant

Schintz, Mike — chief park warden/resource conservation coordinator

Schleiss, Fred — public safety specialist/avalanche forecasting coordinator

Shepherd, Jordy — park warden/public safety specialist

Sime, Jim — chief park warden/resource conservation coordinator

Skjonsberg, Earl — park warden/dog handler

Smith, Dave — mountain guide/park ranger/avalanche technician

Smith, Dave — park ranger/park warden

Sparks, Jenny — park warden/risk management specialist

Spear, Peter — mountaineer/ski patroller/instructor

Srigley, Howard — RCMP officer/ski area manager/air search and rescue

Staples, Frank — park warden

Statham, Grant — mountain guide

Stethem, Chris — avalanche consultant

Stinson, Darro — park warden/public safety specialist/park superintendent

322

Tasker, Peter — park warden/photographer

Tilson, Derek — park warden/public safety specialist

Vedova, Dan — park warden/public safety specialist

Vockeroth, Don — mountain guide

Volkers, Dianne — park warden

Vroom, Mo — warden secretary

Wackerle, John — park warden

Wallace, Brian — chief park warden

Ward, Scott — park warden/dog handler

Waslenchuk, Bill — park warden

Waters, Don — park warden

Watt, Bruce — CARDA dog handler

Wedgwood, Rupert — park ranger/park warden/public safety specialist/mountain guide

West, Ric — park warden

Wiebe, Doug — RCMP dog handler/RCMP dog trainer

White, Brad — park warden/public safety specialist

White, Cliff — park warden/forest management coordinator

Whyte, Peter — chief park warden

Wiegele, Mike — heli-ski operator/mountaineer

Willis, Terry — park warden/public safety specialist

Winkler, Max — chief park warden

Woods, Percy — park warden/public safety specialist/mountain guide

Zimmerman, Chris — park ranger

Zinkan, Charley — park superintendent

NEWSPAPERS

Calgary Herald

The Banff Crag & Canyon

OFFICIAL RECORDS

Alberta Parks and Recreation—Case Reports.

Calgary Mountain Rescue Group—Case Reports.

Parks Canada—Dog Case Reports.

Parks Canada—Occurrence Reports.

Parks Canada—National Parks Warden Service Search and Rescue Reports.

Royal Canadian Mounted Police—Jasper Case Files.

Index